THE GULAG DOCTORS

THE GULAG DOCTORS

Life, Death, and Medicine
in Stalin's Labour Camps

DAN HEALEY

YALE UNIVERSITY PRESS
NEW HAVEN AND LONDON

For information about this and other Yale University Press publications, please contact:
U.S. Office: sales.press@yale.edu   yalebooks.com
Europe Office: sales@yaleup.co.uk   yalebooks.co.uk

Set in Adobe Caslon Pro by IDSUK (DataConnection) Ltd
Printed in Great Britain by TJ Books, Padstow, Cornwall

Library of Congress Control Number: 2023952223

ISBN 978-0-300-18713-7

A catalogue record for this book is available from the British Library.

10 9 8 7 6 5 4 3 2 1

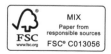

CONTENTS

CONTENTS

ILLUSTRATIONS

NOTE ON THE TEXT

In the main text, I have used today's Ukrainian names for locations within the Ukrainian Soviet Socialist Republic, while noting previous names in endnotes if relevant. A historian might quibble; several cities have cycled through a kaleidoscope of names as various empires took charge in this much-contested space. Ukrainians have already paid enough in blood and treasure for foreigners to begin learning the names they have chosen for their cities and towns.

I have endeavoured to use Ukrainian transliteration for Ukrainian names in the main text, for example Ostap Vyshnia. In the citations I present Russian-language publications by or about Ukrainian authors in conventional Russian transliteration (i.e. Vishnia).

I have simplified Russian names for English readers in the main text (Fyodor Dostoevsky, not Fedor Dostoevskii) and have used the historical 'Soviet' names for cities located in the Russian Federation where this is temporally relevant (Petrograd and Leningrad, not St Petersburg). For citations to Russian-language publications in the endnotes, I use the conventional modified Library of Congress transliteration. Unless otherwise indicated, translations from Russian are my own.

GLOSSARY

bytovik/bytoviki	a person convicted for an 'everyday' (*byt*) offence, such as theft or assault, and in the Stalin era associated with particular decrees (against petty theft in the collective farm; punishing lateness at work); a common criminal
Cheka	Vserossiiskaia Chrezvychainaia Komissiia (VChK) pri SNK, All-Russian Extraordinary Commission attached to the Council of People's Commissars; the security police, 1917–22
chekist	informally, a member of the security police both during and since the Soviet regime
dokhodiaga/ dokhodiagi	'goner': a prisoner suffering from extreme emaciation and associated illnesses; often near death
feldsher	a Russian paramedic, often substituting for a physician in remote locations
Komsomol	Young Communist League; *komsomolka* (f.), *komsomolets* (m.), member of the Komsomol
lekpom	from *lekarskii pomoshchnik*: a medical assistant. A Gulag slang variant is *lepila*

medbrat/medbratia	lit. 'medical brother': a male nurse
medsestra/medsestry	lit. 'medical sister': a female nurse
sanchast/sanchasti	a 'sanitary section' or small medical post which might have inpatient beds, but lacking specialist services and staff. Varied widely in size and shape
Sanotdel	'Sanitary Department', administration of medical services for an entire camp or camp complex. Principal seat of medical authority, usually run by career Gulag employee-doctors. Subordinate in practice and in most regulation to camp commandants and camp internal security police
tufta	Gulag slang for faked paperwork, output figures. In the medical context, faked diagnoses, therapies, cause-of-death certification, or labour-capacity categorisations of prisoners
urka/urki	hardened, recidivist, or career criminals who adhered to 'thieves' law'; typically, they refused to work in general labour and exploited 'political' prisoners to work 'for' their official labour quota
zek/zeks	prisoner/prisoners, derived from the official Gulag abbreviation z/k (*zakliuchennyi*); a slang term used by prisoners

PREFACE AND ACKNOWLEDGEMENTS

This project began in the first years of the twenty-first century when Russia's prospects looked much happier than they did after 2014. The scholarly context was different then too. From the end of the 1990s, new archival evidence about the Gulag, and new scholarship based on it, was challenging long-held perspectives about the Stalinist forced-labour camp system. These perspectives were established in the 1970s with the publication of Alexander Solzhenitsyn's *The Gulag Archipelago*.

In March 1974, as a 17-year-old high-school student I travelled to the Soviet Union for the first time. Just a month before, Solzhenitsyn was stripped of his Soviet nationality and expelled from the USSR; his name was everywhere in the press. In Moscow and Leningrad, the Intourist guides responded brusquely to our questions about Solzhenitsyn: he was a traitor, someone who had enjoyed the high esteem of the Soviet state as a writer and now dared to return the favour with lies and calumny. I was intrigued by the fierceness of their contempt for a man who was being hailed in the West as a truth-teller, and once back home in Canada I read the first volume of his history of the Gulag with deep fascination. My introduction to Soviet history came through this extremely singular channel, a bitter and excoriating indictment of Soviet power and at the same time a compelling human story of death, suffering, and survival against a brutal authoritarian regime. Later, in the early twenty-first century, as a lecturer in Soviet history at Swansea University in Wales, I returned to Solzhenitsyn's text as the new Gulag scholarship was emerging. I began assigning *The Gulag Archipelago* to students and thinking about the history of medicine in the Gulag as a prospective research topic.

The project evolved substantially from its original conceptions, as I describe in the Introduction. Eventually, it found the shape of the book you have before you – an attempt to capture how Gulag doctors and medical workers acted inside the camps, as well as a reflection on how they remembered their activities there and are remembered by Russians today. Finding the will to write this history after Russia's increasingly vicious assaults on Ukraine has been taxing. Pursuing a project that might be said to put Soviet Moscow's labour camps 'in a good light' thanks to the medical services that operated there seemed ill-advised, even if my intent was never to soften the Gulag's image or present it as more humane than it was. Of 18 million inmates who passed through the gates of this institution between 1930 and 1953, it is estimated that no fewer than 2.5 million died deaths attributable to the malnutrition, exhaustion through forced labour, and egregious and preventable disease that prevailed in the system.[1] Experts far more capable than I still do not agree on the death toll, which varies according to the selection of Soviet statistics, their interpretation, and more elaborate 'algorithms' for calculating how many victims of the system's 'release-to-die' practices there were. What I can say with certainty is that Gulag medical care was a drop in the ocean of need generated by forced labour under Stalinist rule. Readers should keep the estimated death toll in their minds as they read these stories of prisoner lives 'saved' and conscientious medical duties fulfilled. As I have written these chapters I have tried to do the same and query the sources that celebrate these achievements behind barbed wire. I have also tried to bring the non-Russian protagonists in my stories to the fore, the better to see the imperial Soviet gaze in the Gulag. It was a police colony that shifted populations across continents, shunted indigenous peoples aside to make way for mining, forestry, and construction projects, and viewed awe-inspiring extremes of climate, geology, flora, and fauna with all-too-human swagger and contempt.

In developing and completing this project I was generously supported by the Wellcome Trust with grant no. 085948 ('Medicine in the Gulag Archipelago', awarded 2008–11). A British Academy grant supported a month's research in Georgia in 2011. In 2021–22 the Leverhulme Trust supported a year of writing, which greatly assisted me in completing this book. I am grateful to these organisations supporting research in the humanities in the UK. My agent, Andrew Gordon, shepherded this project through several transformations, and I am grateful to my Yale University Press London editors, Robert Baldock and Heather McCallum, who have always been encouraging, and most of all, patient. At Yale I am indebted to Katie Urquhart for patient assistance with the illustrations; and Lucy Buchan, Rachael Lonsdale, and Robert Sargant for their expert eyes on the text.

The Russians who assisted me in excavating material and sharing their knowledge and perspectives on the Gulag were legion. Kirill Rossiianov trawled the archives of the central Gulag administration for me in 2008–10, greatly assisting me to see the outlines of the story of medicine in the labour-camp system. We were both helped by the professionalism of the late Dina Nokhotovich at the State Archives of the Russian Federation and her colleagues. The Russian State Library's professionals facilitated my pursuit of rare printed materials too. In Moscow I was given much courage by Elena Gusiatinskaia, and many helpful tips and favours from Natalia Pushkareva: many thanks.

The Memorial Society in Moscow and St Petersburg (now closed by Putin's 'foreign agents' laws) were always helpful, thoughtful, and generous in their support for this project. Irina Ostrovskaya and Irina Shcherbakova in Moscow assisted me in the reading room and library. Irina Flige opened doors for me in St Petersburg. I had a valuable conversation with Arseny Roginsky, then the director of Moscow's Memorial, about the entire theme of Gulag medicine. The closure of this organisation is a tragedy for Russians, but I do not think they have heard the last of Memorial.

Regional museums and archives were critical sources of local historical knowledge, perspectives, and sources. First, I must thank the curators of the Museum of the History of Public Health in Ukhta, Fyodor Kanev and Tatyana Vekshina, for their warm welcome in 2009, and their generosity in granting me access to their fascinating collections that are of national significance. In Ukhta as well I benefited from the kind assistance of Elena Buldakova and Oksana Gritsenko at the Ukhta Historical-Regional Museum, and Evgeniia Zelenskaya of the History Museum of the Ukhta State Technological University. Zelenskaya very generously took me on a tour of the site of the Vetlosian Central Camp Hospital which became an important focus of this book. In the Komi Republic city of Pechora I was equally fortunate to work with the curator of the city's Historical-Regional Museum, Tatyana Afanasyeva, who kept me going in an unheated office with an endless supply of tea and fascinating documents. Many, many thanks to my Komi colleagues.

In Magadan in 2011 a curator of the Magadan Province Regional Museum, Svetlana Budnikova, kindly gave me access to many documents about medical staff in the Kolyma region. She introduced me to local historian David Raizman, who drew my attention to important scholarship about Magadan and Dalstroi. At the State Archives of Magadan Province Natalia Primenko enabled me to view a range of official documents related to the region's medical services. Colleagues in other Russian cities assisted me at various times. In 2014 Leonid Obukhov in Perm obtained documents from Perm's archives, and he arranged for a visit to the open-air Gulag museum Perm-36, just as it was being converted from an independent Memorial-led institution into a government one with contentious changes to its focus and objectives. In Ekaterinburg my path into the archives was smoothed by Aleksei Kilin, who also kindly invited me to give lectures on the history of the Gulag to students in the Urals State Federal University, again in 2014.

Beyond Russia I also owe many debts. In Amsterdam (2009) Nanci Adler alerted me to a cache of Gulag survivor memoirs at the International Institute of Social History, and we had fruitful conversations about them which helped me at an early stage of the project: many thanks. In Georgia (2011) I accessed documents in the State, Party, and Interior Ministry archives thanks to Timothy Blauvelt, who opened doors everywhere. Col. Omar Tushurashvili at the Interior Ministry allowed me to access the ex-KGB collections there. My Tbilisi librarian-guides were Ninel Melkadze and Natalia Gladchenko in the National Parliamentary Library. In Latvia (2022) the staff of the Paul Stradiņš Medical Museum library and archive, Juris Salaks, Artis Ērglis, and Daina Auziņa, assisted me in identifying valuable holdings in the history of Soviet medicine, as did Jana Klebā at Riga State University library. My friend Ineta Lipša was generous with introductions and advice. Warm thanks to all these professionals!

The interviews I conducted in Russia and Canada were inspiring and humbling. I owe thanks to Aleksandr Tsetsulesku, Yuri Fidelgolts, Tatyana Oleinik (in Moscow), Vanda Trifanova (Ukhta), and Anna Kliashko (Montréal), for their willingness to spend time with a curious scholar and their generosity of spirit. I am indebted to the Memorial members in Moscow who connected me with the Russian interviewees, and to Professor Lilia Topouzova, University of Toronto, who with Ekaterina Kuzmenko helped conduct the interviews with Anna Kliashko.

Numerous scholars of Russia, the Soviet Union, and the Gulag assisted me over the long life of this project to understand the Gulag better. Many organised or participated in seminars, workshops, and conferences devoted to these themes, or shared work with me, or read drafts of this work. Among these I want to mention with gratitude Golfo Alexopoulos, Alan Barenberg, Steve Barnes, Nick Baron, Wilson Bell, Auri Berg, Frances Bernstein, Christopher Burton, Johanna Conterio, Michael David-Fox, Alexander Etkind, Don Filtzer, Susan Grant, Jeff Hardy, the late Philippa Hetherington, Peter Holquist, Emily Johnson, Elena Katz, Nikolai Krementsov, Charlotte Kühlbrandt, Rebecca Manley, Paula Michaels, Guillaume Minea-Pic, Mikhail Nakonechnyi, Susan Gross Solomon, Trish Starks, Lynne Viola, Sarah Young, and Benjamin Zajicek. Dozens of seminar audiences heard versions of this work over the years: thank you to organisers and participants in Manchester, Leicester, Bath, Oxford, Cambridge, London, Southampton, St Andrews, Heidelberg, Helsinki, Tbilisi, Moscow, Toronto, and Washington. Polly Jones and

Judy Pallot at Oxford endlessly pressed me to sharpen my gaze, my questions, and my analysis, and have been inspiring friends as well as colleagues. Christopher Davis generously shared an all-too-rare hard copy of his doctoral thesis and many Soviet medical publications. My students deserve mention including the many finalists who took my Special Subject, 'Terror and Gulag in Stalin's Russia', over the years: Oliver Day, at Swansea University, whose BA dissertation on medicine in the Gulag showed me early on what promise this topic holds; at Oxford Calum Holt, who transcribed a cache of Ukhta medical biographies, and Mikhail Nakonechnyi and Nikolai Erofeev, who helped me with materials about the Gulag. My colleagues at Swansea, Reading, and Oxford universities shouldered burdens when I obtained research leave to work on this book, and their camaraderie and kindness are warmly appreciated. Needless to say, I am solely responsible for the errors and weaknesses of this book.

My friends and family have endured this project for far too long. My dear Toronto friend, Jim Bartley, gave me a critical reading of the first four chapters of this book during the pandemic lockdown, and I am grateful for his skilled author's eye and layman's ability to spot the unexplained in a mess of prose. To have such a loyal friend who has known me from the earliest days of my Russian obsession is a privilege. Another such friend is Bernice Donoghue, a one-time comrade in the travel business, who over the years enjoyed and endured journeys with me to Magadan, Yakutsk, Moscow, St Petersburg, Tbilisi, and Svaneti. I gave Bernice Eugenia Ginzburg's memoirs to read before taking her to Magadan: Bernice's reflections about Ginzburg and the Gulag as we walked the streets of Magadan launched me on deeper investigations.

My sister, Michele Healey, a retired respiratory therapist, generously came from Canada to Cambridge in October 2019 and soothed me, and my husband Mark Cornwall, as we confronted a medical drama of my own. My pulmonary hypertension was treated by an amazing team of medical workers in the Royal Papworth Hospital, led by surgeon Mr David Jenkins. The eight days I spent in Papworth, my first hospital stay since birth, gave me the opportunity to observe and appreciate medical workers close up: from the cleaners, porters, catering, and nursing staff, to the surgeons, anaesthetists, consultants, administrators, and managers. I even gave an interview from my hospital room to the national BBC breakfast show, making a minor contribution to 'sanitary enlightenment'. With this book in the back of my mind I experienced the care in a top-rated National Health Service hospital as a thing to marvel at: the result of a cascade of good historical decisions, and continuing political battles, that makes the best of medicine available free to all.

My final thanks go to my husband Mark. His courage and forbearance are something I scarcely deserve, but I treasure them deeply. Mark unfailingly put wind in my sails, gin in my glass, and hope in my heart. This book would not be here without him.

Oxford & Southampton, August 2023

INTRODUCTION

A 'Ukrainian Mark Twain' and the essence of Gulag medicine

In the 1930s Ostap Vyshnia (pseudonym of Pavlo Mykhailovych Hubenko) was one of the best-known Ukrainian writers imprisoned in the Gulag. He was sent to Ukhtpechlag, a prisoner-built oil drilling complex clustered around Ukhta in the Komi Republic, in the far northern wilderness of European Russia. Ostap Vyshnia was a 'Ukrainian Mark Twain' and one of the most published writers in the Ukrainian language, a member of the generation of the early Soviet Ukrainian literary and cultural renaissance.[1] Arrested in 1933 in Ukraine on falsified charges of anti-Soviet conspiracy and given a ten-year sentence, Vyshnia arrived in Ukhta in April 1934 and was quickly assigned to an unusual sort of 'forced labour': to work as a local historian. The commandant ruling the entire regional camp complex, Yakov Moiseevich Moroz, named him editor of a sprawling, collectively authored history of the camp, due to appear later that year to mark Ukhtpechlag's fifth anniversary. The grandiose project, entitled *Five Years of Struggle for the Riches of the Taiga and Tundra*, was already well advanced.[2] Two years previously a meeting of 'old Ukhta residents' gathered to reminisce and start to write their memoirs, and by now officials confronted a sprawling manuscript. Vyshnia was assisted by another prisoner, the former People's Commissar of Enlightenment of Uzbekistan, Manon A. Ramzi; the history was a project as multinational as the Gulag itself.[3] The Ukrainian writer had trained before the Revolution as a feldsher, a Russian

1

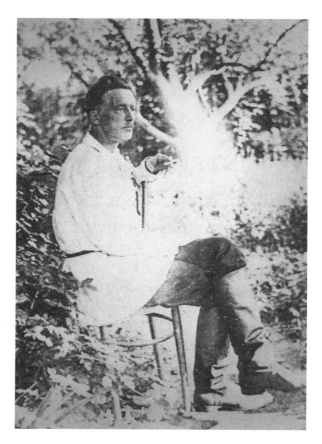

1. Ostap Vyshnia, Ukraine's 'Mark Twain' and forced-labour historian of Ukhtpechlag.

designation for a paramedic, and he had experience during the Civil War of military medicine. Vyshnia contributed his own articles to the 'corporate history' of Ukhtpechlag on the development of its medical services, and a profile of Ukhtpechlag's senior physician, the career medical bureaucrat Yakov Petrovich Sokolov, as well as other sketches and interviews.[4]

Luckily, the archives of the Komi Republic preserved a manuscript of this corporate history of the early Ukhta camps, which never saw publication. In 2005, local historians edited and published extracts, including the medical sketches written by Vyshnia. These texts are filled with puzzles and misleading evasions. Vyshnia's profile of Ukhtpechlag's senior medical official Yakov Sokolov lacks any factual concreteness; it is a hymn to his supposed healthcare achievements in broad-brush 'socialist realist' style. The facts of Sokolov's long employment by the secret police, and commitment to Stalinist methods, go unspoken. Even Vyshnia's longer and more substantial chapter chronicling the early history of medical care in Ukhta's pioneering expeditions and camps is breezy and upbeat. After just five years, he writes, '[a]n entire army of medical-sanitary workers – doctors, medical assistants, sisters of mercy [nurses], orderlies – serve the many enterprises and outposts of the Ukhto-Pechora camp.'[5] Not mentioned is the fact that the vast majority of these 'workers' were prisoners, performing 'forced labour' in their first-aid stations, clinics, and eventually the hospitals that would be established in the camp. Vyshnia presents a picture of robust and cheerfully practical prospectors served by a healthcare philosophy apparently drawn directly from socialist principles:

> ... the main thing was to impart into the consciousness of the entire staff of the expedition that the slightest sickness, however trivial, must not be left unattended, but must be brought to the doctor's attention immediately, so that no further spread of illness took hold. The expedition found itself in exceptional conditions. Every worker, every specialist, was accounted for, at each separate prospecting outpost stood just a single man, and to lose him, even if only temporarily because of illness, would mean interrupting the work of the entire expedition. Therefore, each man looked after his fellows, everyone watched over everyone, for there was nobody to replace even a single worker. The result was a specific form of 'joint responsibility': the health of one was dear not only to the individual, nor even to the doctor, but to the entire expedition.[6]

Socialist values like preventative measures, rapid first aid, and mutual surveillance for the collective good were, supposedly, scrupulously observed by these expedition 'workers' in an exceptionally isolated wilderness. These prospectors and their support teams were in fact made up mostly of prisoners, and not all were dutiful in listening

3

to medical instructions or monitoring each other's health for the earliest signs of influenza, typhus, or worse. Some attempted escapes in the tundra; others succumbed to illness and perished before making it to Ukhta. Yet nobody dies in Vyshnia's sketches of early medical care in Ukhta. Plainly, this first corporate history of a Gulag camp sanitised the reality of early labour-camp forays into the vast wilderness of northern Eurasia along ideological lines to disguise the coercive nature of these enterprises, to hide the collusion with secret police institutions, and to smooth over the unpleasant fact that not all prisoners were rational and obedient servants of the construction of socialism.

The puzzles found in Ostap Vyshnia's history of Ukhtpechlag are similar to those explored in this book. Who in fact were the doctors, the nurses, feldshers, and medical bureaucrats who practised medicine in Stalin's Gulag? How was it that some actually chose to work for the labour-camp system? What was the purpose of the medicine they practised in this huge penal institution, one that has become a byword for lethal exhaustion through hard labour? Medical professionals working behind the barbed wire of the camps were caught between their duty as healers of individual patients, and the stark fact that their patients were prisoners. Many doctors, nurses, and feldshers were themselves prisoners, caught in the precarious tier of Gulag professional and specialist 'forced labour'. Their loyalties were divided: first to their professional discipline, but secondly, and more starkly, to their local camp commandant and the demands of the Gulag machine. Navigating the tension between what medical workers ought to do, and what Gulag officials required that they do, was never straightforward – and seldom reflected upon. This book illuminates many moments when that tension came to light. Finally, how did the Gulag's medical workers remember their extraordinary years in the penal medical service, and how are they remembered in Russia today? To explore these questions, I turn to the biographies of doctors, nurses, and other medical workers in the Gulag medical service. Before diving into these compelling stories, some background is needed on the Gulag, its 'sanitary' service, and the ways in which the Gulag has been commemorated since Stalin's death in 1953, in order to bring the world of these medical workers in focus.

Medical care for Stalin's Gulag

Alexander Solzhenitsyn, in his landmark history of the Gulag camps, dismissed the medical care available within them as malign. 'Like every branch of the camp administration, the Medical Section, too, was born of the devil and filled with the devil's blood.'[7] A former Gulag prisoner, who had suffered eight years in confinement, including time in infirmaries for the removal of a tumour, he had good cause to complain that medical bureaucrats and camp commandants worked hand in glove. Drawing on the reminiscences of 257 Gulag survivors, his otherwise encyclopaedic, three-volume *Gulag Archipelago* treated the 'Medical Section' with withering and dismissive brevity. (The Medical Section he refers to is both the Sanotdel, a medical bureaucracy running from the central headquarters of the Gulag in Moscow down to the lowliest camp subdivisions in the farthest reaches of the Soviet Union; and also, the 'sanchast' or local camp clinic, infirmary, or hospital where medical treatment was dispensed to inmates.) In a few bitter pages Solzhenitsyn dismissed evidence of 'good doctors', practising medicine conscientiously such that they 'could still be doctors' in a professional sense. He argued that subordination to the Gulag machinery of camp commandants, internal surveillance, production managers, and medical bureaucrats, meant that doctors, however noble, could only comply meekly to serve 'the common purpose' of squeezing the maximum labour out of the 'sloggers' – prisoners in hard labour in the system's mines, construction, and timber-felling tracts. It was virtually impossible to stand up to the camp authorities with medical arguments, he claims. Any positive acts accomplished by so-called 'good doctors' were undermined by the contention that they had to 'sacrifice others' to save a given individual. Moreover, Solzhenitsyn claims, it was almost impossible to do good in the medical sections: doctors lacked adequate resources, thanks to webs of criminality and the camp bosses' own corruption.[8]

For Solzhenitsyn, Varlam Shalamov was the chief source of 'a legend about the benign camp Medical Section'.[9] Also a Gulag survivor, between the 1950s and 1970s Shalamov wrote the six-volume story cycle *Kolyma Tales*, depicting Gulag life in a bleak modernist prose style. Shalamov spent longer in the camps than Solzhenitsyn, enduring three separate sentences totalling approximately fourteen years between 1929 and 1951, and sinking to the condition of a 'goner' (*dokhodiaga*), an emaciated prisoner on the edge of death. Shalamov recovered in a Gulag hospital, and arguably survived his last sentence when in 1946 a prisoner-doctor enrolled him on an in-house medical course for feldshers. One might understand Solzhenitsyn's mistrust: in his eyes Shalamov had climbed aboard the sanchast life raft and escaped hard labour. (Solzhenitsyn had found his own life raft in a Gulag *sharashka*, or research institute staffed by prisoner-researchers, but that is another tale.[10]) In reality, Shalamov's own experience of illness and work in the Gulag medical section was harrowing and mixed with dark and light elements. His reminiscences are filled with portraits of corrupt, abusive, and malign doctors as well as turning points where other medical staff enabled him to survive. In his 'documentary fiction' Shalamov painted Gulag medicine in similar shades; he was no advocate of a rosy view of the sanchast.[11]

For generations since the 1970s these two giants of Gulag letters have dominated our impressions of what doctors did in the Gulag and how they thought. In fact, until recently, historians of the Gulag have avoided tackling the subject of its medical services, finding their presence in the camps confusing and contradictory.[12] Solzhenitsyn's brisk dismissal of the medical sections casts a long shadow. Behind the discomfort of historians of the Soviet labour camps as they confront Gulag medicine lies an uneasy awareness that Soviet gulags and Nazi concentration and death camps are equated in the public mind. This popular equivalence prevails even though the two historical cases, as understood by academic and public historians, were distinctive in their ideological character, temporal duration, geographic extent, resourcing, staffing, and much else.[13] How is it possible that the Soviet forced-labour system that worked so many prisoners to emaciation or death, in some of the most extreme conditions on the planet, also had sanctuaries of warmth, better nutrition, clean sheets, and a ration of medical attention? A partial answer can be found in the origins of the Gulag as a thirty-year experiment in 'police colonisation' of vast and often remote regions of Soviet territory. As a form of colonisation, the Gulag required a labour force at minimum free of epidemic disease and capable of toil.[14] That colonial project is outlined in this Introduction. Moreover, looking past Solzhenitsyn's long shadow requires new perspectives. A fundamental argument of this book is that historians must search more widely for more voices to appreciate the nature of the Gulag's medical service and its staff. In part, that means listening to the people who served as doctors, nurses, and feldshers in the labour-camp medical service. Their voices are explored later in this Introduction. But first the Gulag's medical service and its evolution within the wider frame of the history of Soviet medicine need to be explained.

To understand why Stalin's camps had medical sections, we have to listen to his bureaucrats, and take seriously what they said. The Gulag's Sanitation Department, or Sanotdel, was no ordinary medical service, but an 'embedded' one, devoted solely to the penal system's prisoners and free employees. From its earliest days, the Soviet system parcelled out healthcare provision bureaucratically. In addition to a general medical network run by the People's Commissariat of Public Health for the civilian population, the state created integrated 'medico-sanitary' services for key institutions: 'embedded' clinics and doctors served in the Red Army, the Navy, the railway network, and not surprisingly, the Kremlin. The Gulag labour camp network, as part of the security police apparatus, had its own dedicated medical service. All of these 'departmental' or 'embedded' medical services adopted the militarised or bureaucratic hierarchies, and the distinctive internal cultures, of their host institutions.[15] The Gulag as host institution evolved over the course of the 1930s in ways that shaped its medical service and determined its unique character.

Following Solzhenitsyn's landmark study, the Soviet term 'Gulag', an acronym for the 'Main Administration of Corrective-Labour Camps', has come to stand for the entire forced-labour camp system, established in 1929–30 as Stalin launched the First Five-Year Plan.[16] The Gulag was a strange blend of Imperial Russia's exile and forced-labour system, early Soviet experiments in penal reform, and Stalin's drive to industrialise at break-neck speed. From tsarist patterns of repression, it inherited the enormous geographic sweep of the Eurasian continent and the conundrum of how to develop what seemed to Russians an 'empty' territory. Siberia, the Far North, and the Pacific coast were inhabited by indigenous peoples, subjects of the tsar, and needed to be subjugated and colonised. The Russian Empire had to exploit and occupy these territories to save it from incursions by rival powers. Penal practice – exile and forced labour in Siberia – was harnessed to colonial, economic, and security imperatives. Prisoner toil in mines and factories endured from the seventeenth to the twentieth centuries. By the nineteenth century Siberia became a place of exile for political rebels of all stripes; and a dumping ground for criminals who it was hoped might one day after release from confinement settle down and become 'colonists'.[17] In fact, many criminals became a burden on the local Russian and indigenous populations thanks to chronic maladministration, underresourcing, and neglect.[18] Imperial Russia's historians wrote of Siberia as Russia's 'colony', even arguing, like Vasily Osipovich Kliuchevsky, that '[t]he history of Russia is the history of a country which colonises itself'.[19]

The revolutions of the Russian Empire in 1917 brought first the abolition of Siberian exile and forced labour in February under the liberal-democratic Russian Provisional Government; and then a radical, self-proclaimed Marxist revision of penal ambitions under the Bolshevik (Communist Party) regime from October of that year.[20] These penal ideas, such as the establishment of improvised and deadly concentration camps, forced labour as a means of punishment and sometimes redemption, co-existed alongside summary trials and executions, during a bloody series of civil wars that reconstituted Russia's empire as the Union of Soviet Socialist Republics. During the early Soviet years, experiments in penal reform reflected both the ruthless nature of the new regime, and the utopian aspirations of one of the world's first self-proclaimed socialist regimes.[21]

From this ferment a competition between Soviet institutions for control over prisoners, prison camps, and state investment developed. By the late 1920s, the secret police (then known as the OGPU) won that competition as rival commissariats (Soviet 'ministries') dropped out of the running. The OGPU had run forestry camps in Karelia, and devised productivity-squeezing rations-for-work schemes on the distant White Sea island-camp of Solovki in the 1920s; it successfully embroidered this cruel regime with socialist ideology about reforging the criminal through labour. Its eye-catching plans for road, railway, and most notably canal construction as well as mining for precious ores chimed with Soviet dictator Joseph Stalin's political turn towards a policy of rapid industrialisation with his First Five-Year Plan (1928–32). The Gulag, as an institution of the secret police, was formally established on this basis in April 1930.[22] It grew at an astonishing rate and, with it, the industrial enterprises that the penal system ran using prisoners to perform manual labour. From a prison and camp system that housed 179,000 inmates in 1930, it grew to a population of one million by 1935 and topped two million by 1948; at Stalin's death, in 1953, the Gulag held almost 2.5 million people.[23] Eighteen million people passed through its jurisdiction in these years, of whom no fewer than 2.5 million died.[24] The Gulag's 'economic model' presumed that prisoners were cheaper to settle than free employees, could be moved at will by the OGPU's economic planners, and could be sent to remote places where free employees were extremely costly or impossible to attract.[25]

'The history of the Gulag, the history of the development of the corrective-labour policy of the Soviet state during the entire period of its existence, is the history of the mastery and industrial exploitation of the remote regions of the state.' So wrote an administrator in 1950, summarising the Gulag's development, perhaps consciously echoing Kliuchevsky's observation about the history of Russia.[26] The rationale of 'police colonisation' drove Gulag expansion. The story of the Gulag's multifarious activities fell into two patterns: the 'pioneering' prospecting and construction work of mobile prisoner-brigades in relatively temporary camps; and the more deliberate selection and construction of permanent settlements around an industrial, mining, or transportation hub. The showpiece White Sea–Baltic Canal 'demonstrated' to Stalin and the Party leadership the apparent efficacy of rapid pioneering 'assaults' by mobile contingents of prisoners who could then be moved on to other projects.

The expeditions that opened up the Ukhta, Pechora, and Norilsk regions of the Far North, and the special arrangements for the Kolyma gold fields in the Far East, showed the colonial impulse in the Gulag at its most ambitious. In the 1930s the secret police acquired an industrial-penal empire, its own 'internal colony'.[27]

The prospecting and geological expeditions that arrived in these regions very rapidly established temporary and more permanent settlements. In the Far North of European Russia, the Vaigach expedition set up 200 prison camps in just four years.[28] Camps were subdivided and spawned new offspring – *podlagpunkty, komandirovki, podkomandirovki* ('sub-camp stations', 'expeditions', 'sub-expeditions') – until what we know as 'camps' were in fact entire complexes covering vast regions. To 'open up' (*otkryt*) and 'master' (*osvoit*) new territory, this first stage of the Gulag 'assault' often focused on building roads and railways. In the early 1930s, in the Komi Republic, 780 kilometres of roads were built in the Ukhta-Pechora camp complex alone.[29] In the same region entire camp complexes were devoted to railway construction projects.[30] In Kolyma the infamous 'road of bones' linked the 'capital' Magadan with the gold fields of the Kolyma River basin; by 1952 the Kolyma Highway would be over 1,000 kilometres long.[31] Such projects were built hastily, wastefully, and sloppily. Mortality rates for prisoner-labourers on them were very high, and the model of rapidly deployed mobile labour meant that their living conditions were among the worst in the Gulag: unheated tents or dugouts in the middle of winter, poor supplies of food, clothing, fuel, and tools. Medicine and medical care were also in short supply.[32]

The urbanisation of the Gulag followed. The biggest central camps, hubs of entire regions, became administrative and economic centres of development. They might be based at important transportation hubs, as in the case of the Pacific Ocean port of Magadan, with its harbour at Nagaevo, or, more often, be established at the site of major mines, as were Norilsk, Ukhta, and Vorkuta. From their rustic offices in these new 'capitals', Gulag bosses issued their orders to advance the project of economic construction, of 'internal colonisation' we can say, in their regions.[33] The classic wooden structure that housed the Kolyma gold-mining administration in the 1930s became the heart of the new city of Magadan; it was only torn down in the 1960s, to be replaced by a white-stucco modernist office block. During the 1930s these 'towns' became increasingly sophisticated and complex settlements, composed of zones of freedom, where *vol'nonaemnye* (free employees) lived, and zones behind barbed wire for prisoner-labourers in transit or servicing the mines and infrastructure of the 'camp'. Later, in the 1940s and early 1950s, ever larger numbers of non-prisoner inhabitants, free to use emerging civilian amenities such as shops, clinics, and cultural facilities, lived in these centres. Non-prisoners included various kinds of contracted employees and their dependants, and former prisoners themselves, confined by administrative exile to the region, with the families they attempted to form after release.

In the eyes of their police promoters, the forced-labour camps needed a medical system to protect their economic empire's productivity, not to care for prisoner health. The camps' health service grew on a scale commensurate with the continent-wide expansion of the secret police empire, mirroring the institution itself. The Gulag Sanotdel's central Moscow office was run by a physician-bureaucrat who directed a sizeable cadre of doctors and lay bureaucrats acting as medical inspectors, sanitation specialists, and statisticians; on the eve of the Second World War, they constituted 8.6 per cent of Moscow's central Gulag personnel.[34] By 1939 the Gulag Sanotdel network in the camps counted 1,171 infirmaries, clinics, and hospitals with 39,839 beds, for a population of 1.6 million prisoners. During the Second World War it expanded to 165,000 beds (in 1943, when the population was just under 1.5 million) and, by 1953 on the eve of Stalin's death and the subsequent release of millions of prisoners, the Gulag medical service had 111,612 beds at its disposal for its 2,468,524 prisoners.[35] These were enormous bed numbers per capita by comparison with civilian medical services, likely exaggerated by local camp administrators who could redesignate whole barracks as 'sickbays' at the stroke of a pen.[36] The secret police's medical leadership in Moscow expressed a sense of entitlement to Gulag spending when justifying the high bed-count; a logical result of the 'departmentalisation' of medical systems. However, the statistic also pointed to Soviet habits of using statistical indicators of 'progress' by any means necessary.[37] The fetish for counting hospital beds, as we will see, was also a feature of a wider truth about Soviet medicine: there were precious few modern medical treatments and drugs available to the average labour-camp doctor, and a stay in hospital with bed rest, clean linen, and relatively regular food was often the limit of a Gulag physician's therapeutic arsenal.

As the camp system expanded, its appetite for medical professionals grew inexorably. The Stalinist fear of enemies of the state furnished a steady supply of prisoners from the ranks of healthcare workers from feldshers to university professors, with the majority of educated ('intelligentsia') victims accused, usually on fabricated grounds, of political opposition to the Soviet regime under the criminal law's infamous article 58 on anti-Soviet activity.[38] Prisoner-physicians were plucked from transports and put to work as medics, thereby avoiding life-exhausting 'general labour' in the Gulag's mines and forests; such was demand that prisoner-medics were formally allowed to use their professional skills more often than convict-engineers or other skilled technicians.[39] They were supervised locally by 'freely hired' doctors and medical bureaucrats like Yakov Sokolov in Ukhtpechlag, who were Gulag Sanotdel employees. There were 'middle'-level free medical workers too. From 1938 Gulag representatives recruited newly qualified doctors, nurses, feldshers, dentists, and pharmacists directly from the graduate work-assignment commissions of medical institutes and training colleges.[40]

In 1939 the Gulag was served by 2,459 qualified doctors, and another 7,290 nurses, feldshers, and pharmacists worked in the system; in that year 39.9 per cent of the doctors and 42.1 per cent of the mid-level medical staff were prisoners, and the rest, freely hired employees.[41] Again, this was a strikingly high proportion of staff to population, over double the number of doctors per capita than in civilian services.[42] Many prisoners were trained as paramedics and nurses in the Gulag's in-house courses, which varied in quality across the system.[43] Prisoners taught themselves medical basics and forged careers in the camp infirmaries.[44] The medical service was a variegated and dynamic element of the Gulag system, distinctive from Soviet civilian and other institutionally embedded, 'departmental' medical systems because of the prisoner status of most of its patients and many of its workers.

The Gulag's medical personnel answered to two types of authority, each expressing objectives for this penal medical system that were paradoxical, contradictory, and challenging to reconcile. This dual loyalty was the essence of Gulag medicine. The first set of authorities, and most immediate and familiar, was the medical hierarchy in the hospital, clinic, infirmary, or medical station. Mid-level medical staff such as nurses, feldshers, laboratory assistants, anatomists in the morgue, and orderlies, were subordinate to physicians, and physicians answered to more senior doctors in the most complex institutions (directors of hospitals, chief doctors of hospital departments or specialist facilities like radiology cabinets). These personnel could be a mixture of prisoners and 'free' employees. It was often the case that unfree doctors were older, more experienced, with academic training, and they were often seen as more knowledgeable in matters of medicine than the younger, more 'Soviet-minded' doctors who managed them. Hospital and clinic directors answered to senior medical bureaucrats in the camp administration, tasked with implementing the orders of the Gulag Sanotdel from Moscow. This was a hierarchy that ostensibly reflected a technocratic, expertise-led, rational medical and sanitary service, albeit one that served a penal system. Thus, a traditional medical hierarchy ran from the top Gulag Sanitary Department leaders in Moscow down to the lowliest nurses, porters, and feldshers in remote camp infirmaries thousands of kilometres away.

The second authority that Gulag medical staff answered to was, of course, that of the camp commandants and their penal personnel. Directors of entire camp complexes, commandants like Yakov Moroz in Ukhtpechlag, were the ultimate arbiters of order in their fiefdoms; they answered to Moscow's Gulag directors, and pliable state auditors and judicial officials, but had considerable leeway on the ground, and this relative 'freedom' could be reflected in local camp environments. As the Gulag matured, some commandants found resources to fund medical research or cultivate particular medical experts from among the prisoner population (as in Ukhta, Pechora, and Norilsk in the 1940s).[45] Others prioritised football teams and musical-dramatic theatres, and some found money for scientific development and enter-tainment simultaneously.[46] That both outcomes existed points to the free hand commandants enjoyed as directors of a 'colonial' enterprise. Commandants furthermore had an entire penal infrastructure to enforce their rule and the various branches of the penal regime and administration impinged on Gulag medicine at every turn. The camp's internal security police ran networks of informers among prisoners and staff, keeping watch for insubordination.[47] Supply managers controlled the distribution of food, bed linen, soap, medications, and equipment; and financial managers constrained expenditure on sala-ries (for free employees) and clinic budgets. Most intrusively for the Gulag's medical staff, the production and technical directors of the camp's principal industrial, mining, or construction operations viewed the prisoners as a labour pool that must be optimally mobilised to achieve targets and plans. Sickness depleted that labour pool, and the Gulag's medical professionals were always constrained by quotas on the numbers of prisoners to whom they could grant work-release certificates. When food supplies and living conditions were especially poor, prisoner health deteriorated but production managers insisted the plan must still be fulfilled. The emaciated and injured whom pris-oner-doctors might view as obviously in need of rest and therapy were denied this care because of the power of production managers, of the economic plan, and the penal goals of the Gulag. Health and medical care for prisoners was decidedly a second-rank priority when stacked against meeting production targets.

Generations of Soviet doctors

The doctors who worked in the Gulag were the products of a succession of Imperial, revolutionary, and then Stalinist medical policies. Furnishing the Russian Empire, or later the Soviet Union, with a modern network of doctors, clinics, and hospitals, was a daunting aspiration. On the eve of the 1917 revolutions, modern scientific medical care was concentrated in major cities and provin-cial towns, where research institutes, universities with medical facul-ties, nurse and feldsher schools, and the largest hospitals clustered. In

14

St Petersburg and Moscow, centres of teaching and research rivalled Europe's best.[48] Yet 80 per cent of the empire's population were peasants in rural districts, where medical services were provided by local-authority (*zemstvo* or council) physicians, employees of the state's lowest level of administration. They served enormous districts in dire conditions, and their peasant-patients were suspicious of modern biomedicine unless other avenues like the bathhouse, herbal remedies, and midwives had been exhausted. Rural doctors dreamed of a 'universal' medical-care network to wean the peasants off folk-healing, reach the remotest settlements, and improve popular health and hygiene.[49] Their analogues in the rapidly industrialising cities, 'district' (*uchastokovye*) physicians who served workers and the poor, had similar visions of social improvement for the towns.[50] Before 1917 their dreams were unrealised: finance was lacking, and political will was adrift, as ministers disagreed over priorities while the tsar's autocratic rule stymied change. Tsarist Russia lacked a ministry of public health, with the Ministry of Internal Affairs, the police, in charge of this brief.[51]

In 1918 the Soviet government established the People's Commissariat of Public Health, Russia's first health 'ministry'. (Soviet branches of government were called 'people's commissariats' until March 1946, when the Stalinist revival of imperial pomp led to their rebranding as 'ministries' with 'ministers'.) The first People's Commissar of Public Health, Nikolai Semashko, a Bolshevik physician, was determined to define modern medicine in a distinctively socialist way. Modern healthcare, free to all at the time of need, was a touchstone of the socialist programme.[52] Like tsarist medical professionals, the new commissar continued to dream of a 'universal' healthcare network. And yet the reality in the decade after revolution and civil wars did not favour a radical extension of healthcare to all. In the peacetime 1920s Soviet healthcare was highly unequal: medical staff huddled in the biggest cities, while 'insurance' medicine covered only the most privileged urban workers and rural clinics struggled with minuscule resources. A striking statistic encapsulates the dilemma: in 1926–27 per-capita spending on civilian healthcare in the Russian Soviet republic was 3.67 roubles, but this masked great disparities, with uninsured rural citizens receiving 1.08 roubles, while their insured urban working-class comrades enjoyed 21.85 roubles in expenditure.[53] The persistence of 'departmental' or 'embedded' medical systems in the military, secret police, railways, and other branches of the state – a legacy of the old regime, and judged indispensable in the period of civil wars and ever afterward – heightened inequalities. We know little about these subsystems' budgets, but they certainly veered towards the higher urban expenditure seen in the civilian healthcare system. Per-capita expenditure in the foremost secret police concentration camp, the White Sea Solovki island complex, in 1926–27 was about 6.00 roubles, and administrators were keen to reduce that figure.[54]

'Socialist' medicine in this period also emphasised specific values. Semashko talked expansively of the prevention of illness as the socialist solution to the 'bourgeois' focus on therapeutic medicine. These were utopian words that launched experiments in 'social hygiene' – public health programmes designed to nip illness in the bud, or prevent it in the first place, via mass health screenings, sanitary 'enlightenment' and drives for clean workspaces and housing.[55] Another theme focused on the doctor–patient relationship. The capitalist model of payment for service was a remnant of the old regime that distorted the doctor's care for the patient, and the patient's willingness to turn to the doctor. The Communists tolerated private medical practice but hoped it would eventually disappear in the Soviet Union. It never quite did, although eventually a massive expansion of the state sector under Stalin, and his proclamation of the 'victory of socialism', would put residual private practice under a cloud.[56] Medical confidentiality was another area where socialist policy chipped away at the autonomy of the physician. Secrecy between doctor and patient that put society in danger – the example of sexually transmitted infection that endangered wives and children was the usual one aired in these discussions – was impermissible in Soviet society.[57] Yes, Soviet doctors should command popular trust, but confidentiality must defer to social needs, Semashko argued. The Hippocratic Oath – in pre-revolutionary Russia a moral rather than legal undertaking – was for Semashko a dangerous relic of that professional autonomy that obstructed society's interest in the doctor–patient relationship. Soviet authorities scrapped the Oath in medical education, although generations would still learn of it via lectures in the history of medicine.[58] Politically, Semashko and Communists more generally feared that the medical profession would be disloyal to the Bolshevik project, despite the apparent co-incidence of aspirations between rulers and experts. The Soviet regime banned self-governing professional associations inherited from the tsarist era, most notably, the vocal Pirogov Society, and Soviet doctors were subsumed into a state-controlled trade union for medical workers without distinctive professional representation.[59] Formally at least, in Soviet healthcare, collective and social priorities trumped the interests of the individual doctor and patient. As Stalin concentrated power in his own hands by the late 1920s, Soviet medical politics would shift even farther from Hippocratic ideals.

The signature policies of the Stalin 'Great Break' of 1929–32 were forced collectivisation of agriculture, to secure control of the grain supply, and break-neck industrialisation, co-ordinated through grandiose Five-Year Plans. Stalin abandoned the mixed-market economy of the 1920s, and in its place the state built a non-capitalist, 'command-administrative' economy through central planning in Moscow of industrial investment and production, distribution of supplies, control of retail trade and services, and assignment of personnel. Enormous upheaval in towns and especially in the countryside ensued; peasants flooded into the cities to escape collectivisation and dekulakisation, adding 10 million to their population by the end of the First Five-Year Plan in 1932. Famine caused by collectivisation killed an estimated 6 to 9 million in Ukraine, Southern Russia, and Central Asia. In the towns, housing grew overcrowded, living conditions deteriorated dramatically, and supplies of food, clothing, and soap plummeted – but workers were fed, while peasants starved. The towns of the Soviet Union triumphed over the countryside and grew at its expense. In this dramatic period, Stalin's lieutenants reconfigured the People's Commissariat of Public Health and recast its priorities.

In late 1929 the Communist Party decreed that the health commissariat's plans must align more closely with Stalin's exacting demands for the First Five-Year Plan, with the commissariat showing 'an appropriate class line' on healthcare. By January 1930 Semashko, associated with the old 'universalist' dream of healthcare for all, was replaced by a Stalin loyalist, Mikhail Vladimirsky, a medically trained Communist, with extensive experience in Party and government audit and planning institutions.[60] He promoted a 'productionist' or 'industrial' emphasis on key workers whose toil was critical for the success of the Plan. Healthcare for workers was to be provided not in universalist, 'territorially' based clinics, but in factory 'industrial health stations' (*zdravpunkty*), which now received significant investment. Soviet medical policy would see-saw between 'industrial' and universalist 'territorial' priorities over the next three decades. Only in the 1960s would a modern 'universal' system win out.[61] Peasants too got differentiated healthcare access based on their role in the new economy.[62]

The Stalinist medical system now enthusiastically embraced inequality – previously seen as an unfortunate necessity – as a key value: the more productive a citizen was, the more investment flowed towards his or her medical care and, conversely, the less valued one's contributions, the less one received. In essence, this policy led to greater investment in urban, industrial-oriented healthcare and a targeting of key groups in agriculture. Medicine was 'mobilised' to serve the Plan and the Soviet economy in unapologetically discriminatory, collectivist, ways. Dependants, the elderly, and workers in low-priority sectors of the economy would suffer under Stalinist healthcare priorities. Gulag prisoners, as social outcasts, sat somewhere near the bottom of this ladder, but paradoxically the labour-camp economic model, and the industrial activity of the penal system, intended to contribute to the overall Soviet economy, meant that a significant outlay for sanitary and medical services was always part of the penal budget.

Furthermore, medical education expanded dramatically as a result of the Stalinist mobilisation of public health. Decrees in 1930–31 restructured the education of physicians and called for a doubling of their numbers from a 1928 base by 1932. In fact, from 63,000 in 1928, the number of Soviet doctors grew to 142,000 in 1940, from 4 to 7 per 10,000 of the population.[63] Doctors' training moved from universities controlled by the commissariat of enlightenment, to 'medical institutes', vocational schools run by the health commissariat. A drastic experiment in crash-course education for physicians followed. Admissions were opened to all without prior qualifications; the course was shortened to just four years; curriculum downplayed theoretical and scientific issues, with the exception of compulsory Marxism courses. Students were sent to work in hospitals and clinics, from orderlies in first year to assistant- then full mid-level medical staff, and finally to the position of probationary doctor in their final year. By the mid-1930s, the health commissariat rolled back this alarming experiment. Candidates for medical school after 1932 had to have a secondary-school education; eventually, a fifth year of study was reintroduced; theoretical knowledge was revived along with the use of Latin terms in the classroom, and examinations strengthened.[64] Only during and after the Second World War did Soviet health authorities recognise that medical competence had so deteriorated that the state compelled all practising doctors to submit to a process of re-credentialisation in the late 1940s.[65] It also overhauled the curriculum, adding a sixth year of training, which drew on the example of American science-enriched teaching, to deepen students' understanding of the processes behind medical care.[66]

The Five-Year Plan changes led to an increased proportion of new doctors drawn from 'new' social groups promoted by Communist affirmative action, i.e. women and nationalities of the peripheral Soviet republics. Jews continued to be significantly overrepresented among medical professionals compared to their strength in the general population: medicine was one of the traditional professions open to some Jewish entrants, and families seem to have passed on a legacy of interest in medicine to the next generation.[67] Examples of this family legacy among Jewish doctors appear in this book. Mass training on the cheap, detachment from the university system, and the influx of disadvantaged social groups led, for good or ill, to falling status for doctors. Some of that loss of status came from residual Russian prejudice against subject nationalities and women more generally, but the dilution of medical education, and the 'mobilisation' of medicine, had a negative impact on these new entrants. Observers of Soviet medicine discerned a process starting in the 1930s of 'deprofessionalisation' and 'proletarianisation' among physicians as an occupational group. Yet the experience of service during the Second World War, plus the review of credentials and other post-1945 reforms, improved matters. Undeniably, Stalinist restructuring of medical education did produce cohorts of new doctors who indeed behaved more like an 'employee group' than a Western or tsarist-era 'free profession'.[68] Given that the Stalinist economy 'mobilised' medicine for industrial productivity, new doctors seemingly entered a career that treated them more like factory technicians responsible for repairs rather than professionals practising a rare form of highly respected expertise. Some certainly viewed a career in medicine instrumentally; for them it was 'just a job' and a salary, and these doctors thought very little about its social significance.[69]

However bleak this picture was, many Soviet doctors of the 1930s generation certainly still evinced a degree, even a high degree, of professional idealism, as this book will demonstrate. There was a widespread camaraderie among this generation of doctors, inspired by the Five-Year Plan narrative of selfless service to a country in transformation. The same generation showed a lively awareness of the residual prestige of the profession and its value to society. These values were transmitted from earlier generations of doctors in medical institutes, in hospital practice, and in mentoring relationships: Stalinist transformation did not impose a complete break with the past. As in so many other areas of social transformation in the 1930s, medical traditions like the use of Latin, and expectations that physicians should have a hinterland of wider knowledge, reasserted themselves after the feverish radicalism of the 'Great Break' subsided. The older generation's clinical experience and deep erudition continued to command the respect of Five-Year Plan medical graduates, and young doctors often idolised and sought out the advice of senior figures. The Gulag created a specific kink in the relationship between generations. Younger doctors from 'new' backgrounds and Soviet crash-course training (many of them women) were often the freely hired hospital bosses and medical bureaucrats running the local camp medical system; while the senior old-school medics and professors (almost always men) were prisoner, or ex-prisoner, ward doctors and clinicians, owing the younger bosses obedience and fearing dismissal to 'general labour' if they put a foot wrong.

Medical values and ethics under Stalin were thus the product of several diverse influences and currents. It would be a mistake to see Stalin's new cohorts of Soviet doctors as nothing but tools of Communist ideology, 'proletarianised' and deprived of humanistic values by a diminished education. The romanticised memory of *zemstvo* and urban 'district' medicine was an important residual influence upon thoughtful young idealists, and Soviet medical students responded to the powerful expressions of this memory in Russian literature. In this literature, the doctor who served the common people, practising far away from big-city academies or prestigious university posts, was the quintessential intelligentsia hero. The medical version of the intelligentsia ideal of service to the people and a critique of tsarism's failure to provide adequate medical care was well established in the short stories of Anton Chekhov, the highly influential young doctor's memoir of Vikenty Veresaev, and after the Revolution in the sequence of young doctor's stories by Mikhail Bulgakov especially.[70] Indeed, Soviet medical polemics tended to co-opt this literature to argue that the new regime was tackling the problems that old-regime critics flagged up. The Five-Year Plan narrative of a country transforming itself adapted and modernised this heroic story. Medical authorities – with the correct ideological framing – invited identification with the intelligentsia heroes depicted in the classics of Russian doctor's writing.[71]

The Gulag doctor in public and private memory

As the example of the 'forced-labour' historian Ostap Vyshnia suggests, this book is not only about establishing what Gulag doctors did in the Stalin-era labour camps. It is also about how their labours have been remembered. It celebrates the work of local historians, and the anti-Stalinist activists who supported them after the dictator's death, in regions where towns and cities were built by Soviet prisoners. This book argues that the memory of the Gulag doctor and medical staff has been an important part of how regional Russian historians have processed the Stalinist experience. In Ukhta, Pechora, and Magadan, among other Gulag places, stories of the founding of local medical institutions and biographies of medical 'heroes' have served to explain the travails of colonisation, and the painful transition from a forced-labour camp to an 'ordinary' civilian Soviet city. The irregular cycles of memory politics since the death of Stalin created ebbs and flows of this historical work. A complex and shifting trail of remembering can be traced within the biographies of doctors, nurses, feldshers, and other medical staff told in this book.

In the Soviet 1950s and 1960s, Party leader Nikita Sergeevich Khrushchev set in motion 'de-Stalinisation' as official policy. The authorities endorsed a limited and ill-defined public exploration of the legacies of Stalinist violence against the multifarious categories of Soviet citizens and annexed peoples who were victims of deportation, exile, imprisonment, and execution. Gulag survivors began to meet, discuss their experiences, and write their memoirs.[72] The great exemplars were Moscow intellectuals, some of whom managed to see their Gulag-themed writing into publication despite Soviet censorship and political constraints demanding no departure from loyalty to the Communist Party. Solzhenitsyn published his famed novella 'One Day in the Life of Ivan Denisovich' (1962) in the era's most 'liberal' literary journal, *Novyi mir* (New World). Another leading figure in camp survivor literature was the Gulag-trained nurse Eugenia Ginzburg, a university history lecturer before arrest, whose memoirs remained unpublished in the USSR until the late 1980s, but circulated widely before that in 'samizdat'. (Forbidden works were 'self-published' in multiple typewritten copies passed hand to hand at some risk of police harassment and arrest to the typists, editors, and readers.[73]) Finally, another survivor, Varlam Shalamov, who trained as a feldsher in the camps, wrote searing 'documentary fiction', short stories that distilled Gulag existence in terrifying but often vivid fragments, including several stories illuminating the role of medicine in the camps. These, too, were deemed unpublishable and both Ginzburg and Shalamov's work was smuggled abroad and

published in the West. Similarly, Solzhenitsyn's great 'literary investigation' of the Gulag's history, *The Gulag Archipelago*, was too excoriating of all variations of Soviet Communism to see publication in
the USSR. After the first volume appeared in Paris, and an English
translation in Britain and the USA, he was stripped of Soviet citizenship and expelled from the USSR, in February 1974.

Indeed, by the late 1960s Khrushchev was out of power and the
new leadership under 'neo-Stalinist' Leonid Ilyich Brezhnev slowly
strangled the policy of de-Stalinisation, smothering it in a vast cult of
the more positive side of the presumed legacy of Stalin – victory in
the Second World War.[74] During the 1970s and early 1980s it became
far less possible to publish 'Gulag'-themed works in official Soviet
media. No monument to the victims of Stalinist violence, promised
by Khrushchev, was built in Moscow. Soviet public culture fell silent
about Stalin, the Great Terror of 1937–38, and the Gulag camps
until the last Soviet leader Mikhail Gorbachev's 'perestroika' (restructuring) policies after 1987 returned to an examination of the past.
Public memory in the 1970s and early 1980s confined itself to 'veiled
monuments' with ambiguous meanings in the Gulag-built regions,
and historical investigation by local historians and journalists who
wrote in Aesopian terms (if published) or more frankly for the desk
drawer (if not).[75] A de-Stalinisation-era history of the building of a
modern healthcare system for Magadan Province, published by a
one-time NKVD career medical bureaucrat, simply failed to mention
the prisoner status of several heroes while discussing their contributions to local medicine. The surgeon-author's pen was still governed
by a non-disclosure pledge he signed before accepting a Gulag
contract in the 1930s, a promise not to reveal any state secrets about
the nature of the labour-camp environment.[76] Later commemorative
volumes in Gulag towns spoke of the 'achievements' and notable 'citizens' of the foundational decades of the 1930s–1950s, without
hinting that terror, imprisonment, and political stigma lay behind
these triumphal phrases, often using an airy passive voice so beloved
of late Soviet editors.[77]

The late-1980s renewal of debate and disclosures about the
Stalinist past was followed by the 1991 collapse of the Soviet Union

and the opening of considerable archival access in Russia in the 1990s. A 'democratic era' in Soviet and then Russian politics enabled serious historical inquiry until the hardening of President Vladimir Putin's regime in the early twenty-first century. At the forefront of investigation into the Soviet past was the non-governmental organisation, the Memorial Society. Founded in a series of activist conferences in Gorbachev's increasingly unruly Moscow between 1987 and 1989, this grassroots campaigning movement spread across the country.[78] A hunger for authentic, non-ideologised knowledge about the Stalinist past swept through generations of intellectuals and ordinary citizens: surviving victims of Stalinism whose stories lay in desk drawers or had never been written down; people in middle age who sensed a realisation of the promise of the Khrushchev era; and younger activists inspired by awareness of private family tragedies or triggered by older relatives' stonewalling about the Stalinist past (a common dynamic). The most visible and vocal Memorial branches were in Moscow and St Petersburg. They assembled impressive archives documenting the Stalinist past, including very significant collections of Gulag survivor memoirs. Less noticed by most observers were the autonomous local branches of Memorial in Russia's distant regions – many in places founded by the Gulag and built with prisoner labour. These varied widely in membership, activities, and objectives.[79] Provincial activists – many of them museum staff, cultural workers, and amateur historians, some affiliated with local Memorial branches – produced a diverse and still little-understood landscape of memory projects about the Stalinist experience. Included among them were many local museum collections and permanent exhibitions that chronicled the history of the district. With the archival and site-specific research of locally based Memorial activists, some of these expositions now explicitly presented the Gulag as a formative institution for their regions and cities.[80]

Yet these activist and Memorial-led provincial Gulag-town exhibitions could present a narrative in tension with the histories told in Russian metropolises. In the same 'democratic era', big-city museums devoted to the Stalin terror and Gulag appeared, most notably the State Museum of the History of the Gulag run by the city of Moscow's department of culture. A small, obscure museum when it opened in 2001, it was replaced by a larger modern facility in 2015, the same year in which the Russian government adopted a 'roadmap' (*kontsept-siia*) for the commemoration of victims of political repression. The Moscow Gulag museum, with its pretensions to national leadership in framing the story of political repressions, is committed to the compelling narrative of the victimisation, deaths, and survival of the intellectual (and to a lesser extent, the ordinary citizen) in the Gulag.[81] In the same way, scholarly historiography, until 1991, was also tied to these narratives as the principal prism through which we could see and attempt to understand Soviet forced labour. The terrifying story of the individual unjustly arrested, interrogated, sentenced, deported, and wasted in apparently pointless police-empire construction projects ('roads to nowhere') determined what Western and dissident Soviet scholars could examine when they looked at the Gulag. The story of overwhelming waste and injustice has dominated accounts of the Gulag for public audiences in the West and in metropolitan Russia.[82]

In Gulag-built towns and cities, however, museum curators and Memorial history activists confronted a more complex story to tell. How could they describe the emergence of local industrial complexes – hydrocarbon extraction, coal, gold, and rare mineral mining, railways and canals, and manufacturing industries – and the cities that supported them, without acknowledging the original sin of Gulag origins, recognising that, in essence, the Gulag established their city or region? How could they do justice to the wasted lives, and at the same time the constructive actions, of so many prisoners forced to inhabit their region and make of it a 'home' even if only for the time of imprisonment and exile? There were no easy answers in the diverse narratives they settled on.

In 2009–11, to study the history of Gulag medicine I travelled to the cities of Ukhta and Pechora in the Komi Republic, and to Magadan in the Kolyma gold-mining region of Russia's Far East. I soon found that the commemoration of the Gulag was a conundrum with great significance for regional centres built on prisoner labour. In each city, museums wrestled with the dilemmas of memory in various ways. But they all included material about the construction of their localities and the figures who enhanced the life of the region thanks to their professional and intellectual talents. Unquestionably, these 'builders' of the local colonial project were outliers, prisoners and ex-prisoners who often enjoyed better rations, better housing, and more respect, than the average prisoner condemned to 'general labour' in forests, mines, and construction sites. Finding a way to tell these stories in a respectful balance was challenging. The Magadan Province Regional Museum offered the visitor two rooms: a bright one presenting the normal Soviet 'public face' of Dalstroi, the 'trust' that ran the gold mines in Kolyma region in the Stalin era; and a second, darker room explaining how prisoners toiled, suffered, and often died at the hands of Dalstroi's institutional shadow, the Administration of the North-Eastern Corrective-Labour Camps, or Sevvostlag. Visitors were implicitly invited to synthesise the light and the dark for themselves. In Komi, the Pechora Historical-Regional Museum told the story of the rise of the city, acknowledging its construction by prisoners. It included many photographs and biographies of prisoner-medics who helped found medical services there. The museum's curator had assembled extensive archives of interviews, documents, and photographs of the regional Gulag's doctors, nurses, and health-care workers. The History Museum of the Ukhta State Technological University, which focused on the techniques of oil extraction developed in the region, devoted a major proportion of its exhibition to the malign influence of Stalin, represented in a giant portrait in oils, and illustrated the anguish of prisoners in letters to family and inscriptions in the houses they built for 'free' workers. In the same city, the Ukhta Museum of the History of Public Health – an institution that caught my eye thanks to its website, which led to phone calls and a rewarding visit when I began this project – blended the forced-labour origins of the region's medical services with the achievements of its prisoner-protagonists in an unapologetically heroic style. The museum, and the literature derived from its collections, passes quickly, uneasily, over the free-contract doctors and bureaucrats who voluntarily served the secret police while running the Gulag's medical organisation, like the husband-and-wife team of Yakov Sokolov, the early director of the local Sanotdel profiled by Ostap Vyshnia, and Sofia Viktorovna Sokolova, a physician who ran a camp infirmary. No single museum that I visited found a 'correct' way to present this history, and indeed, how could they? What was compelling, to my eye, was the way in which they looked to reconcile the familiar metropolitan story of the Gulag as nothing but a waste of lives and producer of roads to nowhere, and the complicated local story of tragic separation from home and loved ones, combined with a determination to create something of lasting value in the place of confinement. It was in this space that my interest in the Gulag doctor grew.

Finding the voices of Gulag medical workers

I began this project by looking at the archives of the central Gulag Sanotdel administration, part of Moscow's Gulag head office. These official papers offer an important, but necessarily one-sided, view of the medical infrastructure of the forced-labour camp system. Through them it is possible to see the 'aesthetic planning', as Lynne Viola describes it, of the central Gulag bureaucracy – the self-deluding intentions and aspirations of Moscow officialdom, with rather less of the harsher reality reflected in reports from the camps themselves.[83] Historians, notably Boris Nakhapetov and Golfo Alexopoulos, have made great use of these materials to write valuable histories of the Gulag medical service, giving us a sense of the corporate mentality of the comfortable desk-physician far from the camps but close to the Gulag brass, and by extension to Stalin and his team.[84] Originally, I was captured by the 'corporate' mindset of the central Gulag Sanotdel, and my earliest seminar papers and writing about the Gulag reflected a certain naivety about this bureaucracy's freedom to manoeuvre and benign facade. After receiving some salutary knocks on the conference circuit, I turned to other kinds of source material to reflect on the Gulag from perspectives closer to the camps, and closer to the medical workers who worked there. The memoirs of Gulag doctors became a window into this world.

The Gulag doctor's memoir is a hybrid that combines the story of a professional life, the evolution of a career in medicine, with the story of an encounter with an extreme environment. Most of the doctors who chose to write about their experience in the Gulag were prisoners; only a handful of memoirs were apparently written by freely hired doctors.[85] I look at memoirs written between the 1950s, after Stalin's death, and the present; the majority were written during the 'democratic era' in the late 1980s to the early 2000s. The rarity of the Gulag employees' memoirs as a whole is easily explained: during a time when denunciation of the secret police and its Gulag raged in public debate, who would willingly speak about their complicity with a repressive system? The few authors that did presented themselves as outliers, indeed, as failed examples of the career NKVD doctor. The employee memoirs display forms of 'shielding' from complicity with violence and criminality, in euphemism and simple blindness to suffering. Another form of shielding is the claim made by these ex-employees of the Gulag that they were young, green, and essentially playthings of circumstance, not responsible for their environment. Others insist on their staunch defence of medical values for prisoner-patients, in the face of harsh Gulag commandants indifferent to the welfare of their inmates. In these memoirs such positions are literary strategies, adopted well after the events described, a retrospective accounting for past behaviour that reflects these writers' awareness of their association with an ambiguous 'grey zone' (between perpetrators and victims) of a now-discredited institution.[86] While the freely hired doctor's reminiscences may be rare, and their perspectives problematic, they do offer useful material on the young graduate physician's pathway in medicine and her understanding of its application in the penal setting.

The prisoner-doctor's notebook of reminiscences is more prevalent, and less subject to 'shielding' in the narration of brutality and deprivation witnessed by the author.[87] Such a memoir blends features of the prisoner autobiography with the more romantic intelligentsia traditions of the doctor's notebook as social and political critique. Like the usual Gulag prisoner's memoir, it depicts the trajectory of a literal and metaphorical journey across space, and through the typical prisoner's 'stages' in experience, learning, and the struggle to survive. The prisoner-doctors combined that 'sharp trajectory' (to paraphrase the title of one famous memoir, *Krutoi marshrut*, by prisoner-nurse Eugenia Ginzburg) of arrest, deportation, and confinement, with the intellectual Bildungsroman tradition of the physician coping with new and unfamiliar patients, disease, and illness, in this case behind barbed wire.[88] The most detailed of these prisoner-doctors' reminiscences are vivid accounts in the tradition of the social and political critique commonplace in Russian medical writing, of how medical care was often distorted or abused in the camps. While these doctors recount copious evidence of Gulag neglect and abuse of prisoners, and egregious misrule and corruption on the part of commandants, they virtually never approach the level of horror that sets apart prisoner-doctors' reminiscences about the Nazi death camps.[89] As prisoner-nurse Eugenia Ginzburg exclaimed when a German prisoner-patient rumoured to be an SS officer, and deranged with remorse, begged her to euthanise him using a syringe, 'You're mad! We're not fascists. We don't murder our patients, we treat them.'[90] At the same time, there is often a fair degree of professional pride in the prisoner-doctor's memoir, as he or she recounts how, against all odds, humane medical values sometimes triumphed over the brutal realities of the camps. In this way, these reminiscences inscribe their authors into the history of their Soviet century, a common desire among Russian intellectuals approaching the task of memorialising their lives in narrative form.[91]

To test the veracity of these perspectives the historian needs to refer to sources beyond the voices of these doctor-memoirists. This book draws upon a wealth of central and local archival and museum collections to weigh and compare the perspectives of the medical staff in the Gulag. I have already hinted at the weakness of central Sanotdel records, that present the view from Moscow. These papers, held in the State Archive of the Russian Federation, reveal the activities and aspirations of the Sanotdel bureaucracy, reporting to secret police bosses and to Stalin's Politburo. Golfo Alexopoulos has shown how these papers are redolent of the institutional culture of the Gulag and its embedded medical service. From these records a bureaucratic and detached, dehumanised, approach to the prisoners as patients is impossible to miss. Patient-prisoners viewed en masse from these bureaucrats' desks in the capital were reduced to an 'inferior workforce'; medical administrators called them 'contingents', 'human raw material', and drily described mass illness and mortality in the pursuit of maximum productivity. In Alexopoulos's words, doctors 'behaved like typical bureaucrats within a hierarchical system. Their actions were motivated by a desire to comply with the rules of the system, rather than by a distinct hatred towards prisoners.'[92]

Local archives of the Gulag camps bring us closer to day-to-day operations and the preoccupations of camp commandants, and their Sanotdel managers within individual camp complexes. Recent scholarship has profited from these regional collections, showing the emergence of greatly differentiated camp complexes with varying degrees of severity for inmates.[93] They constitute an important counterweight to the comparatively homogenising archives of the central Gulag administration in Moscow. The newest Gulag scholarship unpicks the meaning of contradictory data between centre and periphery.[94] These local state-run archives are scattered around the former Soviet Union; many within Russia itself have become increasingly difficult for foreign researchers to access. During my research, I visited some of these collections, in Ekaterinburg for the Urals region, and the archives of Magadan Province in the Far East of the country, yielding valuable material; I also consulted archives in Tbilisi, Georgia for their discussions of camps and colonies in that Soviet republic. Colleagues have shared materials from other local collections. As well, local scholars have published valuable collections of key documents about the camp complexes in their regions, drawn from official archives, constituting an important source of perspectives from the local camps.

An extremely valuable set of sources for this study comes not from the state's official archives, but from historical-regional museum (*kraevedcheskie muzei*) collections. Gulag people and institutions left a store of materials of regional significance that merit examination, despite the ideologised mindset that gathered and organised them. Working in the collections of the Magadan, Pechora, and Ukhta regional museums proved particularly rewarding for the personal archives of doctors, mid-level medical staff, and prisoners they held, and the fine-grained detail they could reveal about daily life in camp complexes. The unique Ukhta Museum of the History of Public Health (*Muzei istorii zdravookhraneniia Ukhty*) gave me unfettered access to the wealth of personal records of doctors, nurses, specialists, and prisoners gathered by an energetic team of retired medical professionals in the 1990s.[95]

Indispensable assistance came from the colleagues and collections of the Memorial Society in Moscow and St Petersburg. Prisoner-doctors, nurses, and patients were well represented in the archives of both cities' Memorial branches, which gave me generous access and advice. At an early stage, I consulted the selection of the Moscow branch's memoirs held at the International Institute for Social History, Amsterdam.[96] The Memorial collections, and the regional museums of Ukhta and Pechora, were my principal source of unpublished biographies of mid-level medical staff: nurses, feldshers, orderlies, pharmacists, and laboratory staff.[97] A few were members of the intelligentsia who wrote their memoirs, but the majority of these lower-level Gulag medical personnel did not; their reminiscences were captured by amateur historians, relatives, and Memorial researchers. These collections also yielded prisoner-patient narratives, which occasionally offer helpful commentary on the actions of my medical professionals. Also during the early stage of this project, interviews with survivors of the post-war Gulag were possible. I talked to a small, but varied, group of witnesses. In 2009 Memorial in Moscow enabled me to interview two former Gulag prisoners, Aleksandr Tsetsulesku, a Romanian surgeon who worked in the Ukhta medical system; and Yuri Fidelgolts, a medical assistant in various Far Eastern camps. From 2009 to 2012 in Montréal, Québec, with the assistance of her family, I conducted interviews with Anna Kliashko about her work from 1948 as a freely hired doctor in the civilian medical service of Magadan region. Finally, I conducted two interviews with the daughters of Gulag prisoner-doctors, one in 2009 in Moscow with Tatyana Oleinik, whose father Lev Grigorevich Sokolovsky served as a psychiatrist in Ukhta; and the other in 2011 in Ukhta with Vanda Trifanova, whose father Emil V. Eizenbraun ran a hospital complex there from 1936. Naturally, these interviews yield materials with their own weaknesses. Among them obviously looms the long interval between event and testimony, and the active operation of memory-reconstruction and distortion. As well, I was aware of the much-'rehearsed' nature of Tsetsulesku's and Fidelgolts's reminiscences; they had testified many times for Memorial's researchers (and in the case of Fidelgolts, recorded them in a short story of 'documentary fiction' that replicated much of our conversation).[98] Anna Kliashko's precise and unrehearsed recollections of her work, never previously tapped, offered an opportunity to test my impressions of life in Kolyma's clinics and hospitals as drawn from memoirs of free and prisoner-doctors and medical workers.

Gulag doctors practising medicine

This book is organised in a series of chapter-biographies, portraits of doctors and other medical workers, exploring their paths to the Gulag and their labours in the medical services there. For some chapters I have combined two, three, or more lives, to draw out contrasts and comparison: prisoner experience versus that of freely hired doctors, the varied environments where medicine was practised in the Gulag, and distinctive approaches adopted by some labour-camp physicians to writing a memoir. I compare their obscure lives, which largely have not been studied by specialists, to those of well-known Gulag survivors whose medical careers in the camps are better known, such as Eugenia Ginzburg and Varlam Shalamov. Overall, these chapters form a rough chronological stream, from lives of some of the earliest 'pioneers' of Gulag medicine, by way of the experience of the Gulag as it expanded in the Great Terror of 1937–38 and responded to the Second World War in the 1930s and 1940s, to the post-war years of the mature Gulag with its established large central camp hospitals and research facilities. The geographical sweep takes the reader from the camps of northern European Russia in Arkhangelsk Province and the Komi Republic to Siberia's far northern nickel-mining centre in Norilsk, and on to the northern Pacific coastal port city of Magadan and its hinterland of gold-mining camps stretching to the Arctic Ocean.

INTRODUCTION

By looking at a range of medical professionals' experiences in a diverse collection of settings, over the lifespan of the Stalinist Gulag, I argue that Gulag medicine deserves deeper consideration as part of the experience of Soviet forced labour. Historians should not dismiss medical care in the Gulag as 'born of the devil', as Solzhenitsyn did; nor should they mine the archive of the Sanotdel for facts but skirt uneasily past the quandary of its historical meaning as too sensitive, or too confusing, to address.[99] The 'medical section' was a part of the Gulag, implicated in the cruel inhumanity of that system, yes – but it was one of the 'grey zones' in the camps where different kinds of power and knowledge met. In the medical 'grey zone' the penal authority to take life or let life continue – Michel Foucault's 'sovereign power' – confronted the power of medical knowledge – Foucault's 'disciplinary power' – to save and sustain lives.[100] That confrontation, which is the essence of Gulag medicine, animates the chapters that follow. A core argument I offer for the toleration of medical expertise inside a place of such destructive punishment is that medical knowledge supported the 'police colonisation' objectives of the NKVD. Nevertheless, the 'medical knowledge' that was given some authority by Gulag bosses was intended to be Soviet, collectivist, and production-focused: it diverged substantially from the Hippocratic values that some doctors still understood and tried to honour in their Gulag healing. It also differs a great deal from the 'medical knowledge' and values most readers would consider 'humane' today: historical study enables us to understand but it does not compel us to absolve. Lastly, I argue that the contribution of Gulag medicine – with all its flaws and distortions – was significant enough in the minds of survivors and successors (memory activists, Memorial activists, local historians and curators) to gain a place as a valued feature of camp life, and indeed of the history of these places. Solzhenitsyn's long shadow on this issue counsels caution, but the esteem in which local medical heroes are held in local histories and museums merits attention too.

Part I introduces several doctors who worked 'inside the barbed wire'. In chapter 1, we meet two contrasting pioneers of the medical service. The first is a prisoner-doctor, Nikolai Viktorov, remembered as the founder of medical services of Ukhta's camp complex. His trajectory exemplifies the experience of unfree doctors working for the early Gulag of long-distance exploration in remote and untracked wilderness. In the same chapter I introduce Yan Pullerits, a career physician for the secret police, who established the medical organisations of Dalstroi in the camps of the Kolyma River basin. The biography of Pullerits illustrates the close ties medical professionals could forge with patrons in the OGPU, and the cost of such alliances. Chapter 2 follows a former OGPU doctor and expelled Party member, Nikolai Glazov, as he pursues a career, or perhaps better to call it a 'non-career', as a Gulag physician. His familiarity with the 'chekist milieu' brought him close to the commandants he served and apparently ensured his survival. At the same time his memoir presents him as a victim of the Stalinist regime and raises questions about how we should read these autobiographies. Chapter 3 looks at the unusual memoirs of two 'freely hired' Gulag doctors. Both young women 'fresh from the benches of the medical institute', Nina Savoeva and Sofia Guzikova were graduates sent to the Gulag as staff doctors, thrown in at the deep end with little awareness or idea of the penal system and its peculiar internal culture. I compare their experience with that of the Jewish, Belarusian doctor Anna Kliashko, another graduate assigned to Dalstroi, working however in the civilian medical service parallel to the prisoners' system. Together, these chapters enable us to see the nature of Gulag medicine. Enmeshed in penal regulation, these doctors were subordinate to commandants and hamstrung by the prisoner status of their patients. They faced extremes of repression, supply shortages, and isolation. Yet they still created hospitals, refed some prisoners exhausted by exploitative hard labour, treated disease, and operated on and 'saved' a proportion of their patients.

Part II, 'Careers in Gulag medicine', considers how some inmates, and 'free' employees, built medical careers as support staff of the doctors and their bosses. Chapter 4 examines two prisoner-apprentices who eventually became medical doctors after a sentence spent working in the Gulag's health network. Vadim Aleksandrovsky was arrested before he could finish his final examinations for his physician's qualification. Under the patronage of a medical bureaucrat in Arkhangelsk Province, a region where medical personnel were thinly spread, his memoir offers a classic Bildungsroman depicting how a raw almost-graduate blossomed into a confident and compassionate physician. The case of Viktor Samsonov offers a contrasting entry point: a youthful prisoner with no medical schooling, he describes his training in one of the best-documented central camp hospitals, at Vetlosian near Ukhta. Chapter 5 is a collective portrait of nurses, both prisoner and 'freely hired'. Olga Klimenko's memoir of her service in the camps as a prisoner-nurse looks back at a career that extended and even stretched her values in un-Soviet ways. Her experience contrasts with a collective portrait of 'free' nurses drawn from the lower ranks of Soviet society who benefited from the unlikely upward social mobility conferred by a career in the Gulag's medical service. Their stories are drawn from an unusual archive of interviews conducted by a local museum curator, Tatyana Afanasyeva in Pechora. Chapter 6 takes us to the central camp hospital of the nickel-mining complex at Norilsk, where we enter the morgue and meet its self-taught anatomist, Moldovan prisoner Eufrosinia Kersnovskaya. Her unusual perspective on life, and death, in the camps reveals the moral universe her doctor-bosses navigated and the scientific uncertainties of doing medicine in the mid-twentieth century in a place far from the medical schools and institutes of Europe. In these chapters, I suggest that some individuals forged a professional life for themselves despite the extreme constraints of the Gulag's penal regime, finding mentorship and guidance as well as obstruction and violence along the way.

Part III, 'Researchers and dreamers', returns to Ukhta's Vetlosian Central Camp Hospital to explore the medical research culture of this peculiar place. Focusing on two Jewish prisoner-doctors who became good friends, the chapters illustrate how scientific curiosity and a desire to envision a future after the Gulag found expression in official and unofficial 'research projects'. Prisoner-psychiatrist Lev Sokolovsky's investigation of prisoners who simulated mental illness enables an exploration of the spectrum of psychiatric disorders that plagued the Gulag prisoner, while also demonstrating how a damning critique of the labour-camp system could be concealed in a few pages of medical case histories. Ukrainian radiologist Yakov Kaminsky's dream of a 'Northern Resort' based on the radium-rich waters of the Ukhta region, a resource tapped by the secret police in their search for rare elements, reveals the strange hold that radioactive bathing had on medical professionals as a therapeutic weapon against a range of diseases. It also tells the story of the poisoning of a community thanks to Gulag planners' negligence and the weakness of experts in the face of supreme power. The paradoxes, contradictions, and significance of Gulag medicine as illuminated in these stories are considered again in the Conclusion, which also returns to glimpse briefly the lives and fates of the protagonists of this book, after the death of Stalin.

PART I
DOCTORS INSIDE THE BARBED WIRE

1

'THEY WERE THE FIRST'
Pioneers of the Gulag medical service

'The first clinic of Doctor Viktorov was on the banks of the Ukhta River, just him on his own under a pine tree: a table, a medicine kit, a doctor ... That's all.' This is how the Ukrainian 'forced-labour historian' Ostap Vyshnia opened his history of the origins of medicine in the Gulag camps of the Ukhta district. He devoted a short chapter to profiling Nikolai Aleksandrovich Viktorov, Ukhtpechlag's first physician.[1] Vyshnia describes how Viktorov journeyed with the first expeditionary party by river barge to Ukhta, heartily dispensing sanitary advice and first aid, treating colds and rheumatism, and single-handedly building a three-bed infirmary.

The story of Nikolai Viktorov, and how he came to set up his impromptu clinic on the banks of the Ukhta River was, of course, far less romantic than this scene of the lone representative of the intelligentsia engaged in selfless service in the wilderness suggests. Viktorov is commemorated today as the founder of the city of Ukhta's – and the surrounding region's – medical infrastructure. An examination of his biography can tell us much about the ways in which doctors became enmeshed in the forced-labour camps, in the Gulag's earliest years of arduous expeditions into untracked regions. The story of this prisoner-doctor illustrates many of the dilemmas facing prisoners who worked in their occupational fields within the Gulag, attempting to exert their professional skills and judgement under the absolute authority of a prison regime. Commandants held him in esteem in the fledgling camp's earliest days and raised him temporarily to director of the medical infrastructure of Ukhtpechlag, but were quick to demote him when the career OGPU physician Yakov Sokolov arrived to take his place. Sokolov stayed less than four years, and commandants turned to Viktorov to direct Ukhtpechlag's medical network until the end of the Great Terror. Viktorov had a strikingly free hand to recruit medical talent from among the zeks, and this chapter introduces some of this book's protagonists who benefited from his patronage.

From the biography of a zek who became a medical pioneer, I turn to examine a privileged professional of the early Gulag sanitary service. Yan Yanovich Pullerits was a freely hired OGPU doctor who eagerly accepted an analogous post overseeing medical services in the fledgling capital of the Kolyma gold-mining camps in Russia's Far East, Magadan. Pullerits followed his boss, charismatic OGPU commander Eduard Petrovich Berzin, from a prototype penal factory at Vishera in northern European Russia, to the distant wastes of Kolyma. The doctor built and organised the region's network of clinics and hospitals, promoted scientific regional studies, and presided over the desperate conditions that prevailed in Kolyma's camps. When Berzin was denounced and destroyed in the Great Terror, Pullerits too was groundlessly accused of counterrevolutionary crimes, and became one of Stalin's millions of victims. A doctor's eagerness to serve a police empire drew Pullerits ever closer to the structures and values of that power, with tragic consequences for him and his family.

Nikolai Viktorov's path to the Gulag

Nikolai Viktorov, born in 1899 into a peasant family in rural Kostroma Province, would seem to have been someone sure to benefit from the socialist revolution of October 1917. His parents moved with their children to St Petersburg before the Revolution, joining the rising tide of peasant migrants settling permanently to become proletarians in the Imperial Russian capital. His father worked in one of the city's booming factories and his mother worked as a

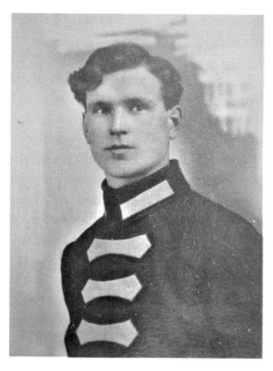

2. Revolution's child: Nikolai Viktorov, student in Petrograd, 1922.

housekeeper, as did his two sisters; a brother worked as a driver back in Kostroma.[2] They clearly had ambitions for the son they brought to the capital. Viktorov, an intelligent boy, completed his gymnasium (academic high school) diploma in 1917. It is unclear from Viktorov's file at the Ukhta Museum of the History of Public Health what the youth did during the turbulent months that followed graduation, when the Bolsheviks seized power and Lenin stripped Petrograd (its name from 1914 to 1924) of its status as capital, moving the Soviet regime's leadership to Moscow. Civil war loomed; Viktorov with his family must have suffered the privations that followed the closure of many factories and businesses, and the uncertainties around food and fuel supply in Petrograd. His father's factory job ended and he got a post as a fireman working for the new city administration. Like his father, Nikolai was certainly adept at finding a niche for himself in the new revolutionary order. In 1918 the son of a peasant made a spectacular leap by securing a place to train as a physician in the Petrograd Military Medical Academy, arguably the nation's foremost medical school.

Nikolai graduated in 1924 and was immediately assigned to service as a junior doctor to the Soviet Red Army in Georgia – then engaged in a bloody campaign to suppress revolts against Moscow's February 1921 annexation of the independent First Georgian Republic.[3] He was needed in the midst of this mayhem. One revolt in August 1924, encouraged by the independent Georgian government-in-exile based in Paris, led to a three-day spree of bloodshed across Georgia, with mass shootings by Soviet forces killing almost 1,000 members of the country's intelligentsia and nobility. The Red Army and OGPU fought ruthlessly to impose Soviet rule in Georgia and were opposed by exiled remnants of the independent regime scattered around Europe: their cause was backed by Polish covert operations intended to harry the Soviets, while in the streets of French and German cities OGPU hitmen hunted and killed Georgian Menshevik opponents.[4] During 1924–25, young Viktorov served an internship in the Tbilisi Military Hospital in the capital of Soviet Georgia; from 1925 he held junior then senior army doctor posts in the Sixth Caucasus Rifle Regiment. He said nothing in a 1934 'Autobiography', handwritten at the request of his bosses in the Gulag, about what he saw during this formative period in Georgia.[5]

Viktorov spent his first furlough from the Caucasus in his home-town, now named Leningrad, in the spring of 1927. Over fifteen days he met friends, wandered through his old haunts, and relaxed as he told stories of his adventures in the Caucasus. This loose talk about a trouble-spot on the sensitive Soviet borderlands where foreign forces were actively conspiring against Moscow was unwise. The 'revolutionary' Petrograd of his student years was now a more Stalinist fiefdom. His tales of adventure led to what Viktorov later called a 'false denunciation' – he was arrested on charges of espionage and divulging state secrets. Within two weeks an OGPU court (*kollegiia*) sentenced him to three years' imprisonment, and he was sent to the OGPU camp complex at Solovki. There he worked for two years, not in hard labour but as a staff doctor, then a manager of the camp's 'Central Hospital', finally as a 'sanitary doctor of the camp'.[6] Viktorov's father launched an appeal against the OGPU's original sentence, in September 1928, perversely yielding a worse outcome – the young doctor was sentenced to be shot. The supreme punishment was commuted to ten years' imprisonment; and later Dr Viktorov was successful in having this reduced to a five-year term. However, by the time of his second year in Solovki he had tasted denunciation and trial, deportation to the country's most forbidding concentration camp, and the threat of execution. His fortunes were at a low ebb.

The Ukhta Expedition of the OGPU

In 1929 the OGPU got the green light to expand its labour-camp system. Drawing upon the resources of the Solovki complex, officials organised an 'expedition' to establish a base camp at Chibyu (renamed Ukhta in 1939), in the heart of the Komi Republic.[7] The purpose of the 'Ukhta Expedition' was to search for and inaugurate the exploitation of oil, gas, radium water, and coal, known to exist in the region from pre-revolutionary prospecting. At the heart of the expedition were forty geologist-prospectors, of whom thirty-six were prisoners; in total, the expedition initially counted 139 prisoners and a handful of OGPU officials. Having deliberately arrested Nikolai Nikolaevich Tikhonovich, the key geologist who had led a pre-1917 trek to Ukhta, the OGPU followed his advice (offered to police planners while under arrest in Moscow's Butyrka Prison) and elected to approach Ukhta by sea. A ship would carry 'everything [necessary for the trek] down to the last nail' from the White Sea to the Barents Sea, then upstream via the Pechora River and its tributaries southward to the destination at Chibyu, near the site of an old prospectors' base.[8] Dr Nikolai Viktorov was assigned to the expedition as its physician, one of its contingent of prisoner-specialists.

The Ukhta Expedition set off from Solovki's mainland port at Kem on 6 July 1929, using the camp's steamer *Gleb Bokii* as far as Arkhangelsk.[9] At this port prisoners transferred the load from the OGPU steamer to another ship, the *Umba* – and two prisoners made a successful escape, the first of several attempts en route. OGPU reports suggest that the specialist-zeks did not seek to flee; escapees were prisoners attached to the expedition as guards, cooks, and labourers.[10] The *Umba* reached the mouth of the Pechora River by 13 July; the sea-going vessel was swapped for a river-steamer, the *Soviet Republic*, and at the Izhma River, to proceed farther south, prisoners once again had to transfer the cargo. Anna Kaneva, historian of Ukhta, describes the toil that followed:

Having loaded the cargo (75 tonnes) on to fifteen large Komi-style fishing boats, [...] they moved up the Izhma River. The whole caravan was divided into six divisions. Convoys guarded the head and tail of the caravan. They proceeded by hauling these barges using ropes passed from hand to hand. Only on 3 August did they have the chance to wash themselves in the bathhouse of the village of Izhma and get long-awaited letters. Ahead lay the hardest part of the route through the Izhma rapids. The expedition only reached Chibyu on 21 August. Later, many more parties arrived this way.[11]

In his 'Autobiography' Viktorov claims to have been assigned involuntarily to the expedition as its chief medic. In the Gulag, work assignments were seldom freely chosen. Nevertheless, Viktorov's youth, vigour, and his military service record in the Caucasus would have weighed in his favour as a candidate. Caught in the grip of waves of typhus epidemics in the late 1920s, Solovki's camp authorities would not wish to release any of their experienced medics, and in Viktorov they took the opportunity to sacrifice a less-seasoned doctor under the cloud of a commuted death sentence. Viktorov was strong enough to have a chance of surviving the expedition, experienced enough in military medicine to handle the challenges expected, and habituated to army discipline.[12] As the writer Vyshnia noted, Nikolai Viktorov was 'a military doctor for whom life on the march was, as it were, second nature'.[13] Only two days after arrival in Chibyu, the OGPU confirmed Viktorov in the post of 'director of the sanchast' (short for 'sanitary section') of the expedition.

His first duty was ominous – a long way from Vyshnia's clinic under a pine tree. Just three days after the expedition arrived and set up its first five tents, and only a day after Viktorov was appointed sanchast director, a cook, Krivonogov, fled and hid in the woods 25 kilometres from Chibyu. Guards in pursuit shot him. 'It was only after four days of travel to the place of death that Dr Viktorov was able to conduct the medical examination of the corpse', the expedition leader reported to OGPU headquarters.[14] As the camp was more firmly established, prospector-geologists set out in work parties to map the area and look for places to sink oil wells. Viktorov instructed a member of each party in first aid, and doled out medical kits from a precious, dwindling, store of supplies to accompany them. In emergencies he often had to follow the prospectors to their bases to care for sick prisoners. According to Vyshnia, who himself had medical training, Viktorov tried to promote and explain the routines of preventative medicine, so central to Soviet healthcare principles. If a man went down with illness, there was no one in the expedition's small team to replace him; Viktorov sought to encourage an 'all for one and one for all' attitude towards health, founded on the old Russian peasant principle of 'joint responsibility' (*krugovaia poruka*).[15] He had not had the chance to conduct a medical inspection of the expedition party before it departed from Solovki, and crew reassignments, escapes, and, one presumes, accidental deaths or punitive killings, took a toll on this first group. Despite the expedition leader's complaints about the advanced age and poor fitness of about half of the prisoners he took to Ukhta, 125 out of 139 arrived there in August 1929.

Within one year the camp held almost 500 prisoners, with new seasonal convoy parties arriving by the sea and river route, or overland on foot.[16] It grew rapidly thereafter, from 824 prisoners on 1 January 1931 to 9,012 in 1932; and 20,886 in 1933. The population rose dramatically during the Great Terror, from 31,035 on 1 January 1937 to 54,792 exactly a year later.[17] To match this growth, in June 1931 the OGPU converted the 'Ukhta Expedition' into 'Ukhtpechlag' (short for Ukhta-Pechora Camp complex) and Viktorov's humble 'sanchast' became a fully fledged 'Sanotdel' – a 'Sanitary Department' which would run a network of clinics, including some with beds for inpatients. Viktorov briefly became its 'acting director' until August when a young OGPU loyalist, Yakov Petrovich Sokolov, just out of medical school, arrived to take over as Sanotdel director. Prisoner Viktorov was downgraded to sanitary inspector of the Sanotdel, a post he held until the end of 1934.

A prisoner-doctor in Ukhtpechlag

With a burgeoning population composed of prisoners arriving exhausted from forced marches or laborious river journeys to Ukhtpechlag, Viktorov witnessed at first hand one of the key features that would mar inmates' lives in the Gulag throughout Stalin's life-time: transport from urban prisons to isolated camps across vast distances took a fierce toll on health. Food and drink en route were often inadequate and lacked vital nutrients; sanitation was poor; shelter and clothing, improvised.[18] Half of one early party of prisoners, having trekked from a transit camp in Kotlas, 551 kilometres south-west of Ukhta, arrived emaciated or so ill they were unfit for heavy labour. Viktorov could offer little to improve their condition: perhaps some bed rest for the worst affected, along with enhanced rations.

With Sanotdel director Sokolov in post, Viktorov's freedom to act was significantly curtailed. One can imagine his frustration. The seasoned military doctor was now subordinated to a greenhorn 'straight from the medical school benches'. This was an inversion of the traditional medical hierarchy where experience usually commanded respect: typically, in the Gulag the freely hired physicians could often be fresh-faced graduates, supervising more senior medical experts, even former professors or health commissars, who were prisoners. Sokolov is described as 'a doctor-administrator' in his secret police file, which also tells us that as a student he volunteered to work for the OGPU and requested a secret police assignment when he graduated in 1931.[19] He directed the Ukhtpechlag Sanotdel until 1934, and local historians deem him an important early organiser of Ukhta's medical infrastructure, although their silence about his actual activity and his evident overpromotion seems eloquent.[20] More striking is their foregrounding of the poor state of prisoner health on his watch. According to Viktorov's recollections, Sokolov the administrator presided over malnutrition leading to scurvy and pellagra, while clothing shortages and exposure created high rates of frostbite, rheumatic and respiratory illnesses. Of course, these conditions lowered the immune systems of these weakened prisoners, leaving them vulnerable to more serious illnesses. Lice infestation, Viktorov remembered, was widespread in these years and epidemics of typhus took many lives in Pechora and Usinsky subdivisions. Kaneva notes how bitterly Viktorov recalled the starvation and hypothermia he witnessed among prisoners even once they settled in the camp complex.[21]

How Viktorov reconciled himself to Sokolov's leadership is unknown; other prisoner-doctors in similar positions kept their heads down, performing their roles as best they could without getting into trouble. (Dr Glazov, subject of chapter 2, would be a textbook example of this attitude.) Yet it is intriguing to think that Viktorov co-authored with Sokolov and a third colleague a brochure about treating malnutrition and starvation-related conditions, entitled *Scurvy, Emaciation, Oedematous Disease*, for the camp's medical workforce.[22] (No copies of this work appear to have survived; indeed, 'emaciation' later became a virtually banned word in official Gulag medical terminology.) As 'sanitary inspector' Viktorov's role was inherently invidious. He was an observer and deliverer of bad news about prisoner health and living conditions, a flimsy part of the bureaucratic checks and balances that kept Soviet institutions from total stagnation. He was fortunate that his sentence ended in December 1934; but he suffered a typical ex-con's fate: he was refused permission to leave Ukhtpechlag for home. His internal passport 'tied' him to the Gulag. He became, instead, Sokolov's deputy director of the Sanotdel, as a 'free' employee of the Gulag. With Sokolov's departure, Viktorov served as full director from 1935 to 1938.

'Ukhta-Shockworker' to civilian doctor

Viktorov experienced a turbulent three years as Sanotdel director. As a recently released prisoner, he was far from secure in his post. The camp's internal secret police conducted an inquiry into high prisoner mortality and morbidity in September 1935, accusing him of failing to inform authorities of real conditions. Viktorov, by now adept at writing petitions and protests, managed to get the local courts to investigate; they threw out the case as lacking in substance.[23] He petitioned the Ukhtpechlag director Yakov Moroz repeatedly, asking to be relieved of managerial duties and returned to clinical work; the director refused. In the inverted world of the Gulag, it was not unusual for some doctors to seek less responsibility, to avoid career progression, or to ask for transfers downward in the hierarchy of medical facilities. This could be a means of distancing oneself from doing active harm or drawing so close to police authority as to compromise one's medical conscience, or indeed one's personal security. It also dodged responsibility for failures of healthcare that were inevitable in the Gulag's model of exhaustion through forced labour.

Whatever Sanotdel director Viktorov's motives were, he somehow avoided the worst during the Great Terror. On the eve of Terror, in 1936, he was awarded an 'Ukhta-Shockworker' medal, with Moroz's blessing, and NKVD head Nikolai Yezhov mentioned him in an April 1937 decree listing Ukhta freely hired employees meriting the expunging of criminal records and awarding of prizes (guns and watches in this case).[24] Only in late 1938, after the execution of over 2,500 Ukhta camp prisoners by roving NKVD plenipotentiaries and their firing squads, did Viktorov's association with the now-disgraced camp chief Moroz, arrested in August, lead to demotion. Viktorov was reassigned to direct Ukhta's Vetlosian Hospital – the town's major prisoner medical facility; after two years he slid further down the ranks, sent to run a local camp division sanchast where he worked until January 1942.[25]

In these more modest roles Viktorov was remembered by colleagues as someone who was 'courteous and generally made a good impression on us'.[26] Arriving in Ukhta in 1938, an experienced radiologist, prisoner Yakov Yosifovich Kaminsky, initially felt demoralised to think that he would end up in general labour. He was surprised to discover that Viktorov would soon have a vacancy for an X-ray specialist; Viktorov prevented Kaminsky from being sent

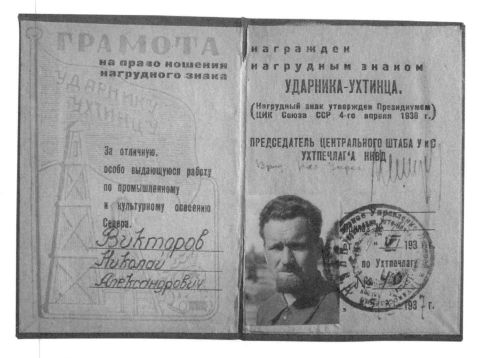

3. *Prisoner no longer: Viktorov's 'Ukhta-Shockworker' passbook, 1937.*

farther north, by giving him a generalist's assignment in Vetlosian's unit for invalids and weakened prisoners. Eventually, prisoner-doctor Kaminsky conducted research as well as serving the patients of Vetlosian, becoming the prisoner-hospital's director in 1943.[27] His story is told in chapter 8.

Viktorov did not restrict his kindness to senior medical specialists. An 18-year-old prisoner, a geology student arrested in Petrozavodsk in December 1937, Viktor Aleksandrovich Samsonov spent most of his first two years in the Gulag struggling to escape exhaustion and starvation-related illnesses because of hard labour. After short hospital stays at Vetlosian to patch him up, including some time working as an orderly and observing autopsies in the morgue, work-assigners judged him able-bodied, and sent him to a timber-felling brigade where the toil took his condition to new depths. An encounter with Nikolai Viktorov at Vetlosian in 1939 saved Samsonov and launched a lifelong passion for medicine. The

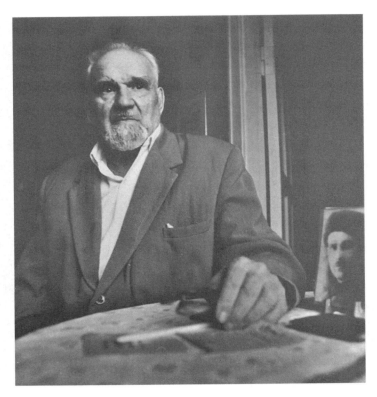

4. Survivor and witness: Viktorov in old age.

young man asked Viktorov, who was treating him, if he could get a
job in the hospital – by then a large establishment with hundreds of
beds – and Viktorov, after learning about Samsonov's attendance at
autopsies, and getting favourable reports from colleagues, bypassed
the work assignment office's opposition to a transfer by hospitalising
Samsonov and simultaneously attaching him to the surgical ward as
an orderly.[28] The young man began a career in medicine which
continued beyond barbed wire into the twenty-first century; his story
is told in chapter 4.

Viktorov's risky wartime resignation from his camp sanchast post
in 1942 was motivated by love. His wife Edit Fedorovna Antipina
(Runge), a gynaecologist, was a Soviet citizen of German nationality.
She worked in the same camp; however, when the war began, she was
forced to 'resign' and given twenty-four hours to leave Ukhta. In a

demotion intended to humiliate the 'German', Antipina was directed to work in an isolated village southeast of the Komi capital, Syktyvkar, far from roads or railway lines. Viktorov 'at his own request' left his job and accompanied her. In 1946, at the invitation of the Komi Republic's Ministry of Public Health, they moved to Syktyvkar and worked in hospitals there, each in their specialist areas. In 1961 Viktorov was designated 'Honoured Physician of the Komi Autonomous Soviet Socialist Republic'. Edit Fedorovna predeceased Nikolai Aleksandrovich; they had no children. Dr Viktorov survived to be interviewed by Anna Kaneva, who wrote the first modern history of Ukhta, under conditions of Soviet censorship that made discussion of the camps all but impossible, in 1970. Nikolai Viktorov died in a nursing home near Syktyvkar in 1980, soon after retirement.[29]

Yan Pullerits goes to Kolyma

Nagaevo Bay, September 1932. A windlass lowers an 8-year-old girl from the deck of a Japanese ship over a frigid Pacific Ocean to the small boat beneath. After a long voyage below decks in the 'primitive' vessel this girl, Margarita Yanovna Pullerits, is enjoying this precarious flight through the fresh sea air. Margarita remembered that her mother, Elena Yakovlevna Pullerits, did not enjoy being winched to the smaller vessel. But when they finally made landfall, they were equally happy to be reunited with her father – Yan Pullerits, director of the Sanitary Department of 'Dalstroi', a socialist enterprise like no other.[30] Dr Pullerits was another Gulag medical pioneer, and Dalstroi, a vast fiefdom of the OGPU where the principal pursuit was gold-mining, and the principal workforce, prisoners. The early arrival of family dependants Margarita and Elena signalled the pioneer-doctor's high social status in the small but soon-to-mushroom settlement of Magadan by Nagaevo Bay. Pullerits was a freely hired employee of the OGPU, a key specialist needed for the establishment of Dalstroi's network of mines in the Kolyma River basin.

Dr Pullerits's career in the OGPU was closely tied to that of Eduard Petrovich Berzin, Dalstroi's first director. Berzin's military service record included unmasking the 'Lockhart Conspiracy' against

Soviet power in the Bolsheviks' desperate summer of 1918; he joined the Party and the chekists that year.[31] In 1926 Berzin took charge of an OGPU project using prisoner labour to build a chemical, cellulose, and paper manufacturing base in the Urals north of Perm. After a sluggish start, with First Five-Year-Plan investment, he led construction of the Vishera Cellulose-Paper Complex in just eighteen months, in an isolated site, out of the limelight compared to the early Gulag showcase-prototype camp at Solovki. In the 1920s Solovki was publicly celebrated in film and journalism as a place for the reforging of the regime's enemies.[32] Meanwhile, in Vishera under Berzin's rule, prisoners were worked to exhaustion and, in some divisions, to emaciation and the edge of death: according to local archival researchers Vishera created more registered invalids than any other OGPU camp at the time. The complex swelled to several sites and over 39,000 prisoners by 1931, while its hospital for inmates had just 40 beds.[33] Moscow gave Berzin a new assignment on the heels of completing the Vishera complex; in November 1931 he was made the director of Dalstroi and dispatched to the Far East. Yan Pullerits, an OGPU medic who since 1926 had served Berzin as chief doctor of the 'Red Vishera Therapeutic-Prophylactic Organisation', and who had seen at close quarters how prisoners received 'therapy', accepted a commission to follow him to Kolyma in December 1931. They both arrived in Nagaevo Bay early in February 1932.[34] Thirty-four-year-old Estonian Pullerits was one of many non-Party members on the tight-knit team of specialists, many of Baltic origin, that Berzin brought with him from Vishera to set up Dalstroi's industrial operations and infrastructure.[35]

Pullerits was immediately made director of Dalstroi's Sanotdel. In the first weeks after arrival, Pullerits oversaw the requisitioning of the existing local authority's small hospital and all medical supplies in the name of Dalstroi, setting up a clinic in Magadan for the administrators and military personnel.[36] Within a year, Berzin reorganised the growing camp administration, designating its medical heart the Nagaevo-Magadan Therapeutic-Prophylactic Organisation, under the direction of Pullerits; it later became the Sanitary Administration of Dalstroi. Magadan's hospital opened new wards, and a polyclinic, for non-prisoners, also opened in 1933.[37] Such was the importance Stalin and the Party assigned to gold production by Dalstroi, that it was free to expropriate the modest pre-existing 'cultural bases' established by local authorities in this far-flung region, and Berzin had a high degree of autonomy in determining its priorities for investment and growth, so long as the gold kept coming in. And it did. In Berzin's first year as Dalstroi chief executive, he delivered half a tonne of gold; the rates climbed dramatically in the mid-1930s, until in 1937 alone Dalstroi gave 51.4 tonnes to the Soviet state.[38] Dalstroi's gold fed Stalin's Five-Year-Plan hunger for imported Western technology to fuel industrialisation. It also fed the Berzin team's love of flashy cars: the Dalstroi chief drove a Rolls-Royce, and other officials brought – to this roadless corner of Eurasia – at least one all-terrain Citroën and a Mercedes. Yet as late as 1939 Magadan's Sanotdel only had one automobile at its disposal for ambulance duties.[39] Despite his privilege, and a plausible case for requiring motorised transport, Pullerits did not rate a vehicle of his own. Yet Berzin personally rewarded his chief doctor in 1933 by giving him a Zeiss camera, purchased on one of his trips to Germany to buy equipment for Dalstroi.[40]

Dalstroi produced its gold at enormous human cost. Pullerits presided over Dalstroi's practices, familiar to him already from Vishera, and prevalent around the expanding penal system, of underfeeding and overwork; he witnessed the system's creation of plenty of malnourished, sick, and work-depleted zeks. From 1932 to 1956, the Gulag sent a total of 876,043 prisoners to Dalstroi's camps; of these, a total of 127,792 or 14.6 per cent died officially registered deaths inside these camps. Of the rest, 546,972 were released 'at the end of their sentences', and this figure must include an unknown and fluctuating proportion of the severely ill who died soon after early release on medical grounds.[41] By the mid-1930s Dalstroi was actually sending prisoners back to the 'mainland' (as the rest of the Soviet Union was called) in remarkable numbers: as much as 25 to 33 per cent of its 'stock' of total prisoner population in any given year. Some were healthy prisoners whose sentences were finished, but many of these were transfers of weakened and invalid prisoners, sent to lower-priority camps in 'mainland' Siberia.[42] While the network of hospitals, clinics, and medical stations grew under Pullerits's direction of the Sanotdel, it is clear that services fell well short of the need suffered by prisoners who toiled in Dalstroi's camps. In fact, in this early period it is difficult to untangle Pullerits's activity as director of the camp medical network, and his construction of a parallel network of clinics for freely hired Dalstroi employees. Retrospectively, in a 1936 history of the region's medical services, he celebrated the resilience of the first expeditionary teams of doctors in characteristically 'socialist realist' fashion:

Medical work in the taiga [...] has its peculiar character. From the conditions of Soviet clinics and hospitals of the big cities, the work of the doctor is transferred to a tent or a barracks built on the permafrost. Knowing how to orient and adapt to these new circumstances plays a significant role in determining the quality and scale of medical service to individual districts. The good taiga-dwelling doctor must show particular imagination and the capacity to create hygienic conditions for a therapeutic establishment regardless of the circumstances (in a tent, a corner of a barrack on permafrost, in the yurt of a native inhabitant). Knowing how to adapt to any conditions, this doctor should be highly demanding and at the first opportunity demand the construction of good clinics, hospitals, and exemplary children's nurseries.[43]

Such facilities were imagined for non-prisoners: the geologists, prospectors, machine-operators, and other technicians hired by Dalstroi. As Dalstroi grew, higher-grade services were created for non-prisoners, and distinctions between prisoners and civilians proliferated.

Pullerits would be summoned to the Kremlin to receive the Order of the Red Banner of Labour in 1935. This honour came on the heels of his work on the problem of vitamin C deficiency, scurvy, in the Kolyma camps.[44] Pullerits encountered high rates of the condition when he came to Magadan, and in 1932 alone he sent 1,500 prisoners with scurvy back to the 'mainland'. From the region's growing medical staff, Pullerits set up a 'scientific association of doctors' to study how scurvy might be prevented using local resources. The pine

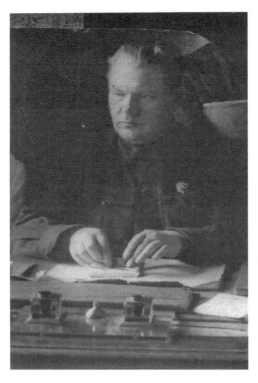

5. *Adapting to conditions: Yan Pullerits, medical administrator, 1936.*

needles of the subarctic creeping cedar shrub (*stlanik*, Lat. *Pinus pumila*) were popularly known, probably from indigenous peoples, as a source of vitamin C.[45] Pullerits led the development of an infusion from needles to be given to prisoners as a supplement. His association of doctors even published a volume entitled *Scurvy and the Struggle with it in the North*, in co-operation with the country's leading vitamin specialist, Leningrad biochemist, Aleksandr Aleksandrovich Shmidt. It was an extraordinary book project, juxtaposing Shmidt's academic prestige with contributions from at least two prisoner-doctors. Berzin wrote a preface for the volume and Dalstroi co-sponsored publication with the national medical publisher. The book circulated within the Gulag's medical network but probably later disappeared from accessible library catalogues.[46] Their pine-needle infusion apparently did something to reduce scurvy, although historians and memoirists dispute the effectiveness of this and subsequent versions of the detested evergreen extracts.[47] The prisoner-feldsher and Gulag writer Varlam Shalamov recalled how the pine-needle drink was produced in the Kolyma camps:

> The needles are prepared at so-called 'vitamin' camps, with their meagre rations, where 'dokhodiagi' (goners) pluck the needles and stuff them in sacks, adding a few stones to make up the weight. Hundreds of starving harvesters, fulfilling, or not fulfilling the plan. The most monstrous thing is that this bitterest of revolting extracts was forced upon everyone everywhere, and yet it contained no vitamin C at all. For decades they tormented people: it was forbidden to give out the midday meal until after the 'medicinal' dose was taken, and then, after all that, they said it wasn't a medicine. Therapy itself they turned into torture. The smarter, more honest doctors knew this.[48]

Such was resistance to the pine-needle extract, and the continued prevalence of vitamin deficiency, that later Dalstroi commandants had to restate orders for compulsory dosages of the bitter drink before prisoner meals.[49] The extract became a commonplace measure to prevent scurvy across the northern camps of the Gulag.

'An amazing man, doctor, and scientist. Died for no reason!'

In the late 1950s and early 1960s (the era of Khrushchev's de-Stalinisation), a Magadan writer, Nikolai Vladimirovich Kozlov, started to gather documents and testimony for a novel about the first pioneers of Kolyma. His central hero would be Eduard Berzin, whose rehabilitation he sought. The end of de-Stalinisation in the late 1960s put paid to this project, and after his death Kozlov's archive of documents eventually passed to the democratic activist and publisher Semyon Vilensky.[50] Among the papers on the history of Dalstroi assembled by Kozlov was a terse 1955 certificate from the KGB, explaining the fate of Yan Pullerits during the Great Terror, with the exclamation of respect and despair that opens this section inscribed in Kozlov's hand.

Pullerits, like his patron Berzin, was arrested and shot in the Great Terror of 1937–38. Margarita, the doctor's daughter, recalled how her father had a period of leave in 1937 and took his family to Moscow; they were living in the capital in a special apartment building for Dalstroi employees. Soon an uncle, Ernest Lapin, also a Dalstroi official, staying in the same flat, was arrested, and Margarita remembered how the police searched his rooms in the middle of the night. She could not sleep, and witnessed him being taken away, 'white as a ghost and with a look of distraction in all his features'. They never saw Lapin again. Margarita's father naively declared, 'No, I know Ernest like I know myself, Lapin isn't guilty, they'll let him go, he's been arrested by mistake.'[51] It is unclear when Yan Pullerits realised that a similar 'mistake' threatened to engulf him. In December 1937 on arrival in Moscow Berzin was arrested, and barely a week later Pullerits himself was being denounced in Magadan in absentia, in a meeting of the medical workers' trade union that dragged on over two nights. On 4 January 1938 the city's newspaper, *Soviet Kolyma*, branded the now ex-director of the Sanotdel an 'enemy of the people'.[52] Soon after, in February 1938 a Berzin associate denounced Pullerits saying he 'conducted hostile work, turned all of the medical personnel against [the denouncer], drove one woman-doctor to suicide. Pullerits gave preference to prisoners ahead of freely hired workers, named them to responsible posts and in general created better conditions for them.'[53] It is impossible to know if these were fabricated accusations or genuinely reflected Pullerits's actions. Given the energy he devoted to establishing higher-grade facilities for Dalstroi's free employees, and his distance from the rank-and-file medical teams in the spreading network of camps and outposts, it seems uncharacteristic that he indulged prisoner medics unduly. And yet, the logic of Gulag medicine – with experts among the prisoners and apprentices dominating the free medics – forced him to favour zek-doctors and nurses more often than not.[54]

It is also unclear how far Yan Pullerits was aware of these accusations arising a continent away in Magadan, while he was on leave in Moscow. Pullerits, however, did decide to leave his family in Moscow and move to Saratov, perhaps naively thinking he could escape detection. There he planned to live with his in-laws and work on a thesis based on his studies of scurvy conducted in Magadan. His old professor supervised the work and arranged for a Saratov University post for Pullerits upon defence of the thesis. Evidently, Pullerits wanted to detach himself from Dalstroi and seek refuge from the Terror in academia: it was a desperate manoeuvre to evade his connections with Berzin's patronage network. Margarita recalled the moment when such hopes crumbled: a telegram arrived in April 1938 from her grand-father, with the news of her father's arrest, on charges of anti-Soviet activity, supposedly inspired by the Berzin circle in Magadan.[55] The NKVD confiscated his papers, including photographs of Gulag pris-oners used in his research.[56] Within two months, police arrested Elena Pullerits as a 'wife of a traitor to the Motherland' and she was given an eight-year sentence. She spent that time in the special camps for such 'wives' in Karaganda; although she was a qualified nurse she worked in agriculture, tending sheep, which as her daughter recalled, she later said saved her life. Margarita was fortunate to be taken in by her mother's relatives in Saratov, where she survived 'cold and hungry years' during and after the war. Margarita did not see her mother again until 1946.

After Khrushchev announced his de-Stalinisation policy at the Twentieth Party Congress in 1956, Elena Pullerits sought rehabilita-tion for herself and her husband. In 1989 Margarita's dignified and brief memoir noted that her mother was rehabilitated in October 1960; her father's certificate was issued posthumously in January 1961. 'On the death certificate it says, "Died 16 June 1938". The cause of death is struck out.'[57] In 2012 Kozlov's archive revealed a little more about the fate of Yan Pullerits. An extract from his KGB case file, seen by Kozlov, described how in prison he initially denied the charges of anti-Soviet activity of any kind. However, a scant month after arrest, Pullerits testified that Berzin had recruited him to commit crimes against the state. The former Dalstroi Sanotdel director was tried individually in person in a Military Collegium of the Supreme Court, a procedure conferred only on the foremost victims of the Great Terror, when most victims were convicted in absentia on paper. On 16 June 1938 in court Pullerits repudiated his 'confession' extorted in prison and branded as 'false' the testimony against him given by others embroiled in the Berzin Affair. The court ignored his protests and sentenced him to the supreme measure of punishment. He was shot that same day.[58] His boss would soon follow him. In July 1938 Stalin signed Eduard Berzin's death warrant, and Yan Pullerits's patron was executed on 1 August 1938.[59]

'Knowing how to adapt to any conditions . . .'

Adaptability was a keyword in the careers of these two very distinctive doctors. The ability to practise healing skills, and to organise medical care facilities, in extreme conditions was a common skill shared by both of these 'pioneers' of Gulag medicine. Both doctors confronted the contradictory impulses of doing medicine in a penal setting, but their responses to this focal conundrum of labour-camp healthcare were markedly different.

For Nikolai Viktorov, a prisoner raised to responsibility in the Gulag's fresh expeditionary network of wilderness outposts, adapting 'to any conditions' literally entailed running clinics from scratch in the open air, and doling out fearsomely short supplies of medicine from barges and tents. Compulsion pressed upon him from expedition commanders and later camp commandants; he was no free agent and yet his medical expertise and initiative were harnessed to the founding of clinics and infirmaries in a territory where the Gulag rapidly colonised a region previously only sparsely inhabited. Adaptability did not mean complete abjection – Viktorov could challenge secret police charges and petition his bosses for changes to his roles, and sometimes win – but he was shrewd enough to choose his battles wisely, navigating the precarious phase of the Great Terror. He was unable to save the mass of prisoners who suffered from malnutrition and exhaustion, but he demonstrated compassion and generosity in the cases of Samsonov and Kaminsky. Strikingly, his most dramatic gesture of adaptability came years after the official end of his sentence, with his resignation during the war to join his politically suspect wife in her administrative exile. Having married someone under political stigma, he embraced a share of that stigma. This characteristic decision marked a determination, long in the making, to escape the orbit of the Gulag and to seek a measure of civilian normality – a goal that Nikolai and Edit achieved.

Pullerits, the medical bureaucrat, was a very different navigator of the contradictory pulls of penal medicine. As director of the 'Red Vishera Therapeutic-Prophylactic Organisation' he tailored his medical training, and values, to suit the requirements of a secret OGPU penal facility and his patron Eduard Berzin. Vishera produced a huge quantity of paper, and invalid prisoners, under the physician's adaptable gaze. That ability to tolerate huge suffering in prisoners served Berzin's gold-mining enterprise at Dalstroi, which yielded a fantastic supply of precious metal for the Soviet state. At the same time, from the directorship in Vishera of modest healthcare facilities, Pullerits established an expanding, and geographically vast, network of medical stations, clinics, and infirmaries in Kolyma that became an impressive empire of penal medicine in its own right. This ambitious empire-building matched that of his patron Berzin, who just before his downfall authored a grandiose ten-year plan for the colonisation of Dalstroi's territory – terrain that encompassed 10 per cent of the USSR's landmass by 1940.[60] Yet there was perhaps a naivety to the Kolyma Sanotdel director's willingness to dance to the tune of Gulag bosses, when followed by his bid to fade into academe in sleepy Saratov during the Great Terror. Adaptable Yan Pullerits enjoyed the fruits of privilege bestowed by a flamboyant patron, but there was no escape for the medical bureaucrat when Berzin's star fell. By the time he repudiated his compliant testimony in court, it was too late.

2

'A NIGHTMARE PARALLEL WORLD'
A chekist in the clinic?

Baku, 1924. A naval medical officer and Communist, 24-year-old Nikolai Aleksandrovich Glazov, is 'not surprised' when a commissar from his own ship approaches him with a proposition. The medic, whose class origins are less than ideal under Soviet power, is told that he should come and work for the OGPU as an informant on the 'intelligentsia circles you frequent'. 'I turned down his proposition,' Glazov recalled over sixty years later:

> He started to rebuke me for not wanting to serve the Party and work for the Cheka, to which I replied that I did not want to work in secret. He presented me with some kind of card identifying him as a special plenipotentiary of the Cheka with the right to mobilise any Party member at his discretion. I asked him if we could discuss it tomorrow, and the next day, when we met on the staircase, he could see from my face that I would not agree to work for him. He told me sharply, 'Very well. If you don't want to you don't have to. But keep in mind that from now on we'll be watching you!' And not waiting for an answer he pushed past me.[1]

Glazov's brush with the secret police in 1924 was not his first, nor would it be his last. Imagining himself able to choose his own path in life, the young feldsher was hoping to upgrade his medical training and become a physician. Ironically, the military institutions that sponsored his doctor's qualification would become so enmeshed in the security police in the 1930s, that Dr Glazov would have no choice but 'to work for the Cheka' after all. He served the medical services of the security police before his arrest and sentence in 1936 to five years' imprisonment for 'counterrevolutionary Trotskyite activity'. Nikolai Glazov worked as a Gulag prisoner-physician in the camps of Ukhta and Vorkuta for eight years, only achieving release in 1944, because like many 'political' prisoners his term was extended during the war.

The challenge for the historian of Gulag doctors is to decide how to interpret Nikolai Glazov's account of his life and service as a physician behind barbed wire. Who was this 'chekist' doctor, and how did his security-service past, and possible 'present', affect his medical practice once in the camps? Unlike Drs Viktorov or Pullerits, hailed as 'pioneers' by local historians, it is fair to say that Dr Glazov left little trace in the memory of the Gulag towns where he worked. Apart from his own memoirs, written with the help of his daughter just before he died in 1989, and published in a tiny print run ten years later, we have scant documentary evidence to corroborate his testimony.[2] Few patient-prisoners who survived to write memoirs recall him. He remained a low-level sanchast physician throughout his prison term. In part, Glazov's obscurity is explained by the fact that the Gulag authorities moved him around the system so often: as a prisoner from 1936 to 1944, he was transported to a new camp, and put to work in a new medical facility, not less than ten times. Such 'perpetual motion' was more typical of the average prisoner trapped in back-breaking general labour than of a privileged zek working in his or her professional field, and it distinguishes him from many prisoner-doctors behind barbed wire.[3] They made themselves indispensable in their posts and did what they could to minimise the arbitrary transfers that constantly threatened all Gulag prisoners.

Other factors may explain Glazov's obscurity and his 'perpetual motion'. We can dismiss the suspicion that he was an incompetent or demoralised doctor; he had scientific interests and publications, and his military discipline apparently did not flag while he was in captivity. That said, his memoir is less a medical Bildungsroman and more a mid-career physician's story of tribulation: it exposes the moments when his medical self-esteem ran up against the demands of the camp bosses. In his Gulag account, Glazov's 'passive-aggressive' attitude towards authority, his awkward philosophy of survival, becomes readily apparent, and suggests that commandants found him difficult to manage. His chronic heart condition may have contributed to a certain obstinacy that explains why commandants put his name down for transportation so frequently. At the same time, in many posts, Glazov got close to the authorities and gained their trust and confidence, often through treating them for illness. Why they relied on this prisoner-doctor remains unspoken in his memoir. His familiarity with the security-service culture may have engendered their trust, and as we will see, he knew how to ingratiate himself to commandants when it proved useful to do so. His memory, as preserved by his daughter, is unambiguously that of a 'victim' of Stalinist repression – which by any reasonable measure, he was. Nikolai Glazov was unjustly imprisoned, as his rehabilitation in 1957 confirmed. He was in no way a committed oppositionist to the Soviet regime, but rather, he was someone from the wrong class who scrabbled to overcome that obstacle in the new society. At most, he flirted with opposition ideas while studying medicine in the late 1920s in Leningrad, but the language of his reminiscences betrays no love of anti-Stalin rhetoric, in the past or in 1987–89 when his memoirs were composed.

Whatever his actual relationship to authority, Glazov's account abounds with the ambiguities and shortcomings that historians have recognised in memoirs written by 'Gulag bosses'. This prisoner-doctor's memoir offers the mix of 'tangled interweavings of fact and self-representation' more typical of the genre of 'bosses' memoirs', as Cynthia Hooper has explained. Comparison of his account with others, where possible, offers one means of discerning his motives. As well, we need to check our expectations of Glazov as 'victim'. Our desire to find an articulate 'liberal subject' espousing Western values in his text may blind us to a conformity deeply entrenched in someone whose life was spent working in Soviet institutions.[4] An attentive reading that reflects on the prisoner-doctor's actions and their consequences, and compares this experience with that of others, can suggest how an ex-employee of the OGPU, familiar in its ways, might become entangled in the chekist milieu in the Gulag. That he did so, and survived the Great Terror in the camps, is worthy of consideration as an example of the confrontation between Gulag authority and medical expertise. Glazov's practice as a prisoner-physician and determined survivor becomes an even more puzzling feat in the violent and unpredictable context of 1937–38. After presenting a summary of Glazov's life, I turn to explore his relationship with the 'Gulag bosses' and the internal security police; his medical practice and professional attitude; and finally his understanding of mass mortality in the camps.

Perpetual motion: The chekist-medic's Odyssey

Nikolai Glazov was born in 1899 into a lower-middle-class family of Polish origins. He studied in St Petersburg's Military Feldsher School. Even before graduation in 1917, young Nikolai volunteered on an army sanitary train; he was decorated for saving an officer. But in the ferment of revolutions and civil wars Nikolai's taste for adventure led him to seek new opportunities. He took a course in hydrometeorology, and later in 1917 joined an expedition to Dikson Island in the Arctic Ocean. Civil War in Russia eventually became inescapable – the Dikson expedition relied upon White forces which controlled Arkhangelsk in 1918. Glazov was appointed to the Whites' sanitary administration; when he refused to accept the commission, for fear of falling into Red hands, a patron sent him back to Dikson. Yet on return to Arkhangelsk in spring 1921, Nikolai found the Reds in charge. They made him director of a sanitary station of the Soviet northern navy. The Soviet Cheka noted his 'White' past and kept him under surveillance. His was already a 'spoilt biography' in the eyes of the new regime.[5]

After his strange isolation from Russia's tumult, Glazov's response to events on the mainland seems ruthlessly pragmatic. He petitioned repeatedly 'to be sent to the front' to fight for the Reds in the Civil War, and to join the Bolshevik Party. He was rebuffed; 'later I learned that they thought I was "sucking up" to the new powers-that-be.'[6]

Perhaps he was. When his Party application was finally accepted, in 1922, he gave his sole motivation as 'Conviction of the inevitability of world revolution'.[7] A Party card brought advancement: the feldsher was sent to the Caspian Sea fleet to manage medical services. He lived a bohemian life in Baku, where he found many sailors used illicit drugs – cocaine, morphine, and especially opium, which he says it was legal to smoke. 'I tried that rubbish myself once, but immediately gave it up,' he recalls, displaying curiosity, bravado – and discipline. After an abortive and romantic bid to study history at Baku University in 1923, Glazov was accepted to the medical faculty to train as a doctor. It was during his first year of study that the OGPU tried to recruit him. Glazov's petitioning and Party work nevertheless helped him get transferred, in a striking promotion, to study in Leningrad. He began a physician's training at the city's prestigious Military Medical Academy in 1924 and graduated in 1929 – just as Stalin launched his First Five-Year Plan.

Glazov wanted to return to the navy, but the newly minted doctor was allocated to Soviet border forces in Central Asia: Party members were needed in the region, he was told. There in Tashkent he met and married his wife, Olimpiada Giorgievna Kolchina, a feldsher in a military hospital. Soviet border forces, conventional Red Army troops led by specialised OGPU forces, were then engaged in pitched battles to staunch *Basmachi* (local anti-Soviet) revolts and to stop the exodus of migrants from Soviet territory, driven away by the regime's collectivisation drive.[8] According to Glazov, he saw action as a Red Army medical officer in several raids against *Basmachi*. His own health deteriorated with the onset of endocarditis, and while the army gave Glazov leave for hospitalisation in Leningrad, the OGPU refused to release him. He remained in Ashkhabad but eventually his illness was recognised, and in 1932 he was transferred to work as a 'therapeutic inspector' for the OGPU's Sanitary Department in Moscow. Precisely *when* Nikolai Glazov became an employee of the security police, or realised he had become one, is difficult to tell in his memoirs; he merely says that his regiment began taking OGPU orders around this time, and his transfer to Moscow was the result of an OGPU command.[9] In his account, the doctor-memoirist sidesteps any suggestion that he *chose* to work for the security police; the OGPU (from 1934, NKVD) appears from the wings as an irresistible force. And yet in 1929, a graduate with a Party membership card was expected to shoulder significant responsibilities, and the OGPU had already tried to recruit Glazov once. It is historical fact that when he was assigned to border force work in 1929, he was already in a chain of command dominated by the OGPU.[10]

Glazov quickly adapted to the life of an OGPU employee in Moscow, by his own admission. He worked in the Sanitary Department of the secret police in various posts from 1932 to 1935, enjoying access to well-stocked official canteens and special closed shops. He had joined Moscow's privileged elite while the peasants of Ukraine and Central Asia suffered acute famine imposed by Soviet rulers.[11] Admiring the OGPU/NKVD's organisation, military discipline, weapons training, and stock of 'theatrical costumes' for plainclothes surveillance operations, he willingly served as a pretend-civilian covertly monitoring Red Square during the funeral of German Communist Clara Zetkin in June 1933.[12] Yet with his heart condition he became unwilling to accept difficult tasks and he rebuffed any move from Moscow. In 1935 he turned down an assignment in the western borderlands, where police were imposing a tighter regime. His political reliability came under scrutiny; only intercession from luminary Emelian Yaroslavsky saved his Party membership. The NKVD discharged Glazov in 1935 on health grounds, and he refused its offer to continue working for the NKVD as a 'freely hired employee'. Instead, he moved to Leningrad where he ran a civilian polyclinic, earning praise in the local press as a 'Stakhanovite'. However, Nikolai Glazov became a victim of the 1936 'exchange of Party documents': he was ejected from the Party, he recalled in his memoirs, on spurious grounds. He believed too that his 1924 refusal to work for the OGPU counted against him. Loss of Party membership entailed loss of his job, and a slide to a less prestigious factory clinic. Within weeks, in June 1936, he was arrested. Glazov's presence at a 1923 meeting in a Caspian navy Party cell, where internal democracy was discussed, formed the basis for charges of 'KRTD', counterrevolutionary Trotskyist activity. Glazov insists he was loyal to the Central

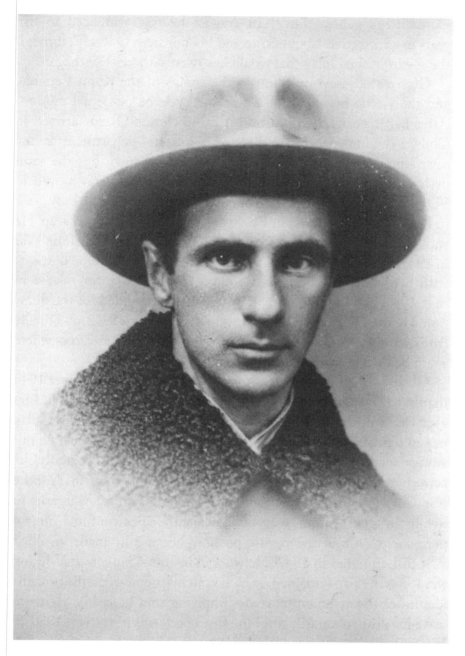

6. *Leningrad healer: Glazov before his arrest in 1936.*

Committee's general line.[13] In August he was sentenced to five years in a corrective-labour camp and his 'northern Odyssey', through the towns of the Gulag that would last twenty-three years, began.

Glazov's odyssey took him to the camps of the Komi Republic and the Arctic beyond it in a dizzying cycle of 'perpetual motion'. After half a year serving in transit camp clinics, Glazov arrived in Chibyu (Ukhta), where he directed a hospital department in the town's growing 'Sangorodok' (literally, 'sanitary town' but the term designated any large hospital complex). In 1938 he was moved to Vorkuta outposts at Vorkuta-Vom and Rudnik; and from 1939 back to Komi where he served in Edzhyd-Kyrta, a coal-mining camp. He was in Edzhyd-Kyrta at the start of the Soviet Great Patriotic War in 1941. In these three camps he directed sanchasti, hospital outposts with beds but few specialist resources. He was due for release in mid-1941, but with the war, his sentence was extended for the duration. He worked in Adzva-Vom invalids' camp from 1942, and finally from summer 1943 in Inta, a large mining and timber camp, where again he directed a Sangorodok department.

Glazov was 'released' from imprisonment early in December 1944 thanks to his good labour record, but he was forced to remain in Inta as a free worker in the same Sangorodok. Throughout his Gulag prison term, Nikolai Glazov was never assigned to general labour but always worked in low-level physicians' postings. Repeatedly, he actively refused greater responsibility. As a free worker in 1946 he was allowed to bring his wife and 12-year-old daughter Margarita to live in Inta with him. Two years later authorities confined him to permanent exile in the North, possibly because he made an illicit visit to Leningrad in 1947. He worked in Inta's Sangorodok during the 1950s; he also remained, as he says in his memoir, 'on the nomen-klatura' of the camp employees – implying that he lacked rights to leave his post voluntarily until the Gulag reforms of the late 1950s.[14] In 1959, two years after his rehabilitation, he returned to his native Leningrad to live with his wife and daughter, remaining there until his death in 1989. In his memoirs he says nothing about his working life after his return to the city of his birth.

Working with the 'Gulag bosses'

In the second half of 1936, prisoner Nikolai Glazov was transported by rail, barge, and on foot from Leningrad to the Komi Republic. His experience of a military physician's 'life on the march' served him well. Guards quickly appointed him 'doctor of the transport' and gave him a ragged sack 'with a few medicines: heart tablets, fever-reducing pills, stomach pills, and a thermometer. This gave me a particular authority not only with the prisoners but among the armed guards too.'[15] Glazov's position as a doctor strengthened with each stage of the journey, and while the regular prisoners' trajectory from Leningrad to Chibyu then took two to three months, he spent about six en route, stopping to set up improvised hospitals at transit camps, while the guards escorted the fitter prisoners to Ukhtpechlag. The diet of salted herring and rye bread, scant supplies of water, and the parlous sanitary conditions weakened many prisoners, and Glazov treated them in makeshift sickbays in the open air, stables, and tents. The prisoner-doctor's work was noticed, and commended, by the deputy director of the Ukhtpechlag Sanotdel who happened to be inspecting a transit camp. It was ex-prisoner-doctor Nikolai Viktorov, by this time a freely hired NKVD employee, although Glazov did not recall his name. From then on, apparently thanks to this chance meeting, the prisoner-doctor would get work that saved him from general labour.[16]

It was late December 1936 when Nikolai Glazov was finally transferred to Chibyu. The trip, from a small hospital 360 kilometres from the Ukhtpechlag capital, was easy enough for the doctor: he was transported by bus and truck with a sack of documents, evidently containing his own prisoner case file. He was to direct the thera-peutic department of Ukhta's Sangorodok, which he describes as 'an entire settlement of wooden buildings, some for hospital wards, [and] specialist buildings: the X-ray department, a laboratory, a pharmacy, offices and living quarters'. It was a typical central Gulag-camp hospital, growing in size and complexity during the 1930s.[17] Like other 'privileged' prisoners fulfilling specialist roles, he was given dedicated lodgings in a house shared by doctor-zeks, a contrast with the usual prisoner barracks. Among his colleagues was a former radiology professor, Boris Nikolaevich Nesterov, previously of the Gorky Medical Institute; he had established the radiology department of the Sangorodok and welcomed the new doctor. Despite a comparatively warm reception, and an initial feeling of liberty 'in his medical environment', Glazov found his fellow prisoner-doctors to be cautious, to judge by their furtive New Year's Eve celebrations. 'Doctors can usually obtain spirits. But our plans for the new year were very modest, limited to tea. As I would later learn, everyone was genuinely afraid of violating the camp rules', including the prohibitions on alcohol consumption and the mixing of the sexes.[18]

Glazov quickly found that some rules were more closely observed than others. His first impression of the therapeutic department he was to run conveys his dismay. The wooden single-storey building had twenty-six hospital wards and he walked right in wearing his outer clothing and camp-overcoat (*bushlat*): no one challenged him. To Glazov it appeared like

> . . . a commonplace barrack. Before me was a long corridor, from which there were doors to wards. In the corridor and in the wards crowds of people gathered, [either] in outdoor clothing, [some] without clothes, [others] in hospital gowns. Those in gowns were wearing bast slippers. In the cots some people were undressed, others were dressed and even in camp-overcoats. Some of the patients had women visiting them sitting on their cots. People smoked in the corridor and in the wards. I walked the length of the building and did not meet a single person in a white coat. There were no signs on the doors, and I could not determine where the doctor's office or the nurse's station were. More than anything else the place was like a railway station during the Civil War.[19]

It is typical of the Gulag doctor to describe his or her first encounter with a camp hospital in similar terms: indiscipline, disregard for basic sanitary rules, promiscuous visitors, and lax control over the wearing of outerwear indoors (a Russian phobia that extends well beyond the medical world).[20]

What is untypical is Glazov's reaction: he asked the Sangorodok's chief doctor *not* to make him director of this department straight away, but to give him time to settle in. Most prisoner-doctors accepted their 'privileged' posts without question. Remarkably, the chief doctor agreed, although Glazov fails to explain why; was this indulgence a mark of respect for the ex-OGPU medical administrator? Initial reluctance to assume responsibility when assigned to it, and a determination to offload responsibility when problems such as soaring sickness and mortality accumulated, became a pattern in Nikolai Glazov's relations with authority.[21] Glazov quizzed the chief doctor about the workload, based on his expectations formed in military or police facilities: what were the bed norms per doctor, how many patients would he be responsible for? 'We don't have any norms here. You will treat as many patients as is necessary.' Glazov would be responsible for sixty-five beds (the norm he expected was twenty-five). The working day ran from 8 a.m. to 2 p.m. and from 4 p.m. to midnight. Already he knew that patient and lower-level staff indiscipline disrupted medical treatment. 'The work of the nurses ... had little effect. The orderlies were irresponsible *urki* [hardened criminals].' The current director of the department neglected his post, and 'there were a lot of fights with the staff and patients'.[22]

Glazov, in his own account, turned things around, once he took over as director of the therapeutic department:

With my military experience I was used to order and discipline. I started by setting out a strict time-regime, which indicated wake-up time, breakfast, doctors' rounds, exercise time, free time, etc. Going for walks was only allowed with the doctor's permission; smoking – only in the smoking room (except for those who could not walk). When I went to the chief doctor to get his signature on the schedule, he refused at first to sign it: 'This is up to you. You sign it yourself.' I managed to persuade him by explaining that it would be easier for me to require obedience if the orders had his signature and not mine.[23]

Enlisting a patient's help, signs were painted to label the department offices and stations, and a library for his wards was set up. Although the Sangorodok had a cinema, amateur theatre, and a hospital library, Glazov felt these amenities for the reforging of prisoners 'all seemed to be in another world'; he personally preferred to read medical literature. Evidently, he thought little of the ideology of reforging. The new director found there were limits to his autonomy; he could not select his orderlies on merit alone. 'They told me that the ones I wanted [to take on] were politicals, and that we should take *bytoviki* [petty criminals] as "socially friendly elements" and re-educate them through labour.'[24]

'The chekist illness' and 'a power stronger than the law'

Nikolai Glazov, the former OGPU medical administrator, found it easy to chat with his patients from among camp officialdom; he knew how to soothe their anxieties. When treating one patient from the administration, the prisoner-doctor urged him to stay in the ward for an extra two weeks to recuperate fully. 'To his question, "with what illness?" I answered that in Moscow they call this in our milieu "the chekist illness", that is working while generally exhausted physically and mentally; you needed "a second wind". He agreed, stayed in the ward for another two weeks, and recuperated fully.' Later, trusting the prisoner-doctor from 'our milieu', this patient showed Glazov copies of the internal security profiles (*operativnye kharakteristiki*) of his staff. Glazov does not conceal that he enjoyed unalloyed trust from the camp security apparatus: 'My security profile was good, it said that I was strict and demanding with the patients and the staff, I was qualified, that with my arrival in the department the treatment improved, mortality went down, that in my personal life I was reserved, did not associate with anyone, did not express my views.'[25] Glazov did try to warn a colleague with a very negative profile, but all this did was upset her, in his account.

Glazov describes in detail the powerlessness of law and medicine in the face of chekist authority. In the summer of 1937, the Great Terror had only just begun, but the camps would soon be swamped beyond capacity. A high legal official, a deputy procurator of the USSR, visited the Chibyu Sangorodok to conduct early release proceedings for prisoners 'suffering from serious illnesses, incurable in conditions of imprisonment', as Glazov recalled. Such releases were, in fact, normally reserved for convicts with a virtually terminal prognosis, and they were a device the Gulag administration particularly resorted to in periods of crisis such as the Terror.[26] Glazov was told to exclude candidates for release with serious anti-Soviet ('article 58') and counterrevolutionary crimes (often denoted by abbreviations like Glazov's 'KRTD'– counterrevolutionary Trotskyite activity; such convicts were known as 'lettered'). He escorted the procurator through the wards, but the official did not turn to acknowledge the prisoner-doctor. Only after the procurator from Moscow met an acquaintance among the patient-zeks, a former Supreme Court judge, and spoke to him at length, did he start to address Glazov. Meeting his colleague in this setting affected him strongly. Next they visited a tubercular ward.

> He stood back from the obviously striking sight of these pale, quietly lying patients, and shielding himself with the door, asked me, 'These are all S-3?' (the code for those with infection in both lungs in the severe stage). 'Yes,' I answered. 'Moribundusy?' (the Latin for 'dying'). 'Yes.' 'Then why haven't you shown me these patients yet?!' 'They are all 58s and lettered,' I explained. 'So what, they're 58s and lettered?!' he cried at me, almost with pain in his voice. 'I was ordered not to show you them.' 'Who ordered you?' 'The Chief Doctor.' 'Present them all to me by 6 p.m.!' He practically tore himself through the doors and then turned to me, 'And are there others like this in the other wards?' 'Yes, there will be.' 'Present those patients to me and you yourself will sign for them.'[27]

Glazov informed the TB patients he was preparing their release papers for a commission of inspection. Their reactions, he recalls, ran the spectrum of emotion: 'one said "At least I'll die at home ..."; another: "Noooo, I'm not going home to die ..."; and still others simply turned over and hid their faces under the bedclothes.'[28] Historian of early release Mikhail Nakonechnyi demonstrates that few such prisoners were able to cope with the physical challenge of leaving camps located thousands of kilometres from home. The released received inadequate rations and clothing for the journey, and in this early period when rail links were incomplete, the trek on foot or by barge was an ordeal even for healthy prisoners.[29]

In the end, the exertions of procurator and doctor to release these patients came to nothing. Only one, an Uzbek student with a spinal infection, was granted a transfer 'to a camp with a milder climate [i.e. not full release from imprisonment]. "And the rest?" I asked. "Refused," they told me. [...] The Procurator left that very day. And we saw that there is a power stronger than the law whose representative he was.'

'You must work! We've shot plenty and we will keep on shooting!'

Nikolai Glazov survived the Great Terror while working in Chibyu and in two brief postings at two Vorkuta camps (Vorkuta-Vom for most of 1938, and Vorkuta-Rudnik until summer 1939). He survived, it seems, thanks to his good relations with the administration, and his ability to navigate situations that might have led to charges of 'wrecking' or 'sabotage'. In the camps, the Terror took the form of execution by quotas established in Moscow and implemented by roving plenipotentiaries with teams of NKVD gunmen.[30] 'Lists' of prisoners to be shot were composed and revised at the regional camp level; Glazov knew colleagues among medical staff who were put on these lists and eventually shot, apparently for close associations with disgraced political figures. In the Ukhta-Vorkuta complex of camps there was a high concentration of genuine supporters of Leon Trotsky, many of whom had participated in hunger strikes in 1936–37. (Glazov tells us that at the Chibyu Sangorodok he refused to force-feed hunger-strikers and authorities directed them to other departments of the hospital where more compliant doctors did. He displays little sympathy for their cause, probably because he was himself imprisoned as a 'Trotskyite'.) The Trotskyites of Ukhta and Vorkuta would be a principal target of the Terror in these camps.[31]

Having received repeated warnings that he would soon be transferred from Chibyu, Glazov already had his bags packed when the order finally came. The Sangorodok chief doctor, Emil Vilgelmovich

Eizenbraun, only recently released from prisoner status himself, regretted he could not keep him in post: 'the circumstances are very complicated', he observed in an obvious allusion to the Terror. Glazov remembered that 'he advised me to keep out of notice as much as possible for my own safety'.[32] After a long transport through a series of camps northeast of Chibyu, Glazov was made director of a sanchast at Vorkuta-Vom, taking the place of a colleague who had been shot. Glazov tried to refuse the appointment, claiming he 'would not manage it', but the chekist who received him explained, ominously enough, that he should be glad of the great trust placed in him. Glazov understood that refusal would be treated as 'sabotage' and lead to execution; he accepted the job without his usual foot-dragging.

Glazov's sanchast was a place for seriously weakened prisoners, set 3 kilometres away from the camp's main Sangorodok.[33] He was not allowed to refer prisoners to the main hospital without himself submitting to interview with the camp's internal security chief, who personally authorised each case. Similar restrictions affected his medical decision-making in his own sanchast. When presented upon arrival with a list of over 100 prisoner-patients in need of milk, of which there was plenty because the site was next to a Gulag dairy, he was required to apply to the dairy's camp commandant. The commandant crossed some 'bastards' off the list who should not, in his opinion, get milk, and added others (including his personal manservant, a prisoner of course) who would. Glazov tells us his philosophy for dealing with official petty obstruction; he arranged to get the crossed-off patients some kind of substitute care, telling his new colleagues, 'The bosses we will listen to, but we will do things our own way. We'll feel good, and so will our "parents". With the bosses there is no need to argue, we just need to "respect" them: agree to what they want, then do things our own way.'[34]

Such tricks enabled Glazov to care for his prisoner-patients while flattering the egos of the 'bosses', many of whom were from his native Leningrad. In Vorkuta several senior commandants were 'outcasts' of the Leningrad NKVD, security police who were demoted to Gulag postings in the wake of the assassination of Party leader Sergei Kirov in 1934. 'Expecting a good mood and softness from such directors was inappropriate.' Yet Glazov again found he could grow close to the chekists he treated for their medical problems. One ex-Leningrad NKVD man, now the director of the internal security apparatus in the camp, required almost daily visits because of a heart condition. Doctor and patient soon relaxed and 'spoke about everything'; but Glazov could do little for the chekist's heart disease – he needed a long furlough in a sanatorium, in the doctor's opinion. Instead, his responsibilities and heavy drinking demoralised him. In the chekist's quarters Glazov had access to media – the press and radio – normally denied to Gulag prisoners, and the security office staff even read him his wife's letter from her exile in Central Asia (he was not supposed to receive correspondence).

More ominous was Glazov's proximity to the plenipotentiary Efim Yosifovich Kashketin, an NKVD lieutenant conducting mass shootings of prisoners during the Great Terror. He had arrived in the region in January 1938 and would be responsible for executions of between 2,000 and 2,500 prisoners in Ukhta and Vorkuta camps.[35] His plane landed at Vorkuta-Vom at the end of March. Glazov recalls in his memoirs that Kashketin asked him to examine him for heart pain, but he could find nothing wrong with the patient. The chekist went to work, cursing local Gulag bosses, and organising the execution of hundreds of prisoners within one week, including several of Glazov's colleagues. Glazov recalls the lists of names of those shot 'for continued counterrevolutionary work in the camp, obstruction, sabotage', posted on the administration door. When it was time to leave Kashketin summoned the prisoner-doctor once more: was he fit enough to fly? 'His heart was significantly worse, but I nevertheless agreed to the flight.'[36] The atmosphere in the camp remained alarming despite the plenipotentiary's departure. In the wake of Kashketin's visit a young Cultural-Education Section activist memorably rounded off a speech with the words 'You must work! We've shot plenty and we will keep on shooting!'[37]

'Tufta, confirmed by a document, ceases to be tufta'

Nikolai Glazov's medical practice and his approach to medical duty in the camps was, if we accept his own account, conscientious in the service of prisoners but alert to the demands of bosses. Certainly, many prisoners passed through the clinics and wards he ran over the years; Glazov does not reflect in his memoir on the injustice of their condition as prisoners and forced labourers. His concern for them takes the form of anxiety about medical statistics: as sanchast director he was accountable for high rates of morbidity and mortality, and he reacted vigorously by protesting to authority, and more rarely, disobeying the 'bosses', when external forces led to sharp rises in these indicators.[38] Glazov employed such dramatic gestures sparingly; during the wartime crisis of high mortality when protest was futile, he worked to save individual patients without protesting against the conditions that starved and overworked them. His response was perhaps typical of the Soviet-trained physician whose work experience was almost entirely within militarised hierarchies as a doctor-bureaucrat. At the same time, he recalls many moments when he discreetly bent the rules, using bureaucratic language and falsifying diagnoses or procedures to satisfy patients or commandants whom he wished to help. Medical 'tufta' – the falsification of paperwork, diagnoses, treatment, statistics, or outcomes in the Gulag sanitary service – was something routine in Glazov's account. Indeed, every memoirist associated with Gulag medicine remarks upon its ubiquity. Glazov was no medical philosopher, and we do not find him puzzling over the ethics of such distortions of medical practice.[39]

A typical example comes from Glazov's encounter sometime in 1939 or 1940 with the Ukrainian poet Volodymyr Zenonovych Gzhytsky, a prisoner at Edzhyd-Kyrta working in the coal mine.[40] Out of friendship, Glazov sought to reclassify the poet as only capable of light labour, to help him escape the mine. The doctor coached the poet to simulate gall bladder attacks; with the first two 'attacks', Gzhytsky was hospitalised for a day of observation. After the third 'attack', Glazov was able to transfer the 'patient' to the light-labour category, and he was then assigned to easier work in greenhouses. The doctor notes that

it was compulsory to register the attacks in the ambulatory journal as the basis for transfer to light labour. Such a notation is already a document, but '*tufta*, confirmed by a document, ceases to be *tufta*' – that was one of the camp precepts. Yet doing such things you had to be very careful. I knew two doctors, who were shot in 1937 for giving a woman-doctor a certificate of invalid-status, freeing her from heavy general labour. She was genuinely ill, but there were insufficient grounds for the [designation of] disability.[41]

Strikingly, this episode of medical 'tufta' is present in the unpublished Glazov manuscript held by Memorial in its Moscow archive, but it does not appear in the book version published by Glazov's daughter ten years after his death. Perhaps coaching a patient to fake an illness seemed to her too great a departure from professional probity; and yet she allowed other cynical examples of 'tufta' to stand.

During the war, when crisis gripped the camps, similar rule-bending and outright fraud were less dangerous for the Gulag doctor. At Adzva-Vom, in 1942, Glazov convinced a veterinarian responsible for the camp's horses to trade medicines with him. He became aware of the vet's ignorance of human dosages after the vet had amateurishly prescribed an equine dose of belladonna to an unwell stable worker; Glazov had to revive the patient who was brought to his sanchast unconscious (he recovered after two days in hospital). From this point on, Glazov obtained extra supplies of morphine, a drug perennially in short supply, from the vet, who worried intensely about these transactions. Glazov had it all figured out: 'I advised him to think up a false history of illness for a horse and record the use of morphine there. That would be a document and, as is well known, "*tufta*, confirmed by a document, ceases to be *tufta*". Aside from morphine, I sometimes got other things for the sanchast from him.'[42] Even Gulag animals could get a false diagnosis.

Glazov was not above using tufta to assist bosses harried by surveillance. At the same camp, he recalls, he was in a meeting delivering a report to the camp commandant and officials, when a prisoner came to tell him there was a man near death in one of the barracks. Glazov sent a dentist to go and tend the prisoner as he could not interrupt his report. When the dentist returned to say that the prisoner had died in the barracks, Glazov's camp commandant became greatly agitated: not because he regretted the loss of the prisoner, but because of *where* the prisoner had expired. The paperwork for deaths outside of hospital was onerous, involving an investigation by internal security police. Glazov grasped this delicate problem; he instructed the dentist

> to move the body to a bed in the hospital near an entrance where it was dark, where few would notice, and give him a heart injection. And turning to the commandant, I said, 'Let him die in the hospital.' It was clear he understood and was relieved. When the meeting was over, I went to the hospital, examined the patient, and realised he was still alive. I gave him another heart injection, and transferred him to another ward, where the attention and observation would be better.[43]

A happy outcome ensued for all concerned, and one which illustrates how Glazov, a prisoner-doctor who understood the 'milieu' of the security police, might win the trust of his camp bosses with a frank resort to artifice.

The other side of Glazov's pragmatic cynicism was a reliance, when it suited his purpose, on the rules, especially those handed down by Moscow that might be used against local bosses. Again at Edzhyd-Kyrta, the coal-mining camp, Glazov had running battles, he recalls, with the commandant in charge of construction of a new mine. Glazov complained that the commandant failed to observe the hygiene standards set by the central Gulag administration in Moscow: canteens were too far from prisoner barracks, and a camp bathhouse, essential to prisoner health, was simply not planned for at the new mine; prisoner-miners had to walk 8 kilometres after a shift, on their own time, to wash. By 'digging about in the decrees of the Gulag' the prisoner-doctor forced the commandant to build makeshift kitchens closer to the barracks (within 500 metres), and to permit prisoners at the new mine to bathe during working hours. The commandant in charge of construction vented his fury at Glazov – 'You were a wrecker when you were free and you're a wrecker here!' – but when the doctor cited decrees by number and date, this boss feared being responsible for mass illness or mortality and approved the concessions.[44]

'Am I dry as dust?'

At Adzva-Vom during the war, Nikolai Glazov enjoyed good relations with the camp commandant Krasnopolsky and his wife, who worked as the camp censor. Glazov treated the wife, whom he does not name, for an illness that required frequent house calls. Glazov found husband and wife to be intelligent, and in increasingly relaxed conversation it emerged that they were 'former people': the commandant had been an Imperial Guards officer, and the censor hinted at having been close to the Imperial Court. As censor of prisoners' mail, Krasnopolsky's wife saw a photograph of Glazov's daughter, and she commented,

> 'It's good that she is being raised without you: you are as dry as dust ...' I replied that I didn't think I was dry with my daughter. She said, 'No, that dryness would come out anyway.' This forced me to ponder. I was not dry, I did a lot for others, but found it impossible to show it. Especially in relation to women: these days people just get married and divorced at the drop of a hat.[45]

It is striking that Glazov includes this bystander's observation about his personality, showing he was perceived as distant and lacking in empathy. Such an assessment also seems to fit with the internal security police profile on the prisoner-doctor: 'in my personal life I was reserved, did not associate with anyone, did not express my views.' How Glazov's dry and distant character affected his medical practice and bedside manner is hard to assess from his own memoir.

However, from the unpublished memoirs of a prisoner-patient we have a rare independent perspective on Nikolai Glazov's medical practice; it comes from Rudnik camp before the war, during 1938–39. Grigory Vlasovich Kniazev was a genuine member of the intra-party opposition of the 1920s, sent to the Gulag in 1936 for this 'crime'. Glazov, unusually for a prisoner-doctor, and possibly a sign of how much commandants trusted him, conducted a 'commission' to classify newly arriving prisoners by their physical capacity for labour. (Such commissions to sort prisoners by their labour capacity and physical condition were routine rituals in the Gulag and mirrored civilian medical inspections of the disabled.[46]) He judged Kniazev fit to work in the Vorkuta-Rudnik mine. Kniazev recalled that he next met Glazov later when he fell ill from exhaustion and malnutrition. He needed a long spell of hospitalisation, but Glazov's ability to grant it was constrained:

My legs were shaking, swollen, I was short of breath. Doctor Glazov examined me in the clinic, the same doctor who on the arrival of our Adak group to Vorkuta had put me down among the 'miners'. He gave me a release from work for several days and ordered me to see the feldsher every evening to have my temperature taken.

'You must get into Dr Galperin's hospital,' Zhitomirsky, the pharmacy worker in the clinic, told me when he heard about my condition. 'Aside from the fact that Galperin is an experienced doctor-therapist, he is also a good person and will help you. But you can only get into the hospital through Dr Glazov who has to write the order for you to be sent there. Glazov has bad relations with Galperin, and therefore no bribe [blat] of any kind is going to help. Now the whole case depends on your temperature: if it stays high for about ten days, then Glazov is obliged to put you in the hospital; he often goes there. Otherwise, he will discharge you, and you go back to your previous work assignment. Glazov does not have it easy, he is under surveillance: the number of those released from work must not exceed the established norm.'[47]

This vignette illuminates the tightrope that prisoner-doctor Glazov walked: he apparently wanted to treat exhausted zeks fairly, by releasing them from work, but he was limited by the 'norm' for release and hospitalisation. At the same time, Glazov's personality or perhaps his chekist affinities meant he was not on good terms with Dr Galperin, 'a good person' who seems to be regarded by the pharmacist Zhitomirsky as the better doctor. Kniazev celebrates Galperin for his generosity, while the best Glazov can say about him in his memoir is that he is 'literate' in medicine, in contrast to other doctors in his hospital.[48] The pharmacist also hints that in other circumstances Glazov might have been susceptible to an exchange of favours (*blat*). In Glazov's bedside practice, empathy was constrained not just by his 'dry-as-dust' personality, but by chekist surveillance, and bureaucratic quotas, too.

Vitamin deficiencies and mass mortality

At Rudnik, in late 1938 or early 1939, Nikolai Glazov, only recently appointed sanchast director, participated in a commission to review prisoner living conditions, conducted by the camp administration, internal security, and Sanotdel officials. The results were dire: tents used as barracks exposed zeks to freezing temperatures; there was insufficient clothing and bed linen to compensate; and as early as November 1938 meat and fish reserves had run out, leading to avitaminosis – vitamin deficiencies. Glazov had encountered the same illnesses early in his career in the border guards of Central Asia, where the diet was equally limited; he now sought to educate his new medical colleagues who 'had never met with these [illnesses]'.

Scurvy, vitamin C deficiency, and pellagra, caused by a B-vitamin shortage, were the main scourges which were hardly new to Gulag prisoners by 1938; but young doctors fresh from the medical institute benches, often freely hired, and older ones who had practised in urban Russia, usually prisoners, were unlikely to have encountered them.[49] Glazov recalls making a speech that failed to convince his sceptical co-workers about the nature of avitaminosis to a Rudnik production conference:

> I explained the threat posed by vitamin deficiencies, about the need for meat and fish, but I got little support from the other doctors. They did not understand that even with sufficient food of a monotonous carbohydrate-based diet – and it was far from a sufficiency – we would not correct vitamin deficiencies. But after that meeting the administration nevertheless began to buy meat from the reindeer-herders and organised fishing brigades from the tundra lakes.[50]

Glazov found two young, female doctors (likely free employees) particularly resistant to the concept of vitamin deficiency: they put a pellagra patient with whom they sympathised on the 'strictest of diets' that only made his condition worse. In a characteristically dry gesture, Glazov suggested to them they grant their 'hopeless' patient 'his last wish': a 'general diet, meat' meal, a consolation to both him and the doctors. The patient began to recover; 'with embarrassment they told me how he was eating eagerly, especially meat, and was noticeably improved. From then on they trusted my experience of treating avitaminosis.'[51]

The prevalence of vitamin deficiencies presaged worse to come during the wartime supply crisis that caused Gulag mortality to jump sharply. Glazov was posted to the invalid's camp Adzva-Vom in 1942, just as prisoner mortality was spiking across the camps. The doctor's memoir approaches the mass death he witnesses dispassion-ately, with no comment on the penal system's lack of food. At this camp 'many died, simply because they were very weak, and the exhausted organism could not resist the slightest disease. People were driven to extremes of exhaustion.'[52] The next camp Glazov moved to in 1943, Inta, a coal-mining, timber and service-farming camp of 9,000 prisoners, was a place where the dying were concentrated, evidently, by the authorities' deliberate design. There were large numbers of tuberculosis and pellagra patients; the only medicine for diarrhoea available was the natural remedy of 'clay and willow bark'; even paper to keep track of patient histories was in short supply. Glazov says he was assigned to direct a department of the Inta Sangorodok housing seventy patients; a local historian records him as deputy director of the Sangorodok, and therefore more respon-sible for conditions there.[53] In Glazov's own words, 'The Sangorodok was not so much a hospital, as a throng of the dying.' A transport of prisoners arrived with many dead, and he notes how their frozen remains made a grim impression:

These corpses were brought to us in the morgue. In the morning we were to conduct several autopsies. We entered the morgue; it was crowded with frozen corpses. Someone muttered 'Auschwitz'.

Some of the dead were standing on their legs and leaned against the warm stove. The sight of reclining corpses surprised no one, but the dead standing on their feet and warming up by the stove was unusual and unpleasant.[54]

This troubling passage, with its reference to the Nazi death camp, illustrates Glazov's attempt to reflect on the mass mortality he witnessed. While Auschwitz was mentioned tersely in Soviet newspapers from June 1941, Soviet media did not describe the death camp in detail until late January 1945. It may be that Glazov had heard of the camp from other prisoners. Its mention here, in a text composed so long after the event, seems less a faithful record of what was said, than a retrospective attempt to process the trauma of this sight.[55] The pages of his reminiscences that follow describe patients he treated in the midst of mass mortality. These cases are presented as memorable because the authorities or other doctors prevented their receiving adequate care, often due to misdiagnosis, while Glazov with his superior knowledge, detective skills, and therapeutic talent, identified the genuine cause of illness and rescued the patient. In one example, a young pilot, diagnosed with syphilis, turned out to be suffering from pellagra once Glazov familiarised himself with the case. He pursued treatment to a successful conclusion, despite resistance from the authorities, who had an animus against the pilot.[56] In the prisoner-doctor's account, the ubiquitous manifestations of mass starvation and mortality evoke little pity or reflection, but instead an assertion of the memoirist's greater scientific knowledge and medical prowess.

Who was Nikolai Glazov?

In 1999 Margarita Nikolaevna Glazova introduced her father's memoir by stating that he had been unjustly arrested on charges 'that bore no relationship to reality'. In the Gulag he met 'many interesting people – from the milieu of old revolutionaries, intelligentsia, citizens of other countries'.[57] The heart of the memoir, in her view, was its record of these encounters. She balances the shade and light of her father's situation in the camps as follows:

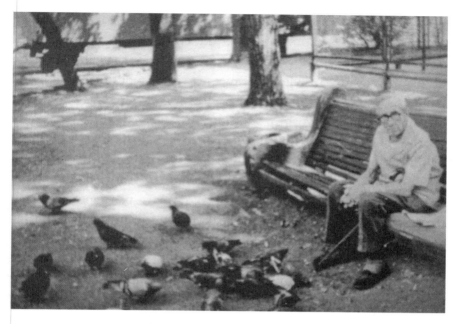

7. The pensioner-memoirist, 1989.

N. A. Glazov survived in inhuman conditions thanks to his artistry as a doctor: he cured not only prisoners, but their guards as well. Even under threat of retribution he helped his comrades in misfortune: he obtained release for the weak from unbearable labour, transfer to lighter regime. The stories of the doctor about his patients are full of invaluable medical experience acquired in the harshest of conditions of labour-camp life. It is the science of survival in the literal sense of the word.[58]

Political victim, committed physician, cultured individual. Having assisted him in writing his memoirs, this was Margarita Glazova's assessment of her father. She understood herself to be a child of one of Stalin's victims of repression and framed his experience accordingly. By framing the prisoner-doctor as a 'victim', this memoir avoided nuanced retrospection; no searching dialogue between the glasnost-era pensioner and his younger Stalin-era self takes place in the text. Instead, 'tangled interweavings of fact and self-representation' remain that raise more questions than they settle.[59]

Puzzled by this arrested retrospection and intrigued by this Gulag prisoner-doctor's relationship with the chekists that spanned three decades, I have read Nikolai Glazov as a survivor as well as a victim of the Soviet system.[60] He was someone with a 'spoilt biography' who joined the Party in 1922 proclaiming his surprisingly instant faith in 'the inevitability of world revolution'. He rejected working secretly for the OGPU in 1924 but by 1933 he was on the OGPU payroll, admiring its discipline, collecting provisions in its closed shops, and relishing his undercover role on Red Square at Clara Zetkin's funeral. When he was cast out as a 'counterrevolutionary' he found his feet in the Gulag as a doctor, and almost certainly survived thanks to his chance encounter with Sanotdel boss and ex-prisoner Nikolai Viktorov. But he also survived thanks to his professional training, his inclination to ingratiate himself to the 'bosses', and his understanding of the chekist milieu. In that milieu rules were there to be bent, broken, or leaned upon according to the situation, and as essential as the morphine purloined from veterinary supplies or the documents that 'ceased to be tufta' once created. In his own prose Nikolai Glazov expresses his pride in his medical skill, implicitly framing his service in the Gulag as honourable because he was true to his scientific training and his 'artistry as a doctor'. 'Dry as dust' he might be, and short on empathy, but his diagnoses were accurate and his prescriptions sound. As a prisoner-doctor he was perhaps unusually compliant and comfortable in the company of the camp commandants. Glazov's memoir offers us Gulag medicine as a precarious undertaking for the prisoner-doctor, a 'grey zone' occupation where solid medical skills were necessary, but not sufficient, to assure survival. An alertness to the Gulag system's demands and constraints, an ear for the chekist milieu and its expectations, were essential too: a doctor's exercise of free clinical judgement in the Gulag was limited by a higher authority. The zek-physician needed an ability to read that higher authority's signals and, when necessary, trim his healing to suit. Glazov, a prisoner-physician who 'does not have it easy' and who was keenly aware of the constraints of his situation, offers a valuable case in the history of Gulag medicine to compare with the 'freely hired' doctors we meet next.

3

'I CHOSE KOLYMA'

From the medical school benches to the hospitals of the Gulag

Sofia Lazarevna Guzikova graduated as a physician from Moscow Medical Institute in the winter of 1940. She was 23 years old. Much later, probably in the 1980s, she recalled how she became a 'freely hired' Gulag doctor:

> A commission to assign jobs to future doctors sat in the dean's office. Students had no choice over their work assignments; the commission allocated them according to its own requirements.
>
> Students awaiting their fate crowded the corridor. Most were downhearted. Where would we end up? The majority of the assignments were in distant corners of the country.
>
> My turn came. I went into the grand room. Behind a massive table sat the representatives of various employers.
>
> The gaze of the director of personnel of the NKVD's Gulag fell on me. She liked the fact that I was an excellent student, and a Young Communist League (Komsomol) member; I ought to be showing a good example. My classmate Olga K. sobbed, begging not to be sent to the countryside . . . She got lucky, her outburst of tears got her a job in the city of Piatigorsk.
>
> They described my work in the godforsaken hole where I would be the only doctor in the district. I thought of *A Doctor's Notebook* by Veresaev, [the medical stories] by Chekhov, and recalled my own grandfather, a country doctor under the tsar.

Romanticism welled up inside me, overwhelming my reserve. 'Send me as far away as possible!' I loudly declared. No doubt I made an impression. The commission looked at me with surprise and fresh interest. And I was assigned to the Far East, to the Lower-Amur Gulag camp.[1]

Sofia Guzikova explained her decision to go to the Gulag as a romantic desire to imitate the classic models of Russian medical intelligentsia service. Perhaps her choice was motivated by grief as well. Her fellow student Yura, 'my first, difficult, love', had died of an unspecified illness less than a year before graduation. She visited his grave to say farewell before departing from Moscow.[2]

Unlike prisoner-doctors who did forced labour in the Gulag's medical service or who sought work in their profession while in captivity, many free civilian doctors apparently 'chose' to work for the forced-labour camp system. A few like Yan Pullerits followed patrons to the camps in the early years of Gulag construction; but these were exceptional cases. The Gulag was chronically short of skilled medical staff as it grew; it recruited 'freely hired' doctors and other medical personnel through multifarious channels in the 1930s. By 1938 a system of graduate assignment, conducted by the medical schools, with oversight from the Party and institutional recruiters, catapulted candidates fresh from the medical school lecture-hall benches to work in the Gulag's 'sanitary' service.

It was almost certainly Gulag recruiter, and later deputy chief of the central Gulag Sanotdel, Liubov Abramovna Chudnovskaya, whose gaze fell upon Sofia Guzikova in winter 1940. This Kyiv-trained medical doctor and manager joined the Gulag in 1938; she apparently had her eye on Guzikova's good marks, her Komsomol membership, and her leadership potential. From 1938 the assignment of hundreds of jobs to graduating classes of physicians was an annual ritual in medical institutes taking several days or even weeks. Commissions, chaired by representatives of the health commissariat, and composed of school directors and Party representatives as well as recruiters from specific employers, spent much time reviewing references and academic results, hearing from Party monitors, and interviewing each candidate separately, discussing three to five prospective assignments with them. Embedded medical services (army, navy, railways, secret police) got first choice of the graduates, with the remainder going to civilian service or post-graduate academic careers. Remarkably, the Gulag, and even branches of its operations like Dalstroi, sent senior representatives to scout for talent. By the time that Guzikova was assigned to Gulag work in 1940, Chudnovskaya's recruitment machine was well oiled, and between 1939 and 1952 it sent 5,359 new doctors to work in the camps.[3]

Almost none of these doctors told their stories in memoirs, and the few who did explained their decision for the Gulag in romantic terms. A Magadan doctor of Guzikova's vintage, Nina Vladimirovna Savoeva, who boldly entitled her 1996 memoir *I Chose Kolyma*, tells a similar story of her decision:

> They offered me four different places to choose from, one of which was Magadan. The commission told me it was a town of prisoners. I made my decision for Magadan. 'Do you have someone there?' asked the chairman of the commission. 'I am an orphan, I don't have anyone out there,' I replied. 'I've only heard about the existence of this town for the first time here. I think I'm needed there more than anywhere else.'

Savoeva was one of at least fourteen Moscow Medical Institute graduates sent in 1940 to Magadan to work in Dalstroi's camp infirmaries and clinics.[4]

Why did these doctors 'choose' the Gulag? Naive romanticism or stirring altruism may appeal in a memoir, but the official archives show that pragmatic bargaining, tears, and grandstanding were at least as prevalent in job-assignment commissions as youthful romanticism.[5] At the same time, the late 1930s was a moment when the Communist Party and state media promoted remote construction sites as exciting opportunities for youth, and there is evidence of some genuine enthusiasm for these prospects, whatever participants may have felt in retrospect.[6] Finally, as unlikely as it may seem, the alternatives to Gulag employment looked much less attractive to some candidates. I asked Dr Anna Kliashko during our interviews in Montréal why she had chosen a job with Dalstroi. A Jewish Belarusian evacuee to Siberia during the war, Anna entered Novosibirsk Medical Institute at age 17 in 1943; she was so young her classmates called her 'The Embryo'. She qualified as a doctor in 1948 and went before the graduate commission; in her recollection, militarised entities like the Gulag had first choice of the graduates, and they offered her a post in the civilian branch of Dalstroi's medical system. She recalled, 'I didn't particularly oppose their [Dalstroi's] selection of me, because other choices didn't appeal to me.' The alternative posts were rural clinics deep in Siberia, and she had seen enough of these wretched villages while on potato-harvesting detail as a student. There would be few drugs, no equipment, scant chance for professional development, and the tedium of isolation. Was the Gulag as unknown to graduates as Savoeva suggests in her memoirs? Kliashko thought so – but she had heard about Kolyma from 'an acquaintance of my mother and father' despite thinking it was 'a blank slate for me until I got there'.[7]

The puzzles explored in this chapter revolve around both the experience of the Gulag's 'freely hired' doctors, and the ways in which their experience is remembered. Few of these staff doctors wrote their memoirs, and the two narratives by Guzikova and Savoeva offer an opportunity to hear what they chose to recall, late in life during the 'democratic era'. First in this chapter, a comparison with what is known about young graduate doctors working for the Gulag, from official sources, allows us to locate these memoirs in a broader context, and justifies the focus on Guzikova's and Savoeva's lives. The mix of 'tangled interweavings of fact and self-representation', as seen with the memoir of Nikolai Glazov, applies with particular force in the autobiographies of these Gulag employees, and a sceptical eye is indispensable for sifting truth from fancy.[8] Second, the ways in which these doctors present their youthful selves working with, or in conflict with, Gulag commandants, while claiming their expertise as professionals, is analysed. What opportunities existed for the free Gulag doctor to act on the Hippocratic medical duty to help the sick and do no harm, when the patients were prisoners in a labour camp? Finally,

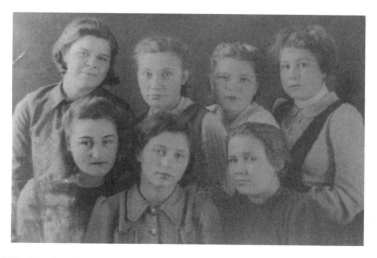

8. 'The Embryo': Anna Kliashko with classmates, front row, centre, 1946.

the chapter examines how these doctors confronted the mass sickness and mortality of the Second World War in the Gulag, and how in their texts they represented their youthful selves as medical professionals encountering extreme situations. These rare, and flawed, sources from Gulag staff doctors remain important landmarks in historical memory, in part because they illuminate the tension between the doctors' sense of professional duty and the allegiance owed to the institution they served.

Who were the Gulag staff doctors?

The Gulag had a voracious appetite for medical staff. As noted in the Introduction, the labour camps' dedicated medical system had twice the number of doctors for its prisoner population compared to the USSR's civilian medical network. In 1939 the labour camp staff had 2,459 qualified doctors of whom 39.9 per cent were prisoners in that year. In 1944 the system supposedly had 3,684 doctors, with 43 per cent from prisoners. The rest were 'freely hired' employees of the Gulag.[9] (Guzikova's case shows how 'freely hired' is a dubious label for Soviet graduate recruitment, but as a status-marker universally used in the Gulag, I adopt it here.) The proportion of prisoners to freely hired doctors varied over the life of the Gulag, and across the diverse camp network, but rules meant prisoner-physicians had a better chance than most specialists with an article 58 conviction to work in their profession.[10] The Gulag-employed staff doctors came from several sources. Some, in towns and cities near construction camps, were seconded from civilian healthcare networks; others transferred into the camp medical service from other 'embedded' medical networks like those serving the railways, army, or other branches of the security police. An unknown number even answered advertisements placed in the medical press for staff to work in the Soviet Union's remote 'construction sites'.[11] In these regions, isolated camp complexes proved difficult to staff, and from 1938 the Gulag and NKVD recruited physicians from graduate assignment commissions at medical institutes. Each subsequent year, the Gulag catapulted graduate doctors fresh from their training into the camp medical service, prioritising Komsomol members.

Typically, Gulag staff doctors were well compensated by comparison with civilian counterparts, and enjoyed wage bonuses, relocation and book-buying allowances, professional development courses, and paid holidays. They normally lived rent-free in barracks for specialists and partook of subsidised canteens. Pay was significantly better than the standard 300 to 400 roubles per month offered according to a law of 1935 to doctors starting off in the civilian healthcare system, from which of course rent and board had to be paid.[12] Liudmila Aleksandrovna Saveleva, in 1940 a new doctor from Savoeva and Guzikova's Moscow Medical Institute, signed a contract with Dalstroi offering a starting monthly salary of 900 roubles (plus a 10 per cent bonus after each six months worked); she immediately received 1,600 roubles for travel expenses. Saveleva's personal luggage allowance from Moscow to Dalstroi territory was 240 kilograms plus more for dependants. She was expected to work the first twenty-eight months of her contract without a break, taking pay in lieu of holidays; but from her third year of employment she would get a three-month holiday entitlement every year.[13] In practice, these cohorts did not take holidays until after the war, often in long stints that dovetailed with professional development courses in Moscow or Leningrad.[14]

The higher pay was not just a reward for remote and tough working conditions but signalled the elevated status of the Gulag as industrial producer in the command economy, and as a department of the security police. 'Embedded' or departmental medical systems paid more generously than Stalin's civilian medical network.[15] Local museum and archival sources show that Gulag staff doctors could enjoy rapid and challenging career advancement. The vast majority of these doctors, like Ukhta's Yakov Petrovich Sokolov, benefited from working for a priority employer in the Stalinist command economy. In a period of rapid promotion of young, politically reliable professionals, Sokolov was made director of the Ukhtpechlag Sanotdel – a remarkably responsible assignment for an inexperienced graduate.[16] When the Gulag was reformed in the 1950s, most of these 'contract' doctors transferred into managerial posts and leading roles in the civilian medical network.[17]

Like other Gulag employees, almost none of these staff doctors told their stories in memoirs. Employees of the Gulag signed non-disclosure pledges which enforced their silence, and the fact that the vast majority chose not to write about their careers that began in labour-camp medicine tells its own story.[18] After Nikita Khrushchev's denunciation of Stalin in 1956, individuals whose early career was formed in the structures of the security police felt confusion, betrayal, and vulnerability. Even if Soviet leaders reversed de-Stalinisation in the 1960s, it was wisest to say little about the past. Historical commemoration in this late-Soviet era was evasive and 'veiled'.[19] Of course, only a minority of doctors chose to write memoirs or possessed the necessary literary skills to do so. But the tradition of doctors writing about the medical challenges they faced was a long and strong one in Russian letters, and the silence of this cohort suggests their discomfort at this story of professional development behind barbed wire.[20]

Sofia Guzikova and Nina Savoeva: Outliers among 'freely hired' doctors

That Guzikova and Savoeva wrote memoirs about their Gulag camp medical journeys makes them outliers among labour-camp staff. It is worth pausing to analyse their biographies briefly and to assess why they wrote reminiscences. They are compared with a handful of other free-doctor accounts. Ultimately, it appears that family interest, or the curiosity of historical activists, in the 'democratic era' of the late 1980s encouraged these unusual Gulag doctors to record their experiences.

Sofia Guzikova's brief unpublished account of her short Gulag career is undated, just twenty-eight pages long, held in the archives of the Memorial Society in Moscow.[21] In relatively unpolished prose, it describes an eventful two-and-a-half years in Gulag service, from late 1940 to February 1943. Guzikova was very likely born in 1917 in Kyiv to a Jewish Ukrainian intelligentsia family, with one uncle a professor of gynaecology. She evidently grew up in Moscow.[22] Perhaps her decision to study medicine had roots in family tradition; yet it would also have been encouraged by the Five-Year Plan policy of promoting women and ethnic minorities into physicians' training. After graduation, she never made it to the Far East posting assigned by the Gulag recruiter in the opening scene of this chapter. Instead, she was reallocated to a dam-building camp near Kuibyshev just before it closed, and from there she 'chose' to go to a canal construction camp near Vyterga in mid-1940. All of this shuffling was evidently the result of bureaucratic caprice.[23] She worked in a camp infirmary, and was quickly promoted to director of the sanchast of a camp subdivision. She also volunteered for emergency operations in Vyterga region to contain epidemics; she herself fell ill with tuberculosis. With the outbreak of the war Guzikova transferred to work in Usollag, to be nearer her parents, who had been evacuated from Moscow to Molotov. After she refused to go 10 kilometres on foot to an outlying camp to inspect prisoner-patients, her Sanotdel director dismissed her for insubordination. She was mobilised into the army in either 1942 or 1943. Guzikova served honourably and ended the war a senior lieutenant of the Army's medical service; it is possible that her Gulag service was deliberately 'erased' in her Army records.[24] She practised in a Moscow clinic after the war, surviving into retirement and depositing her memoirs with Memorial in the glasnost era.[25] Documents from Guzikova's exemplary war record were uploaded to an 'Immortal Regiment' veterans' commemorative website in 2015.[26]

Sofia Guzikova's memoir is written in the present tense and she portrays herself as a youthful, light-hearted, emotionally naive cog in the Gulag wheel, unsuited to the camps' special environment. One of the puzzles of the text is its abrupt end with her dismissal from the Gulag and transfer to army medical service. A continuation of her story would invite comparison between her work in the camps with doing medicine in the army; both contexts must have been hugely challenging for the young physician, but she does not reflect on them. Evidently, this memoir was not meant to remember military medicine. Sofia Guzikova's motives for depositing her short memoir with Memorial Moscow's archives remain unstated in the text and indexing materials of the archive. Rather like the Gulag prisoner and memoirist Tamara Petkevich, whose reminiscences veer between horror and levity, Dr Guzikova apparently wished to bear witness to the Gulag's brutality, but also to a milieu where camp staff conducted romances and socialised while ignoring what the doctor dubbed 'the horrors of the camp'.[27] The impression that Guzikova's memoirs were elicited, perhaps by a relative or Memorial activist, from a subject who had previously been reluctant to write, or who lacked the literary and philosophical capacity to reconcile such challenging tensions, may explain the origin and character of this rare text by a Gulag staff doctor.[28]

We know more about Nina Savoeva, thanks to her 46-page memoir, published in 1996, and from central health commissariat archives, and documents Savoeva herself deposited in the archive of the Magadan Province Regional Museum in 1989. We also have characterisations from well-known Gulag memoirists Eugenia Ginzburg and Varlam Shalamov, from her husband ex-prisoner, engineer, and journalist Boris Lesniak, and from Anna Kliashko, who knew Savoeva as a colleague and a patient. Nina Savoeva was born in 1916 in North Ossetia into a peasant family, one of five girls. Savoeva was the only child sent to school; she finished local schooling and was keen to become a doctor. Nina joined the Komsomol relatively early, in 1931, at age fifteen.[29] More obviously than the comparatively

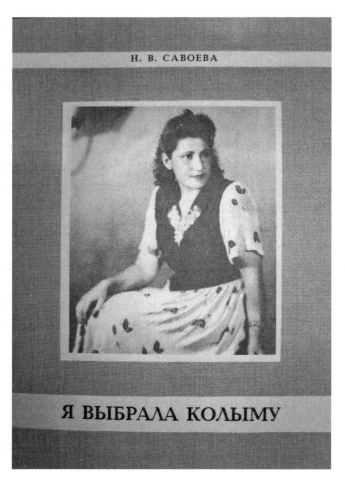

Н. В. САВОЕВА

Я ВЫБРАЛА КОЛЫМУ

9. 'I chose Kolyma': Dr Nina Savoeva's 1996 memoir.

privileged urban Ukrainian Guzikova, Savoeva the North Ossetian peasant woman was a *vydvizhenka* – a promotee of the Five-Year Plan era, selected by the Party for her demographic characteristics (female, peasant background, minority nationality) and offered a pathway to further education. In 1933 she moved to Moscow to take preparatory classes for medical school entry. Graduating in 1940 from the Moscow Medical Institute, Dr Savoeva was assigned to run a clinic in a mining camp north of Magadan (Chkalov Chai-Urinsky mine).

From 1942 to 1945 she was chief physician and director of Belichya prisoner-hospital in the Northern District of the Kolyma camp system.

By 1943, if not earlier, she became a full member of the Party. It was during this period that she sheltered prisoners Eugenia Ginzburg and Varlam Shalamov at Belichya. In 1946 she married Lesniak, an ex-prisoner. She was excluded from the Party in 1949, apparently for this politically disloyal marriage.[30] Savoeva worked in a succession of camp hospitals after the war, and left the prisoner-hospital system around the time of Stalin's death. Eventually, she occupied a senior position in the civilian Magadan Central Provincial Hospital.

In the late 1980s Nina Savoeva first wrote about working as a Gulag doctor, and published excerpts in a Magadan medical newspaper. In 1994 Savoeva and Lesniak met Ivan Panikarov, an amateur historian in Kolyma, an activist-researcher and journalist, who encouraged Savoeva to publish her full memoir as a short book, in 1996.[31] Extracts appeared in the democratic activist Semyon Vilensky's compilation of Gulag memoirs – hers is one of the very few non-prisoner voices in this respected collection.[32] Interest in Savoeva was assured by the fact that she had sheltered famous prisoner-memoirists Ginzburg and Shalamov.[33]

The Gulag's 'specific conditions' and the limits of medical power

Stalinism's explosive economic growth was built on the education and rapid promotion of young graduates into responsible positions.[34] This could be a dizzying experience, challenging in the best of circumstances, for raw specialists. The NKVD's Political Department painted a stark picture of the young graduate in the Gulag for camp commandants in a 1938 instruction: 'The majority of those whom we have sent are excellent students, Komsomol members, young women between 19 and 25 years of age, having no practical life experience and starting their very first jobs in the specific conditions of the camps of the NKVD.'[35] Moscow ordered Gulag commandants to explain their new jobs to medical recruits patiently, to give them work based on their personnel files and even personal preferences, to assure them professional advancement, and to bring the best of the non-Party doctors into the ranks of the Party, all to sustain morale and retention.[36]

Gulag officials feared political and sexual disruption when dropping these tender recruits into the camps. Savoeva describes vividly how Dalstroi chief General Ivan Fedorovich Nikishov, and labour-camp and medical leaders received her cohort on the day after their arrival in Magadan:

> He explained that most of us would be working with prisoners, that these consisted of a very varied collection of bandits, thieves, murderers, dangerous assailants, *bytoviki*, but the majority were enemies of the people: traitors against the Motherland, spies, wreckers, enemies, and terrorists. Therefore, in any dealings with prisoners we must exercise extreme caution, be firm and vigilant. He said that many of these people were capable of base actions, to say the least. And he advised us to always keep that in mind, especially the women among us.
>
> Then our group had a reception with the director of the Dalstroi camp system (USVITL) Lieutenant-Colonel Drabkin and the director of the Sanotdel Sadomsky. Everyone spoke to us as if they were the sighted and we the blind. They warned us not only of the possibility of assaults from the prisoners, but also to avoid their influence.[37]

Clearly, officials believed a degree of political consciousness, and a strong character, was necessary for work in this environment. The recruits' youth, lack of 'practical life experience' and their gender were potential liabilities.[38]

New contract doctors also had to come to terms with the 'specific conditions of the camps' and their role as healers there. These recruits, most with some experience of Party-work in the Komsomol, understood subordination to hierarchical authority well enough; but leading a young Communist anti-epidemic brigade, as Nina Savoeva did in her student years, or enrolling comrades in a 'voluntary' study group in the medical institute was one thing. Coming to terms with the Gulag's chronic undernourishment of prisoners, and the frequent deprivation of the means to save them, especially in wartime when food supply was at crisis point, was something else. It

produced a tension between a commitment to medical professionalism learned in the institute, and the obedience that staff doctors
owed to the camp's commandant and production officials. The
'specific conditions' of life in the Gulag and the limits they placed
on a physician's power, were learned in confrontations with the
bosses.

The limits of medical power: Guzikova's 'crazy risk'

Sofia Guzikova tells us repeatedly that her 'infantile appearance' and
naive attitude towards her duty shielded her from punishment for
failing to understand the 'specific conditions' of Gulag service. 'At
that time, I looked like a teenager: very thin, with my hair cut short,
in a short skirt and blouse. Very straightforward, I took everyone at
their word and was rather modest.'[39] We have few clues by which to
judge these claims. Guzikova's own representation of her professional opinions and actions often contradicts this picture of modesty.
Confrontations with the commandants' power were, in her retrospective view, part of learning the limits of medical power.

At Vyterga, on the eve of the war, while contending with extreme
deprivation and rising mortality among prisoners, Guzikova describes
how she struggled to reconcile official decrees with local realities.
She recalls an episode when she acted on a decree from the deputy
head of the NKVD, Sergei Nikiforovich Kruglov, about preparation
for the coming winter. Kruglov ordered camps to ensure that prisoners had 'warm clothing and good footwear'; however, at Vyterga,
the inmates only had ragged jackets and improvised sandals (wooden
soles with canvas tops) for shoes.[40] The morning after she received
her copy of the decree, in freezing temperatures, Guzikova claims
she refused to permit guards to escort 7,000 prisoners to work. Bosses
in charge of production gave her a dressing down:

I justified my actions by referring to the minister's decree. They
told foolish me that I should have cleared my actions with the
commandants first. 'Seven thousand zeks sitting idle! If anything
like this happens again, you'll never hear the end of it!' That's how

they taught me to live. Apparently, they didn't punish me because they saw my inexperience and sincerity.[41]

Not long after that, Dr Guzikova was instructed to prepare and deliver a report for a production meeting including the Sanotdel director of the entire camp complex, commandants, administrators, and chekists.

> With the figures at my fingertips, I explained how mortality from pellagra was constantly increasing, and I concluded by saying, 'The camp is an institution of education, and no one gave us the right to destroy people through starvation.' My report was used as the pretext for the arrest of several camp employees. I became celebrity No. 1, although at first, I did not understand why. Chekist operatives, unknown to me, would bow to me demonstratively in the street. Which is to say, I was popular. Reflecting on all of this many years later, I realised what a crazy risk I took with that report.[42]

Guzikova's 'crazy risk' led to arrests among the camp employees, who may well have deserved punishment for undersupply of food to prisoners. Officials and prisoners alike stole frequently from food stocks, especially during the war. The traditions of Stalinist blame-shifting required that such an open exposure of failure in the 'public' forum of a Gulag administrators' conference could trigger a chekist search for suitable scapegoats.[43] Guzikova presents herself as a green physician uninitiated in Soviet habits of 'rooting out those responsible' for criminal misdemeanours. And yet she must have witnessed and pondered the arrests and disappearances that took place during the Great Terror in the Moscow Medical Institute while she was studying there. Undoubtedly, she heard the accusations that flew against professors, lecturers, and students in those years.[44] Her self-presentation as 'blind' strains credibility.

Another episode challenges the medical memoirist's self-distancing from the power of the commandants. Dr Guzikova, unlike ex-chekist Nikolai Glazov, conducted at least one force-feeding of a hunger-striker. For Gulag prisoner-memoirists, the hunger-striker enjoyed great moral authority, and doctors' interference to halt strikes was to Solzhenitsyn and others a violation of medical ethics.[45] Guzikova hardly flinches from describing how she willingly presided over the forced administration of an enema on a prisoner in the isolation block ('the prison within the prison'), with the assistance of a prisoner-feldsher and guards who restrained the zek. Apparently, trying to soften the impression of her compliance with penal power, she claims that she subsequently refused to testify to chekists against the hunger-striking prisoner for resisting, and how that refusal earned her respect among inmates and free employees alike.[46]

'More than once I cried, that's how sorry I was for them'

Sofia Guzikova says that she found the initial sight of prisoners shocking, one of many 'difficult impressions' of her first days on the job. 'Often it happened that prisoners passed by on the street under guard. More than once I cried, that's how sorry I was for them.' At the same time, she found their presence and behaviour threatening and 'unpleasant' with columns of zeks hurling 'all manner of criminal jargon' at her, including indecent proposals.[47] As she adjusted to life in the camp environment, the young doctor says that she found compassion for her prisoner-patients. In a typical scene, worth quoting at length, she describes a commission to inspect and classify newly arrived prisoners for their labour capacity.

> At first, arriving transports were allowed to rest, and then they were examined by doctors, who determined which kind of work each of them was fit for. Extra doctors were called in for these duties. Three or four doctors sat behind a long table, filling in a long form for each prisoner. The zeks stood there, humiliated, waiting for their medical examination. Most of them were Uzbeks, Tajiks, Moldovans, or other national minorities. As a rule they didn't speak Russian. Prisoners from the eastern republics, in quilted robes almost to the floor, in skullcaps and torn slippers undressed before the table. Their robes shivered on the surface

with lice. Often, they lacked any underwear. They got completely undressed. We were meant to ask each one if he had any illnesses. Not understanding Russian, the prisoner remained silent. Then a totally idiotic question: 'Does your *kursak* [gut, gizzard in Turkic languages] hurt?' This standard question got a lively reaction, the prisoner would grasp his stomach, showing how much his 'gut' hurt. In broken Russian he would sometimes explain how he had been imprisoned unjustly, how he didn't want to be parted from his herds or other animals as a result of de-kulakisation or collectivisation. It was terribly sad for these true sons of nature, the steppes and mountains, torn from their habitual environment. On these days I got very tired, physically and spiritually. In fact, there was just enough time to determine whether their limbs were intact. There was no time for listening to their heartbeat, checking their lungs or examining their stomachs. They were sorted by two categories of fitness for labour: 'heavy physical labour' and 'light physical labour'. That was the categorisation on the form we filled in. The examination was little more than a farce, an empty formality. For it was apparent that the work was the same heavy labour for all. The earthworks were dug manually, there was no mechanisation to speak of.[48]

Retrospectively at least, Dr Guzikova understood that these 'commissions' of inspection were farcical, and she portrays herself as powerless in the face of the commandants' authority that constrained medical-expert decisions. The work was tiring, 'physically and spiritually', because higher authorities sapped the doctor of her capacity to make judgements in line with her apparent sympathy for these lice-infested new arrivals.

The limits of medical power: 'My sharp character'

Nina Savoeva presents herself in her reminiscences as no plaything of circumstance. Her memoir reads like a chronicle of a 'natural attorney of the poor', to borrow the nineteenth-century German physician Rudolf Virchow's characterisation of the place of the doctor caring for the abject. Indeed, Soviet doctors treating civilian patients often assumed this role, so it was perhaps a logical reflex that some carers of prisoner-patients should advocate for their well-being too.[49] Doctors in the Gulag were enjoined in official regulation to monitor the labour capacity (not 'health') and the sanitary standards of the camps, to assure production and prevent illness and epidemics. Savoeva presents herself as a robust professional advocate for prisoner health. According to Dr Savoeva, her insistent advocacy on behalf of her patients, when combined with her forthright personality, meant that she was unafraid of confrontation with commandants and camp authorities. 'Conflicts with the bosses started almost from the first day', Dr Savoeva tells us, wearing her assertiveness as a talent, not a liability.[50] Battles with authority for medical principles are the central leitmotif of the story she tells of her medical career.

At her first posting at Chkalov Chai-Urinsky mine, Savoeva's battles with authority began over temporary releases of prisoners from general labour on medical grounds. She nearly doubled the existing rates of release, and immediately felt the rage of production bosses. Savoeva passes over how this confrontation over quotas ended, but it looks likely that she lost this first battle. She was still new, inexperienced, and learning the limits of medical power. Indeed, the series of battles in her first job suggests that she had energy but lacked focus: she fought unsuccessfully to fire a brutal feldsher who beat prisoners trying to seek medical care; she campaigned for – and won – cleaner drinking water by having new equipment installed; and she apparently tried to protect patients in conflict with authorities or requiring early release on medical grounds with only limited success.[51] Dr Savoeva's attempts to right wrongs in this first posting included a flurry of report-writing, which she hints was the result of an emotional response to her apparent powerlessness as a doctor.

I felt like I stood on the edge of catastrophe, a nervous breakdown. I wrote reports to all levels of the Dalstroi administration, right up to the director of Dalstroi himself, General Ivan Fedorovich Nikishov, without any success. The camp administration and internal security looked on me with hatred and disbelief.

The director of the camp guard Yurchenko once said to me, 'You're cooking up all this stuff about enemies of our people and our motherland. Watch out that it doesn't end badly.'[52]

By the time her report reached General Nikishov the war had begun and it ultimately yielded a summons to meet him during his inspection tour of the Chai-Urinsky mine. She recalls getting a thorough dressing-down:

'What do you think, doctor, that we don't know how things are in the camp? We know as well as you do. But this is a war about life or death. The country needs metal. Wars are not fought without victims. Don't obstruct the work of the mine. And watch your tongue,' he said, dismissing me.[53]

Finally, authorities evidently decided Dr Savoeva's energy was better harnessed in a different setting. Savoeva's boss, Chai-Urinsky Sanotdel director and freely hired doctor Tatyana Dmitrievna Repyeva, summoned her and spoke unapologetically about the limits of medical authority in the forced-labour camps:

'Nina! You cannot stay in Chkalov any longer. You aren't yourself, you're getting ill, you are on the edge of a nervous collapse. You know, I also sympathise with the prisoners and I do everything I can for them. But we cannot do as much as we wish. I will give you a break from work and send you for two weeks to Talaya, you'll rest, relax and get better, and then we'll see.'[54]

Savoeva's recollection of this conversation considerably softens the usual corporate language of Sanotdel managers, at least as recorded in official archives; however, the message about the constraints on medicine's freedom in the penal setting was the same.[55] Talaya was a hot-springs sanatorium, 265 kilometres north of Magadan, recently opened for Gulag employees. After her rest break, in summer 1942, Savoeva was assigned to run a prisoner-hospital at Belichya, near the Dalstroi settlement of Yagodnoye.

The move to Belichya was a considerable step up from a local camp clinic, for a doctor with barely two years' experience. It was the central prisoner-hospital, with 'several hundred' beds, serving the camp complex of Sevlag (a regional division of the Dalstroi camp system).[56] Prisoner-patients with serious conditions arrived there having passed through first-tier clinics and infirmaries like the one at Chai-Urinsky. The magnitude of this assignment suggests that Savoeva enjoyed a greater degree of confidence among Sanotdel and Dalstroi management than her claims of constant conflict imply.

Nina Savoeva reports that the hospital lacked the 'symbols of a camp': there was no barbed wire, towers, guard houses, and soon, at Savoeva's insistence, we are told, armed guards were withdrawn too. Despite an order to impose these 'symbols of the camp' when the war began, resources and prisoner-labourers were lacking (as was the case across the camp network nationally), and the facility remained unguarded.[57] Savoeva's claims about Belichya's 'non-standard' regime may be soft-focus nonsense, and yet, memoirists with ambivalent views on Savoeva (explored later in this chapter) remember Belichya's special atmosphere. Varlam Shalamov was addressed humanely there: 'Where is the patient?', he heard a doctor ask as he arrived in autumn 1942, '[t]he first time in six years that someone called me a patient, and not "asshole" or "goner"'.[58] Eugenia Ginzburg, whose arrival in Belichya in August 1943 would turn sour quickly enough, still records what seemed at first encounter a stunning degree of normality: the hospital looked like a sanatorium, with manicured flower beds, raked gravel paths, and two-storey buildings reminding her of central Russia. She mentions no guards, commandants, or camp regime.[59]

Savoeva's memoir confidently describes the challenges of running Belichya, and feeding its prisoners in the depths of the labour camps' wartime supply crisis. Conflict with bosses takes a back seat briefly in her account. Indeed, it was in 1943 that she joined the Communist Party as a full member, and evidently being an 'insider' enjoying Party status gave this green physician some authority. The narrative of confrontation with camp bosses only resumes in her memoir as a result of a decision that drastically altered her relationship to the Party. In November 1946 she married the feldsher and recently released

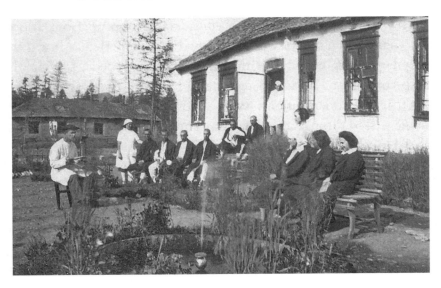

10. 'Cultural organiser' Shalamov reads to patients, Belichya, 1944.

ex-prisoner, Boris Nikolaevich Lesniak. Accused in a Party meeting of a 'failure of vigilance' for marrying an enemy of the people, Dr Savoeva was 'all but told to dissolve the marriage, or "leave her Party card on the table"'.[60] Shalamov says that she decided to quit in a principled decision to choose husband over politics. Savoeva's account is evasive, mentioning her exclusion from the Party in passing.[61] Her career after this inflection point took a knock; she was assigned to a series of run-down camp hospitals where her battles with authorities resumed. Now an 'outsider', the attempts she describes to cut corruption back-fired, with one commandant unsuccessfully framing her for supposed theft of three bolts of calico. Dr Savoeva's final camp-hospital job, in Magadan's prisoner camp, ended in 1952, she tells us, as she embarked on a down-in-flames campaign against a drunk and violent camp director who had her investigated by the Magadan Party organisation. She transferred out of the prisoners' medical system and joined the civilian central hospital in the city, where she spent the rest of her career.[62] 'More than once I was told to my face by friends and foes that I am an extremely difficult person, with a surprising ability to cultivate enemies, that my sharp character and inability to compromise would cost me dearly. There was a lot of truth in those words, but I was unable to change my nature, and I didn't want to either.'[63] Nina

Savoeva ascribes her battles with camp bosses over prisoner health and against corruption to her 'inability to compromise', a formula that glosses over several years when she held a Party card.

The 'horrors of the zone' in staff-doctor memoirs

'We were a merry company, especially those among us who did not have to see the horrors of the zone.' This is how Sofia Guzikova introduces the divide between normal life in provincial Vyterga town – parties with gramophones and dancing, poetry and courtship, friendships with teachers from the local technical college – and the existence of prisoners dying of pellagra, 'a disease of hunger', in the camp where she worked nearby.[64] In fact, several pages of her memoir recount in detail romantic attachments with a succession of freely hired specialists and NKVD officers.

Such juxtapositions of normal and abnormal mark her encounters with mass death. Even before the German invasion of the Soviet Union in 1941, prisoners were starving to death in this camp:

> To help me I was sent a woman prisoner, the eye-doctor Valkhovskaya, a wife of an 'enemy of the people'. Already middle-aged, very intelligent, a quiet, shy woman. A person of the kindest character. I very much pitied her. Each morning we felt the feet of the zeks lying in the bunks in our infirmary: cold feet were the feet of dead patients. These morning hours were very hard, especially for Valkhovskaya. They were dying from pellagra, there was no way to treat them, it was a disease of hunger. [. . .] Every day zeks died. The director of the political department of the camp came, I gave him a report about mortality in the camp and its causes.[65]

The hopelessness of this situation eventually resulted in a mental breakdown for Valkhovskaya, Guzikova writes, while dispassionately describing her own response. She was required to conduct autopsies on many zeks when they died in hospital, to determine cause of death – a fixed bureaucratic ritual of the Gulag medical routine, discussed in chapter 6 – but she found it impossible to move the corpses herself and she had no access to 'non-convoyed' unguarded prisoners for assistance with this grim task. The corpses had to be transported to a city morgue and examined there. A 'free' engineer and keen suitor, Serezha, volunteered to assist her:

> We dragged the corpses out of their coffins, put them on the table and I set to work. A month went by like this. Serezha never ceased to amaze me with his lack of fear and squeamishness. Is there nothing that love can't overcome? He saw me home afterwards. Once, on the way home, he proposed. I did not share his feelings. With my rejection, he stopped helping me on Sundays. From that time I had no help in the morgue.[66]

The morbid juxtaposition of unrequited love and ubiquitous death amplifies the 'horror of the zone'. Another man falls under Dr Guzikova's thinly disguised desiring gaze, a Polish prisoner:

> At the beginning of November [1940] the zone filled up with Poles. They were easily distinguished by their appearance, their own clothing that they wore. Among them a stately, tall, very handsome, young and intelligent man, the picture of health, stood out. He wore a leather sports jacket with a zipper fastener and he was very conspicuous. Soon they brought him to the clinic [...] Examining him I noted his hypertrophied heart, indicating serious sports training. He confirmed that he was a sprinter. After some time, his leather jacket disappeared, and he somehow slipped into the general mass of prisoners. But I always recognised him. He began to change in appearance: the blush left his cheeks; his face grew thinner. Not long after he fell ill with pellagra and was brought to the infirmary. It was impossible to save him.[67]

Perhaps encounters like this led Dr Guzikova to take the 'crazy risk' of declaring to the internal conference of Gulag officials that 'no one gave us the right to destroy people through starvation'.

Wartime conditions in the camps that she saw were even worse. In Usollag she was assigned to a subdivision, Bulatovo, 'called

"Umerlag" [Camp of the Dead]'. 'The zeks there were very sick, mostly with pellagra. As well, dead zeks from other camps were transported there for pathological-anatomical autopsy.'[68] Here she recalls that she also performed amputations without anaesthetic on gangrenous prisoners, and describes how a healthy, fresh-faced young camp commandant kept watch in the entrance hall of her infirmary, kicking article-58 prisoners in the groin if they tried to apply to her for work-release. In Sofia Guzikova's short memoir, the accumulating scenes of cruelty and the limitations to medical power lead to her act of disobedience and her dismissal from the Gulag medical service.

In contrast to Nina Savoeva, who found an interlude of Party membership and 'insider' status at Belichya, free doctor Sofia Guzikova failed to settle into a satisfactory position in the Gulag medical service. Despite an apparent willingness to subordinate her medical skills to authority, she implies that she found the 'horrors of the zone' and the bosses' limits on her medical decision-making during her tenure ultimately intolerable. Her principal self-defence in her memoir, that she was too young and naive to understand the 'specific conditions' of the camps and their clinics, sits awkwardly with episodes that display bold confidence or determination. Another peculiar gap in Guzikova's memory is her unwillingness or inability to compare and contrast her Gulag experiences with her wartime medical service. The war is scarcely mentioned in her short memoir, and it appears that she did not write a memoir about her work in the Red Army. The commemoration of these two major traumas of Soviet experience – the Stalinist penal system and the Second World War – are so incommensurate in the Russian public mind that Sofia Guzikova might be forgiven for not attempting to extend her reminiscences to present her wartime experience.[69] And yet, in the context of describing her career, the ending of her Gulag memoir is abrupt and wrenching.

Settling scores and diverging memories

In her memoir, Nina Savoeva was keen to settle scores as well as recall her medical apprenticeship, and this is where reading the Gulag staff memoir becomes an exercise in comparison and triangulation, pitting the historian's judgement against discrepant witness accounts. Savoeva's 1990s account challenges the earlier memoirs of ex-prisoner Ginzburg. Beyond accepting that the victim of Stalinism's account should prevail over those of her tormentors – a natural reaction motivated by democratic and humane impulses – the historian hoping to decode the specific perspective of Gulag staff memoirs should ask why two such divergent narratives are possible.[70] Discrepancies are likely, given the shifting power differentials between the two memoirists: in the 1940s Savoeva held sway in the camp hospital; while from the 1960s as a survivor-memoirist Ginzburg seized the moral authority. Their investments in very different memory projects, and their varying temporal distance from Belichya of the 1940s, inescapably mould these discrepant accounts too.

Eugenia Ginzburg painted an unflattering portrait of the doctor in her extremely popular, and widely circulated, samizdat prisoner-memoir *Krutoi marshrut* (literally 'Sharp Trajectory') and Savoeva evidently felt aggrieved. Of Ginzburg and Shalamov, Nina Savoeva writes that their presence 'aroused consternation and internal protest among the genuinely hard-working' in her team, becoming 'grit in the eye of the staff [. . .], they were my sore point, my Achilles heel'.[71] In her famous memoir, Ginzburg had condemned Savoeva's personality as proud and abrasive, the doctor's 'terrifying presence' and 'tyrannical and arbitrary instincts'. Mockingly dubbing the North Ossetian chief doctor of Belichya hospital 'Queen Tamara', she claimed Savoeva 'used to order her female acolytes to bathe her and anoint her rather clumsy and shapeless body with various aromatic substances'.[72] Ginzburg's orientalising taunts are compounded by her claims that Savoeva was under the influence of a fellow Ossetian and petty-Stalin, the boss of the district mining camps.

More damning than these personal slights is Ginzburg's claim that 'something like a thousand' tuberculosis prisoners died in her arms as she nursed them while working in the 'tuberculosis block' at Belichya hospital under Savoeva from 1943 to 1946, that 'half-dead' patients were discharged to mines, and that the morgue disposed of bodies with savage disrespect. Belichya's tended grounds, air of respectability, and lack of camp fencing she condemns as a cynical ruse 'to cloak the horror within'.[73] Nina Savoeva's account of Ginzburg's time at Belichya vehemently contradicts almost every accusation, although it does so indirectly, without referring to Ginzburg's narrative. Savoeva emphasises how she distorted her professional values at the request of 'prisoner-doctors, my colleagues' to assist Ginzburg, hinting that she invented a job as a favour to Ginzburg's supporters.[74] The doctor-memoirist contradicts Ginzburg's account of the job Savoeva assigned to shelter her. She says that she posted Ginzburg as a 'nurse-housekeeper' to a 'rest-and-recovery station' treating prisoner-miners; later, in an unrelated passage, she states that Belichya had the lowest rates of mortality of the regional camp hospitals. Finally, where Ginzburg offers a dramatic scene of her 'hysterical fit' at the sight of mutilated corpses handled by thugs running the morgue, Savoeva relates how she ordered dead prisoners be buried in at least underwear (previously, corpses were interred naked) and claims that the patients greeted this as a heartening 'moral victory'.[75] The two portraits of Belichya could hardly be farther from each other, and the discrepancy has not gone unnoticed. As the highly respected anti-Stalinist Magadan historian Alexander Grigorievich Kozlov observed in 1991, Shalamov's and Ginzburg's accounts are very 'subjective', and while they saw many 'horrors of the camps' he argues that they owed their lives 'to the humane attitude towards them shown by people such as N. V. Savoeva'.[76]

To contextualise, if not reconcile, these discrepant accounts we need to look to other documents and recent scholarship. First, while medical statistics for Belichya central camp hospital apparently no longer exist, it is possible to put this institution's mortality in the wider Gulag wartime context.[77] The years when Ginzburg served in Savoeva's hospital were among the very worst for mortality in the camps, according to central records and recent investigations. The Soviet state allocated scarce food supplies grimly in wartime, with camps at the bottom of a merciless ladder of priority. Tuberculosis brought on by exhaustion and malnutrition was prominent among causes of prisoner death.[78] Belichya, however efficiently run by the inexperienced Dr Savoeva, who had only graduated in 1940, after all, could not escape these pressures. New, empirically robust scholarship on informal practices of camp commandants using 'release-to-die' subterfuges to reduce mortality rates in the Gulag, especially in 'crisis years' such as the war, substantiates impressionistic reports from survivor memoirs and implicit hints in the Gulag's central records.[79] Prisoner corpses were frequently disposed of with vicious disrespect by morgue staff across the camp system, and a February 1943 Gulag decree authorised burial in mass graves of unclothed corpses.[80] It would seem difficult to deny many of the claims made by prisoner-nurse Ginzburg, even if her presentation is subject to literary embellishment.

Furthermore, Savoeva's argumentative and defensive language of keen professional striving to meet basic requirements in wartime Belichya sometimes resembles the euphemistic Gulag Sanitary Department discourse used by desk-physicians in Moscow, and regional Gulag medical managers gathered in Novosibirsk for their first conference in September 1945. Using Soviet jargon about the 'contingent' (of prisoners) and 'labour capacity' or 'physical condition', they could both express concern for the preservation of prisoners' lives and dehumanise their patients simultaneously.[81] Savoeva insists that she, along with prisoner-doctors, worked to the slogan 'Everything for the patients!' as she details their efforts to grow their own food to expand the supply, improve sanitation, modernise therapy, and lower mortality. Shalamov in his reminiscences suggests that she also obtained food for the hospital through illegal barter and turned to petty criminals to solve supply blockages.[82] It is striking that Savoeva does not address Ginzburg's charge that she discharged 'half-dead' prisoners to return to work in the mines, nor the charge of criminal morgue staff mutilating corpses. Her gestures in this direction deflect rather than deny the charges (Belichya had the lowest mortality; she ordered corpses be buried in underwear to general approval). Savoeva writing in the 1980s–1990s makes some blustery errors. For example, she claims to have set up the first blood-transfusion station in Kolyma, after taking a course in Khabarovsk, and training Belichya staff including Lesniak. In fact, Magadan's central hospital set one up in 1939, thanks to another young freely hired surgeon and medical bureaucrat Aleksei Fedorovich Khoroshev who opened the region's first transfusion laboratory in 1939, well before Dr Savoeva had even graduated.[83] There is evasiveness and clumsy assertiveness in her bold claims of precocious professionalism. And yet Savoeva commands the respect of local historians who are de-Stalinisers and democratisers. Even if she was a greenhorn physician, overpromoted to hospital director barely two years after graduation, she had considerable help in running the institution from older, experienced prisoner-doctors and specialists. In her own account she admits that she was fortunate to work with these figures who guided her decisions, doctors from among the prisoners like Petr Semyonovich Kalembet, a peasant promoted to professional education like Savoeva, but with a decade's experience in epidemiology and elite clinics. Even misanthropic Shalamov recalled Kalembet with grudging respect.[84]

Choosing the Gulag

Sofia Guzikova and Nina Savoeva were hardly typical of the 'freely hired' cohorts of graduate doctors who worked in the Gulag's medical service. Both had plainly unsuccessful Gulag careers. Guzikova was dismissed for insubordination as her three-year mandatory term of employment neared completion; and in 1953, not long after dismissal from the Party, Savoeva's career in the camp hospital system ended after one too many battles with Sanotdel and labour-camp bosses.

Their career paths look different from scores of others in the cohorts of contract-holding Gulag doctors, like Dr Savoeva's immediate boss at Chai-Urinsky mine, Tatyana Repyeva, or the successful medical manager Aleksei Khoroshev. Both climbed the penal-medical ladder with none of the turbulence described by our doctor-memoirists. Alongside his work in blood transfusion in Magadan, Khoroshev was named the first editor of the region's medical journal in 1945; by 1952 Khoroshev was the 'chief surgeon of Dalstroi' and a member of the regional Sanotdel's scientific council. In 1959 he became Kolyma's first historian of medicine, writing a chronicle, in 'veiled' terms, of the establishment of healthcare services in the region.[85] By 1961 Repyeva's service was recognised with the Order of Lenin.[86] Employment records in Magadan of other freely hired graduates tell a similar tale of respect for medical and Party hierarchy, advances on the career ladder, and politically acceptable family

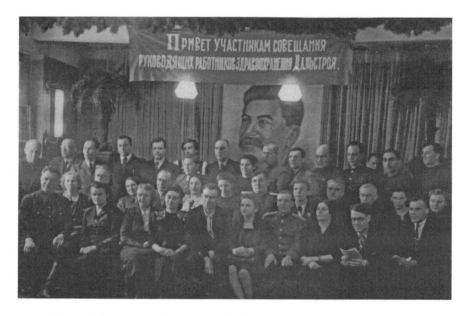

11. Successful careers under a non-disclosure agreement: freely hired medical workers in Magadan, late 1940s.

lives, even as they say little about the ways in which these doctors regarded their duties and treated prisoner-patients.[87] The freely hired doctors of Ukhta, Pechora, and other Gulag towns likewise won awards and got promotions during Stalin's lifetime and afterwards. But they seldom if ever wrote memoirs to describe these careers that began with the original sin of labour-camp medicine. A silent majority of freely hired Gulag doctors tells its own story with its adherence to the NKVD's rule forbidding the disclosure of the penal world's secrets.

Emboldened by the democratisation of the 1980s and the collapse of communism in the 1990s, Sofia Guzikova and Nina Savoeva violated this rule by writing their memoirs. In their stories, they illustrate how the 'choice' of the Gulag came with heavy consequences. Freely hired, newly graduated physicians fresh from the medical institute benches were entangled in Stalin's inhumane labour-camp system. They were answerable to authority for prisoners' 'labour capacity' and yet they were surrounded by what Savoeva called the prisoners' exhausted and starved 'greyish-brown faces'. Even suitably conformist doctors like Tatyana Repyeva felt the burden of this dilemma: 'You know, I also sympathise with the prisoners and I do everything I can for them. But we cannot do as much as we wish.' Their dual loyalties – to their patients, and to the institution that employed them – were an extreme version of the crossfire in which all doctors who worked for embedded medical services in the Soviet Union were caught.

PART II
CAREERS IN GULAG MEDICINE

4

'FEELING MY WAY'
Apprenticeships behind barbed wire

Late August 1949 at Leningrad's Military Medical Academy: professors are examining finalists hoping to qualify as physicians. Vadim Gennadievich Aleksandrovsky is among them, eager to get his diploma. Twenty-five years old, Vadim is already a Navy lieutenant-feldsher, and he has had a good war, serving in the Caspian fleet and earning a place in the Academy in 1944. He is ascending the medical hierarchy from feldsher to physician. Married, an expectant father, and soon to be qualified, a bright future beckons. By 29 August the young lieutenant has passed three examinations and has only five more to go.

But on 30 August the secret police arrest him on charges of anti-Soviet agitation. At first, his classmates are oblivious; the police detain their victims discreetly. But as the examination days go by without Aleksandrovsky and another classmate, Georgy Afanasyev, turning up, and results are posted showing blanks next to their names, students guess the reason for their absence. The 'Leningrad Affair', a campaign of terror focused on Russia's second city, is gathering steam. Vadim Aleksandrovsky's provocative contributions in the compulsory Marxism-Leninism lecture course, when discussion turned to the Party's recent condemnation of the journals *Zvezda* and *Leningrad* for promoting poet Anna Akhmatova and satirist Mikhail Zoshchenko, irked a professor who denounced the finalist. He is imprisoned, investigated, sentenced to ten years, and later that winter he leaves Leningrad in a transport of prisoners bound for the Gulag.[1] Aleksandrovsky's mental state can only be imagined. Of it, he says in his memoir that what disturbed him, aside from the injustice of his conviction, was not completing his exams: 'the most awful thing for me was that I had not managed to get my diploma'. His Gulag journey began, and in a formal sense would end, without his becoming the physician he wanted to be.

Nevertheless, even before he was freed after six years of service in a string of isolated camp clinics in Arkhangelsk Province, Vadim Aleksandrovsky could say he was 'standing on my own two feet' as a doctor. He had met the challenges of bringing his book learning to the extreme realities of Gulag medicine, and he had matured as a physician and as a man despite penal servitude's humiliations. The Gulag turned out to be an unwanted, but effective, 'post-graduate education'.[2]

So far we have met doctors working in the Gulag who had already earned their qualifications in 'civilian' life as free individuals. As such, they enjoyed a degree of professional confidence that Aleksandrovsky ruefully lacked. His experience was not unique, and the fact that the penal medical system fostered and shaped careers in medicine has been noted by famous Gulag memoirists such as the camp-trained feldsher Varlam Shalamov, the self-taught nurse Eugenia Ginzburg, and the feldsher Janusz Bardach, who acquired his medical knowledge on the fly.[3] Little attention has been paid to the environment in which Gulag prisoners acquired and enhanced their medical skills. Some Gulag survivors, notably Alexander Solzhenitsyn, rejected the possibility that Gulag medicine could be anything but destructive. Survivors' claims as witnesses are correct accounts of their own experience – but they cannot tell every Gulag story. There were places in Stalin's penal world, perhaps not always, and not everywhere, but in sufficient quantity nonetheless, where concentrations of personnel, of institutions, and of rational management made the pursuit of a medical career a possibility for nimble and alert prisoners.

Varlam Shalamov took a feldsher course in a hospital at the 23rd kilometre on the Kolyma Highway north of Magadan, in 1946. The course saved him from the debilitating cycles of hard labour followed by hospitalisation and back to hard labour, that marked the previous nine years of his incarceration. He was able to spend the final five years of his imprisonment working in Kolyma hospitals, gaining rich clinical experience which he eventually poured into his stories of Gulag life. Yet when authorities finally permitted him to leave Kolyma for the 'mainland' he discovered that his 1946 feldsher's certificate was useless 'in freedom' – a Gulag 'diploma' was unrecognised by medical authorities and he had to seek alternative employment. The experience bewildered him, as he justifiably believed that the Stalinist state had stolen his youth and, with it, the opportunity to acquire a solid profession.[4] The theft of Shalamov's future contributed to the bitterness that forged his *Kolyma Tales*.

Other experiences of Gulag work and education were possible – if less celebrated for their contributions to Russian letters. The stories that follow present two cases where prisoners were enabled to make lifelong careers for themselves in medicine. They show how prisoners were motivated to acquire medical training – beyond an instinct for mere survival as a *pridurok* or trusty, working in the 'grey zone' of the Gulag's privileged occupations – from an urge to develop their talents, to grow as a person and to 'stand on their own two feet'. These examples demonstrate the possibilities that older, experienced medical professionals grasped to teach and foster humane values and medical knowledge in younger prisoners. They illustrate the crossing back and forth over the boundaries of the Gulag and the non-Gulag in the sharing of medical knowledge between the zek and the freely hired. Finally, they highlight the great variability of Gulag camps and the different kinds of professional environments they fostered. Medical education and training were available in the camps, to very different degrees and in very different settings, depending in part on when we look in the quarter-century-long history of the camps, but also on the nature of the camp complex and the medical institutions it harboured.

Viktor Aleksandrovich Samsonov: A Gulag 'lekpom'

One prisoner who entered the Gulag without any intention of pursuing a medical career was Petrozavodsk student Viktor Samsonov.

He came from a family of enterprising peasants and small-town workers. His father was a railway official in Karelia's Kondopoga; his mother's family farmed and laboured in the vicinity. Viktor completed seven years of primary education in 1934 and gained a place to study land-surveying in the mining faculty of the Petrozavodsk Industrial Technical School. In December 1937 the 18-year-old was arrested in a secret-police sweep through the school; its Komsomol had been wracked that autumn with accusations of anti-Soviet agitation. Samsonov fell victim to this local episode of the Great Terror. After imprisonment and interrogation, a closed NKVD tribunal sentenced him to eight years' imprisonment in March 1938, and by July, after a laborious journey by rail, river barge, and a 220-kilometre march, he arrived in Ukhta's camp complex. He remained a prisoner there for five years – gaining early release – but like others was required to stay in his Gulag post until the end of the war. He worked principally as a feldsher, eventually acquiring enough knowledge to be trusted to run a sanchast and hospital ward independently. A distinctive feature of Samsonov's camp biography is the relative stability of his situation: after early months of uncertainty, he settled into medical work in Ukhta's main prisoner-hospital, Vetlosian, and he remained an employee of this well-documented institution until the camp administration decommissioned him in February 1946. He left Ukhta that summer to enter the Ivanovo Medical Institute, where he qualified as a physician in 1951. In the next eleven years he completed candidate and doctoral post-graduate degrees and had an academic career, teaching medicine as a full professor of Petrozavodsk State University, until retirement in 1989.

Samsonov's life is particularly well documented, largely thanks to his own literary skill and the sequence of nine autobiographical books he published between 1990 and his death in 2004.[5] His writing about his Gulag years in Ukhta constitutes one of the richest sources on Vetlosian Hospital, and on the medical history of Ukhta and region. As well, the holdings of the Ukhta Museum of the History of Public Health contain many references to him by other medical figures, and depictions of the professional environment that formed this inadvertent physician. Samsonov also maintained a brisk corre-

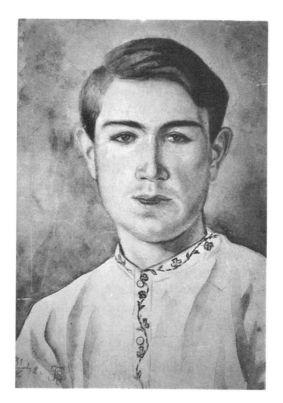

12. An unintended career: Viktor Samsonov, Gulag 'lekpom', May 1942.

spondence with readers and contested Solzhenitsyn's negative view of medical care in the Gulag camps. His story shows how a young man in a major Gulag camp centre in the late 1930s could fashion a career for himself, with the assistance of an entire community of doctors, professors, and medical administrators.

Will life go on?

Viktor Samsonov arrived in Ukhta exhausted and ill. The journey, over some six weeks, deprived prisoners of an adequate diet and the final 220-kilometre march sapped their strength. Samsonov, like many in this transport, came down with night blindness, a vitamin A deficiency that renders the sufferer blind in darkness. He was assigned to general labour, trench-digging, at an oil-extraction subdivision. There he noticed surveyors at work on the construction site and he spoke to them, hoping they would take him on because of his training. The camp work-assigners blocked this precocious attempt to escape general labour. Samsonov would have to dig trenches for another month before foremen reassigned him to the surveyors' brigade. In the meantime he was lucky to have a brigade leader who put him down for a 'lighter' quota (60 per cent of the norm) because of his weakness and youth; and he got treatment for his worsening night blindness in the subdivision sanchast. Medics gave him 'anti-scurvy rations' and eventually fish oil, which cured the night blindness and improved his nutrition at least marginally.[6]

The surveyors' brigade work was varied, at first planning and clearing paths for railway construction without quotas; but later they worked in the oil-sand mineshafts where Ukhta's hydrocarbon wealth was extracted. These shafts were dirty, wet, and Samsonov got an eye infection that was allowed to develop unchecked, despite his regular visits to the sanchast. Medics there got him an appointment with a visiting eye-specialist. She referred him for treatment to the Ukhta central camp hospital at Vetlosian; in late November 1938 Samsonov arrived there and was assigned to a 'weakened prisoners' team' performing various forms of 'light' labour: gathering kindling in the forests, and eventually working in a carpentry workshop. His eye infection was treated every day after work, where he befriended a 'lekpom' or medical assistant, Nikolai Kirillovich Sologub. When the woodworking shop was closed in January 1939, Viktor Samsonov might have been sent to general labour in the forest. Instead, Sologub invited him to come and work as an orderly (*sanitar*) in the eye ward of Vetlosian Hospital. Samsonov seized the chance to escape hard labour: by now he realised that his constant illnesses stemmed from exhaustion and undernourishment and survival depended on finding lighter work.[7]

As an orderly, Viktor had to keep stoves stoked night and day, feed and assist patients with toilet visits and washing, and clean the wards. He took orders from a 'lekpom' named Stevens, who discovered in Samsonov a sponge for knowledge. The boy's responsibilities expanded dramatically; he learned to give patients their medicines, take their pulse, and monitor wards in Stevens's absence.

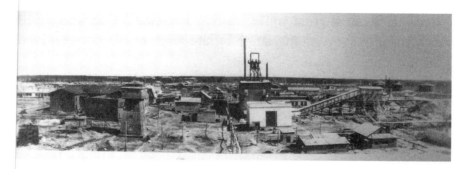

13. Nefteshakht No. 1, the oil mine where Viktor Samsonov's eyes became infected, Yarega, 1940s.

Stevens encouraged him to consider becoming a nurse (*medbrat*), saying, 'He who does not aim to become a general is not a soldier.' Viktor was also encouraged by a nurse who let him shadow her rounds, and by the orderly in charge of the morgue who let him observe autopsies. He scrounged medical textbooks where he could but there were few in this ward. Samsonov would only work here for three months but in his reminiscences at least, these were the months that triggered a love of medical lore and a determination to make a career in the medical section of the Gulag.[8]

The next twist in Viktor Samsonov's fate was decisive. In March 1939 the camp administration dismissed all able-bodied orderlies from the hospital; Samsonov was abruptly sent to timber-felling work. His body wasted rapidly, taxed by the tree-cutting and later log-sawing detail in snow and mud. Attempts to make brushes and brooms in his spare time to exchange for bread came to little. He frequently referred himself to the sanchast for medical attention, suffering from depression and a prolonged bronchial infection. He was referred to a specialist – who turned out to be the chief doctor of Vetlosian Hospital, Dr Nikolai Viktorov, the 'pioneer' who founded Ukhta's medical services. Samsonov told Viktorov about his short apprenticeship as an orderly in the eye ward and his ambition to become a medbrat; he begged the chief doctor for a job. Viktorov made enquiries, learning of Samsonov's excellent record on the ward, but he found the camp work-assigners set against transferring the young man back to hospital work. As a ruse, he hospitalised Samsonov, observing, 'I can see that you're wasting away, lad'.[9] Paradoxically, it was Samsonov's severe emaciation by late summer 1939 that enabled Viktorov to rescue him.

While formally hospitalised, Samsonov worked as an orderly again, this time in Vetlosian's therapeutic ward under the zek-doctor Semyon Ilyich Kristalny. For three weeks the new orderly prepared sterilised bandages, shadowed nurses on their rounds, and read as much medical literature as he could manage to find. Soon he had another meeting with chief doctor Viktorov, who had plainly followed Samsonov's progress and heard good reports of the youth. Viktorov gave him a job as a medbrat. 'And so my dream came true: in October 1939 I put on the white coat of a medbrat for the first time.'[10] Samsonov never saw general labour again.

The Gulag as medical school

Reflecting in 1969 on his education in a letter to former prisoner and leading Ukhta psychiatrist Lev Grigorevich Sokolovsky, the subject of chapter 7, Samsonov acknowledged the peculiar role of Gulag medicine in accelerating his medical career. Life in the camps threw up a challenging array of medical problems, and 'for almost seven years I was trained in Vetlosian Hospital among members of the intelligentsia and highly qualified specialists'.[11] His medical education behind barbed wire had been, arguably, richer in clinical experience and one-to-one contact with learned medical professors than it would be in the civilian medical institute he later attended to obtain his physician's qualification.

In one respect, Samsonov's medical training behind barbed wire was manifestly poorer than it would be in a civilian school: he lacked unfettered access to books about medicine, therapy, and disease. Formally, Gulag prisoners were only allowed to obtain books held in the Cultural-Enlightenment Section (KVCh) libraries, volumes supposedly filtered for ideological rectitude and doled out as a privilege to docile inmates. Reading to improve oneself in the Gulag fell within a political agenda of 'reforging' the prisoner to become a good Soviet citizen. In practice, penal libraries were very uneven in quality and ideological control, and many prison libraries contained proscribed books banned from circulation in civilian collections.[12] A similar unevenness evidently governed the Gulag's technical libraries. Medical practitioners, both freely contracted and prisoners, collected and hoarded personal libraries sometimes consisting of many dozens of titles. Free physicians with their book allowances were able to amass significant collections, and many were generous in lending these to trusted zek colleagues.[13] Samsonov thirsted after medical literature that would explain the phenomena he encountered in the clinic as he shadowed nurses and took orders from lekpoms and doctors. In the eye-diseases ward, he first managed to borrow an old anatomy textbook, from which he drew sketches of internal organs during his spare time; this interest led colleagues to suggest he visit the morgue and study autopsies. In Kristalny's therapeutic ward a nurse lent Samsonov the leading Soviet manual for nurses by M. S. Ikhteiman, and the 774-page tome thrilled him. 'I opened this thick book, and my heart began beating excitedly from joy. Here was every-thing I needed, everything that I had been trying to pull together and understand from snippets in various books and from conversational explanations.'[14] Even if we discount the memoirist's predilection for seeing the past self in a heroic light, Samsonov's appetite for study was prodigious, with medical authorities keenly cited at the bedside at the time (how he must have annoyed the nurses he shadowed!) and in retirement in these reminiscences.[15] Night shifts gave him even more study time: he devoured the 512 pages of Professor Chernorutsky's *Diagnosis of Internal Diseases* by night and tried applying diagnostic logic in the cases he assisted with by day.[16] These textbooks were both comparatively current and important Soviet medical teaching titles, not out-of-date manuals 'relegated' to penal servitude. In 1940 an Estonian freely hired doctor, just qualified from the Leningrad Medical Institute, Edgar Johannesovich Gaav, arrived in Vetlosian and Samsonov helped him unpack. There were tea things, shirts, and 'the rest of the case was filled with books. When I brought in the teapot with boiled water and glasses and saucers, there was a tall column of books standing on the table. Their owner could not help but notice my stolen glances and said, "These are all medical

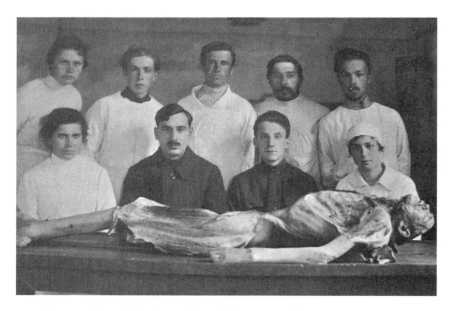

14. Evgeny Kharechko (second from left, standing) with classmates during a study session in the morgue, Kharkiv Medical Institute, 1926.

books".' Gaav lent them freely to Samsonov, and when he left Vetlosian in January 1941, he gave the aspiring medic a copy of A. F. Berdiaev, *Surgery for the Clinical Doctor*, an extremely popular handbook published repeatedly since 1928.[17] In Viktor Samsonov a love of medical books was kindled by their scarcity and was sustained by the kindness of both prisoner and free mentors.

Samsonov's earliest work as a medbrat was in the therapeutic department of Vetlosian Hospital, run by zek-doctors, including Ukrainian Evgeny Ivanovich Kharechko, a graduate of Kharkiv Medical Institute and then medical researcher in Leningrad, before arrest in 1936 on a falsified political charge. He was a natural communicator, later in the 1960s becoming a television host on Ukhta's local channel.[18] In Kharechko's wards, nurses taught the young medbrat how to give injections and medicines independently. Samsonov observed and made notes as Kharechko examined the most interesting patients. A particularly striking case of pellagra, presenting discoloration of the hands (the 'glove' effect noted by Shalamov in a story by that name) caught Kharechko's attention. Samsonov recalls his consultations with other doctors, their scepticism about his proposed diagnosis, and Kharechko's decision to research the disease in depth. As Nikolai Glazov found, doctors with little camp experience had seldom seen advanced vitamin deficiencies. Later, Samsonov witnessed the charismatic Kharechko demonstrating the patient and convincing his colleagues, explaining the origin and progress of pellagra in detail, and advising them to be aware of the disease as they examined prisoners.[19] Samsonov recalls realising, as he learned more about disease from books and doctors, that most tuberculosis patients in this department were incurables, cases so far gone that science could not rescue them. There he witnessed bitter and agonising patient deaths that renewed his commitment to medicine.

Samsonov's experiential learning benefited from his movement around Vetlosian's large range of departments, typical of a central camp hospital. After four months with Kharechko in therapeutics, in March 1940 he moved to the surgical department run by the prisoner Vilhelm Vladimirovich Vittenburg, a Ukrainian professor of obstetrics and gynaecology.[20] Vittenburg became Samsonov's most influential mentor and teacher. He quickly taught the young nurse to improve his patient notes and showed him unusual procedures and patients. The professor encouraged Samsonov's curiosity by coaching him to study scurvy patients and therapies offered in Vetlosian, eventually preparing a conference paper on his observations. He instructed Samsonov in the administration of light anaesthetic in a hernia operation; despite the young man's terror at the prospect of doing harm to the patient, she recovered normally. Vittenburg also encouraged Samsonov to observe autopsies in the morgue; in mid-twentieth-century Soviet medicine, the autopsy was a diagnostic routine central to the scrutiny and affirmation of medical opinions, and they were surprisingly frequent in large Gulag hospitals. Gulag morgues, discussed in chapter 6, also had a teaching role: they were run by medical experts who often led courses for training mid-level medical staff. In the second half of 1940 Samsonov spent so much time in the morgue that by the year's end he was dissecting corpses himself.[21]

January 1941 saw Vittenburg transferred to run the women's department of Vetlosian Hospital, and he took Samsonov with him;

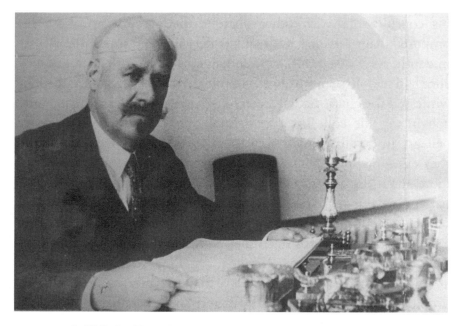

15. Vilhelm Vittenburg on the eve of his arrest in Kyiv, 1938.

it was an opportunity to learn another new branch of medicine from a leading specialist. Vittenburg composed an eight-page programme of study to train Viktor Samsonov, and a second prisoner, Nina (her surname is unknown), in all the subfields of obstetrics and gynae-cology. The course was approved by the hospital authorities, but Vittenburg still had to lend his students textbooks surreptitiously. Samsonov recalls hiding obstetrics manuals by Genter and Bumm under his Gulag-overcoat when he borrowed them to make notes at night.[22] Nina and Viktor made a *fantom*, a doll-model of a newborn infant, to practise delivery techniques. They studied female physi-ology and prepared for seminars with Professor Vittenburg. Samsonov studied in between call-outs to the morgue where he still dissected corpses in post-mortems. His first birth, delivering a healthy infant to a first-time prisoner-mother, went chaotically and Vittenburg had to intervene to repair damage to the womb lining. The next day Samsonov got a classic dressing-down; when he tried to explain himself Vittenburg roared, 'Keep quiet when your seniors are talking!'

The following day the professor apologised and explained that his own son had been sent to the front and no word had been received from him, causing him to lose his temper. Samsonov's second delivery, in January 1942, again to a young zek, went successfully; and soon he and Nina had completed Vittenburg's 'course'. Camp medical authorities permitted them to be examined for a formal certificate of their qualification as midwife-nurses. In May 1942 a commission headed by Vittenburg with three other doctors passed both students. Samsonov recalled, 'I was very glad that I finally had my first document attesting to my study of the fundamentals of medicine.'[23]

'I raise my sail'

Viktor Samsonov's recognition as a Gulag nurse came with virtually immediate reassignment to a busy outpatient clinic in another branch of Vetlosian. His boss was the prisoner-feldsher and Ukrainian writer Ostap Vyshnia, the editor of the suppressed history of Ukhta. Despite his admiration for the senior feldsher, the move was challenging. 'On one hand, it was an attractive chance to broaden my professional training. On the other, the queues of patients frightened me, as did the need to make quick diagnostic decisions. Would I be able to handle it?' Samsonov recalled evening clinics after the working day were thronged with prisoners, and he felt the burden of giving them sufficient attention 'so that we not only relieved them from work at the right moment, but also prescribed treatment or even hospitalised them [in a timely manner]. Otherwise we might have made unforgiveable, unjustifiable mistakes.'[24] Identifying the tipping point when a prisoner's physical condition was greatly deteriorated, but still salvageable, was a delicate clinical and political decision. Signing off zeks from general labour could bring Vyshnia pressure from internal security, who had already accused him of stoking Ukrainian nationalism in the camp.[25]

This hundred-day assignment demonstrated to medical superiors Samsonov's capacity to handle these challenges, not least the life-and-death decisions he was compelled to make at speed. Kharechko and other allies were watching his progress, and successfully requested

Samsonov be allocated to run wards under their command. The young Gulag medic supervised zek and free nurses on his ward, reorganised a bandaging station within the surgical ward, and, in a grim reminder of the hunger disease prevailing at this stage of the war, dealt with a backlog of autopsies. 'Already several corpses had been buried without post-mortems, and the Sanotdel was going to give us hell.'[26] The burden of pervasive and meaningless death in the camps of Ukhta contrasts, in Samsonov's memoir, with the heroic sacrifice at the front.

> In contrast with civilian hospitals, especially in peacetime, among [our] dead there was not a single old man, all were young or middle-aged. Many men of this age were, at this moment, defending the country, dying in battle from bullets and shells. But they knew why they were shedding their blood, and their relatives would receive a notification with the words 'perished fearlessly in the service of the Motherland'. Their parents, wives, children, and grandchildren would know this. They would suffer terribly from their loss, but they could be proud. Among those who died in the camp, 'enemies of the people' predominated. Perhaps, among [these bodies of] nine dead there were military specialists, maybe even scientists, skilled workers, who could have been very necessary for the country in this difficult time somewhere else, on the battlefield, in factories, in the collective farms. Here they were murdered by diseases associated with imprisonment, with heavy, sometimes insupportable labour, constant undernourishment, and crowdedness in dark barracks.[27]

Whatever Samsonov's positive view of his medical education in the Gulag camps, there is no mistaking his disapproval of the systemic injustice behind prisoner maltreatment, a point he returns to frequently in his account.[28]

Amid these changes, Viktor Samsonov's sentence ended in December 1942. He was no longer a prisoner but was tied to his work for the Ukhta Camp Sanotdel until the end of the war. The change of status enabled Samsonov to move from Vetlosian camp to

Ukhta town, and eventually to secure a significantly improved ration, partly by growing vegetables in his own allotment.[29] While continuing work in the wards of Vetlosian, and attending deliveries in town and camp, Viktor, now 23 years old, turned his attention to his studies in medicine. He set his sights first on getting a civilian qualification as a feldsher; his ultimate goal was now to become a physician. The nearest feldsher college was in the nominal capital of the Komi Republic, Syktyvkar, over 300 kilometres southwest of Ukhta. The Syktyvkar Feldsher-Midwifery School accepted him for examination as an external candidate, but it was only with Dr Evgeny Kharechko's direct pleas to the Ukhta camp governor Semyon Nikolaevich Burdakov that Samsonov, still an 'exile' with restricted rights to travel (the more so in wartime), was permitted to make the journey with his notes, meagre rations, and books to the Komi capital for his examinations.[30] In July 1943, over three days, he underwent fourteen oral examinations in obstetrics, pharmacy, pathological anatomy, children's diseases, and the history of the USSR, among other subjects. He was awarded the civilian feldsher's qualification that month. He returned to Ukhta exhausted, drained from advanced undernourishment and stress, which he retrospectively diagnoses in his memoirs as 'neurasthenia'.

Samsonov now realised he had exhausted himself to chase a diploma, and with the help of Dr Kharechko and other allies he devoted the remaining war years to solidifying his clinical, scientific, and organisational experience in the sanchasti and wards of Ukhta's medical network. In summer 1944 Samsonov received a big promotion to director of the sanchast of camp subdivision No. 7 (Vetlosian Hospital's surrounding camps) where he would organise periodic labour categorisation of all prisoners, and monitor outpatient clinics and general sanitary standards. He worked alongside the chief doctor of the Vetlosian Hospital and answered to the Ukhta Camp Sanotdel director, by this time a Ukrainian 'Party-Soviet worker', Nadezhda Adamovna Skakunovskaya.[31] In this post Samsonov frequently fell into conflict with authorities over his clumsy navigation of the bureaucratic maze behind labour categorisation, and he once drew adverse attention from Moscow Gulag Sanotdel headquarters with

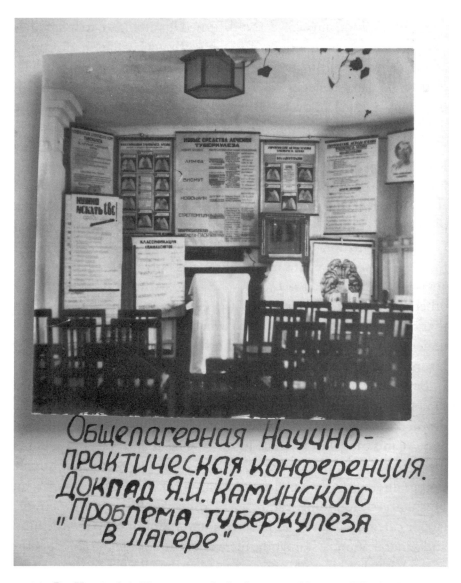

16. *Dr Kaminsky's illustrations for his keynote address on 'The Problem of Tuberculosis in the Camp', 1943(?), Vetlosian Hospital, Ukhta.*

an apparent sharp rise in syphilis cases, the result of mixing 'old' and 'fresh' cases in his reports.[32] Nevertheless, he heard from a friend in the camp governor's office that he was viewed as 'an eager young man' and valued as capable.[33] Samsonov served out most of his term of compulsory attachment (*zakreplenie*) to the Ukhta Camp Sanotdel in this post, apart from brief reassignments to manage a ward in Vetlosian Hospital, and a month-long leave to visit his family in Karelia, in autumn 1945.

An important feature of professional life in Vetlosian Hospital, and its sister-hospital outside Ukhta at the Sangorodok (where Nikolai Glazov worked during the Great Terror), were the many doctors' conferences that stimulated Viktor Samsonov's interest in the science and practice of medicine. In 1941, aged just 21, and only two years into his life as a Gulag medbrat, he gave his first conference paper to an audience of colleagues, mostly zek-doctors, on his treatment under Professor Vittenburg's supervision of patients suffering from scurvy or boils using a vitamin-stimulus therapy.[34] A 'camp-wide scientific conference' of doctors made a big impression on Samsonov in October 1943, with medics gathering at Vetlosian to hear a range of papers from an array of prisoner- and ex-prisoner-physicians whose names are warmly recalled by Ukhta's medical historians. Among these local luminaries were Yakov Iosifovich Kaminsky, who gave the keynote address on tuberculosis in camp conditions, and Lev Lvovich Davydov, who presented an analysis of Ukhta's radium spa waters and their therapeutic effects (described in chapter 8).[35] Kaminsky became Samsonov's line manager and a generous mentor. Samsonov himself prepared and gave a report on abscesses and dermatitis in pellagra patients, a study he conducted from patient histories. These histories were more than paper records for the aspiring medic: 'Behind each of these modest notes a living person, fated to suffer an illness, could be seen.'[36] This work was supervised by Dr Kharechko, by now a well-informed expert on pellagra in the camps; he had just received a copy of the Gulag's instructions on 'alimentary dystrophy' and pellagra.[37]

The conference, and several others like it that Samsonov attended, mixed zek and freely hired doctors and in retrospect were remembered for the fact that, in this environment at least, professional solidarity overrode the penal hierarchy:

> We left reluctantly, wanting to continue our conversations. At least, that's how I felt, having been seized by the liveliest impressions. Here, during the professional discussion of biomedical and social problems the barriers between freely hired and prisoners, the old and the young, were swept away and one felt creative and human solidarity.[38]

Conferences were a frequent feature of many Gulag medical centres, and participants recalled the strength of professional solidarity across the prisoner–free employee divide.[39]

'To start my life from the beginning again'

In February 1946 the Ukhta Camp administration finally released Viktor Samsonov from his tied employment in its Sanotdel and he was free to pursue his medical education – up to a point. He recalls that because of his criminal record, he could only apply to the medical institutes of Arkhangelsk or Ivanovo.[40] Despite having his interrupted training in land surveying, and his full civilian feldsher qualification, to enter physicians' training Samsonov needed to get the Soviet version of a secondary-school leaving certificate. (Like many Soviet technicians, he had entered the land-surveying course at 14, missing out on the three-year secondary diploma.) He spent the next months in night-school courses on mathematics, Russian language, literature, chemistry, physics, and other subjects. Fortunately, these courses were available in Ukhta and Samsonov's Vetlosian Hospital mentor Dr Kaminsky reduced his workload and found him a maths tutor among the hospital staff. In July 1946, having passed these examinations, Samsonov got his leaving certificate. He spent much of the summer arranging to sit the entry examinations for Ivanovo Medical Institute – an expensive proposition requiring him to travel there and spend heavily on room and board while competing for a place in the course. In August Viktor Samsonov was successful; he would enter Ivanovo Medical Institute's six-year physician-training course to start that autumn. This endlessly energetic student returned to Ukhta to say his farewells to the place that formed him. From Professor Vittenburg he received a fatherly embrace and a few words of advice: 'See that you avoid everything that is unnecessary. Don't scatter yourself, eliminate every temptation and second-rate interest. Only then will the way to science open to you.'[41] The Gulag's Vetlosian Central Camp Hospital became in Samsonov's retrospective gaze, his alma mater, and he memorialised it in the many iterations of his reminiscences.

Vadim Gennadievich Aleksandrovsky:
Inside a barbed-wire academy

If the Ivanovo Medical Institute was perhaps among the most basic of post-war Soviet Russia's schools for physicians, the Military Medical Academy in Leningrad was close to the pinnacle. Samsonov's medical career began with a slow, grinding ascent out of the Gulag to gain entry to Ivanovo; Vadim Aleksandrovsky's started with a precipitous fall from a top institution. It was a sensational humiliation to be pulled from final examinations at the Academy, arrested, interrogated, and sentenced for challenging the Party's decree against Akhmatova and Zoshchenko. But such independent-mindedness was dangerous in Leningrad in 1949. Aleksandrovsky's individualistic streak grew from a family background in the intelligentsia: his father had two university degrees and worked in municipal administration; his mother had a pre-revolutionary degree from the prestigious women's Bestuzhev Courses. Vadim's parents were not persecuted in the 1930s, but one uncle, an aviation engineer, was arrested and held in an OGPU research laboratory for two years, and another was detained simply for being the brother of Leon Trotsky's ally Evgeny Alekseevich Preobrazhensky.[42]

After almost six months of imprisonment and transport, the young not-quite doctor spent five years as a prisoner working for the medical network of Kargopol Camp. The Kargopol complex of camps dotted Arkhangelsk Province, not in Russian terms that distant from Vadim's Leningrad home but deep in depopulated forests along a railway line running in a northward vertical from Vologda to the port of Arkhangelsk on the White Sea. The journey from Leningrad to Kodino, Aleksandrovsky's first camp, took a mere seven days by rail: comparatively short and easy by the standards of Gulag transport. The trip illustrates how by the late Stalin era prisoner labour was ubiquitous in the Soviet economy, close to major centres and deployed to assist reconstruction and development after the war.[43] Kargopol's network of camps belonged to the Gulag's in-house timber industry; in Kargopol, prisoners cut down trees, trimmed and transported them to sawmills and factories where they prepared construction materials, furniture, skis, cellulose, footwear, railway sleepers, and virtually anything else that could be fashioned from wood. Three prisoner-staffed state farms serviced a population of 20,237 inmates (1 January 1950).[44] Isaak Moiseevich Filshtinsky, a linguist who served in the same system at the same time as Aleksandrovsky, remembers that Kargopol Camp 'was ordinary', by comparison with remote Kolyma or camps for grandiose building projects. 'By Gulag standards, it was so insignificant that it didn't even figure in the "for service use only" directory of camps.'[45] The 'insignificance' of Kargopol has to be balanced with recognition that conditions were extremely harsh especially in wartime, with very high mortality, exacerbated by the camp's low priority in Gulag supply chains.[46] According to both Filshtinsky and Aleksandrovsky, by 1950 conditions were not so desperate as they had been in recent years, but the impact and memory of ubiquitous death from undernourishment and its consequences was still present in these camps.[47]

Vadim Aleksandrovsky's Gulag memoir is a compact 78-page brochure completed in February 1989 and published seven years later. As a prisoner-doctor writing a memoir during the glasnost years, Aleksandrovsky felt little anxiety about describing his service in the Gulag's medical network for at least two reasons. First, as a prisoner arrested on trumped-up charges, he was unquestionably a victim of the Stalinist system, even if he survived by taking a 'soft' job behind barbed wire and enjoyed the privileges associated with it. He reflects on that privilege retrospectively and his understanding of the

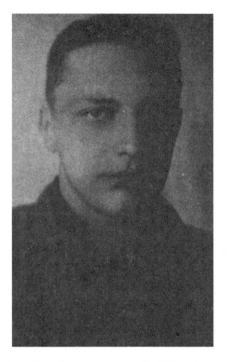

17. Vadim Aleksandrovsky, a green medic fallen from grace (c. 1949).

injustice of Stalin's forced-labour camps is typical of the late 1980s. Second, Aleksandrovsky was very green as a medic when he entered the camp system, and his reminiscences are shaped by the learning curve he confronted upon arrival. Like any rookie doctor's memoir, this account of a young doctor thrown into the reality of practising medicine after years of study relies on the shock of the unexpected and the story of the author's getting of wisdom to gain the reader's sympathy.[48] This rookie-doctor memoirist also shields himself from apparent complicity with Gulag atrocity by demonstrating how little he understood about the world he was in. Although Aleksandrovsky's career and camps are less documented than others, Filshtinsky's reminiscences offer a perspective on these camps even if these two zeks did not meet in Kargopol. As well, historians have studied the forestry-camp system and Kargopol in particular, offering official perspectives gained from Soviet archives.[49]

'We weren't taught this way in the Academy'

Vadim was extremely fortunate to arrive at Kodino station camp with a group of intellectuals from Leningrad; there were no criminals among them to steal their clothing and make life miserable during the 21-day quarantine against typhoid on arrival. Such harassment would come later as this was a camp with a varied population of 'politicals' and criminal offenders. Once released from quarantine, the party was inspected by the camp's administrators, including its sanchast director. Ervin Sigizmundovich Drukker was an Austrian communist who emigrated to the USSR in 1934, only to be arrested as so many foreign communists were, in the Great Terror, on charges of espionage. Drukker had served out his seven-year sentence, remaining in the camp after release working in the Gulag medical network. By profession Drukker was a dental technician, 'clever, with a sense of humour', and by fraternising with medical staff while imprisoned he learned enough about medicine to rise to the post he now occupied as a 'free' worker. He was obviously a natural leader and a capable manager despite his limited medical training: he ran the sanchasti for the surrounding camp subdivisions, overseeing three zek-doctors and three freely contracted ones in the Kodino sanchast alone. Drukker would have a profound influence on Vadim Aleksandrovsky's formation as a physician.[50]

Drukker took note of Vadim's training, and after just a single day of unspecified general labour, he summoned the prisoner to Kodino's fifty-bed central infirmary, where Aleksandrovsky was to work and be housed. The transition to Gulag medical practice was wrenching for Aleksandrovsky, whose training scarcely prepared him for it:

In the academy, for five years they had been stuffing me with grand philosophies and routines of practice that seemed extremely distant from real life, all the more, from labour-camp life. Literally everything (I mean of medical practice) I had to learn from getting bruises and bumps, stumbling at every step, feeling my way, for I had almost nothing to guide me.[51]

Drukker relied heavily on the zek-doctors in this infirmary; the free doctors were busy practising in the civilian hospital beyond the zone, and they only periodically visited to monitor prisoner-medics' work and perform tasks in other camp subdivisions. Drukker evidently spotted an opportunity to expand the ranks of his reliable doctors by recruiting Aleksandrovsky, 'even though I lacked a diploma' as the younger man marvels in his memoir.

The unaccredited physician had not yet recovered 'from the colossal shock' of imprisonment. 'It was still far too great a break between the freedom of the officers' academy and my slave-like situation.' The barbed wire, watchtowers, and guard dogs depressed and repulsed him. His sense of being catapulted into a 'phantasmagoria' assists us in seeing the differences between his academic expectations and the way medicine was done in the zone.[52] Drukker ordered him to observe and assist in his first outpatient clinic, an afterhours evening reception when about thirty to forty zeks would come seeking medical aid, hoping, in most cases, to be released from work. Aleksandrovsky's recollections merit lengthy quotation:

> The reception worked at a furious pace. At the 3rd camp subdivision, one of the doctors or feldshers I have mentioned would preside. Stethoscopes...were rarely used, and seldom were the usual methods of diagnostics employed. The camp doctors developed a subtle feeling – which patient should one treat seriously, and which one should simply be asked, 'What's wrong?' 'Vasya, give him something for his stomach (or head, or loins, or chest).' With serious patients they acted like a proper doctor, but always at a fast pace. Whoever needed it was sent to the infirmary or given a minor operation right there in the bandaging station: draining abscesses, sewing up minor wounds, extracting teeth, giving injections and so on. Sterilisation and asepsis were quite relative, not because the doctors forgot about them, but because of the primitive conditions in general.[53]

Aleksandrovsky quickly learned that in the camp, a moral evaluation accompanied diagnostic practice; not all patients were equally deserving of the professional gaze of 'a proper doctor'.

With my experience in the Academy with its unhurried and thorough analysis of every patient, its exemplary textbook palpation of each patient, it was difficult for me to adjust to this new set-up, to the fast tempo, to the malingerers, the pleaders, the self-harmers, to the very specific dialogues, and the entire basis of camp medicine. With time I got used to all of it, without losing, it seemed to me, my medical and human features. But there were people there who had lost all of that . . .[54]

Fortunately for Aleksandrovsky, his new colleagues treated him, 'green and lost, with sympathy and understanding, and they tried with their advice and their whispered suggestions to help me on my first, uncertain steps in this new path'.[55] The doctors and feldshers in this infirmary respected his learning and guided him with discreet commentary that, they hoped, would help him make the leap into Gulag practice while preserving his authority as a doctor in front of the prisoner-patients.

Aleksandrovsky's induction to Gulag specificities was capped by observing a commission to assign the labour categorisation of all prisoners in this camp subdivision. In March 1950 Drukker and a free doctor conducted this 'komissovka'; they assigned categories (capable of heavy, light, or no labour) as a zek-doctor escorted the prisoners before them and reported on their 'purely medical' assessment of each case.[56] Again, Aleksandrovsky was struck by the rapid pace, superficiality, and apparent negligence of this procedure, which boiled down to a medical inspection of the stomach and buttocks of each man. Doctors sought to identify the cases of malnutrition that could benefit from medical care – and to limit the number seeking such privileges.

The method was quite exact and was an echo of recent times when hunger and dystrophy were rife in prisons and camps, and people died like flies from emaciation and exhausting work. So, the doctors' hands flashed rapidly, feeling the naked zeks by the stomach or the buttocks. It was unusual and surprising to me. We weren't taught this way in the Academy. [. . .] This work went on for several hours. The forms were filled in with the work categories: some were selected for recuperative rest, some for two weeks of POO (station of convalescent rest [*punkt ozdrovitel'nogo otdykha*]), some were sent to the hospital, and some were sent packing with swear-words for faking illness. The machine worked flat out.[57]

After a month working in camp subdivision No. 3 alongside Drukker and his comrades, Aleksandrovsky was judged ready to work on his own in the Gulag environment. Not long after the 'komiss-ovka' Drukker assigned Aleksandrovsky to camp subdivision No. 6, a 15-kilometre walk away in the woods, accompanied by two bored armed guards taking potshots at crows and telegraph-insulators.

'My independent career began'

At subdivision No. 6, Aleksandrovsky was assigned to run the sanchast, supervising two prisoner-feldshers. Vadim quickly became accustomed to the sanchast doctor's routine: 'My independent career in camp-medicine began. Receptions, examinations, treatment, sanitary inspec-tions of the barracks, kitchens, privies, telephone conversations with Drukker, obligatory dealings with the authorities, increasing interac-tion with the prisoners: that was everyday life.'[58] Aleksandrovsky raised the number of day-releases from work for prisoners, but with Drukker's supervision he managed to persuade the camp's work-assigners that these concessions were legitimate. In just two months, after a visit from Drukker, who went over Aleksandrovsky's medical notes, the sanchast director sent his apprentice-doctor to 'Kliuchi' camp subdivi-sion No. 1, which was the oldest in the complex and even farther from Kodino. Again, it lacked a doctor, and its sanchast 'was in total disarray, mixed up, a mess. I looked at it and threw my hands in the air – let it stay like that: apathy and indifference had not yet left me.'[59] The facility had a reception room for evening clinics, two 'wards' of three beds each, and a tiny room with a cot for Aleksandrovsky's lodgings. He had two feldshers and two orderlies, plus a 'statistician' who kept records, to supervise. Vadim Aleksandrovsky would spend nine months running this sanchast, and he underwent an epiphany that burned away the 'apathy' he felt when he first set eyes on this wretched clinic.

Aleksandrovsky's energies, rather like Savoeva's in her first posting, were scattered between a cascade of challenges, but in contrast with her expressions of boundless self-belief, the product of her 'free' status and retrospective editorial gaze, his reactions came quite reasonably from the depression and disorientation he felt as a prisoner. He became fixated on taking inmate blood pressure, something familiar from Academy lessons but (he observed) neglected by Gulag physicians. As a result, referrals of patients to Kargopol's central camp hospital shot up, and 'Drukker was unpleasantly surprised' because this led to more work-releases, and thus pressure from commandants.[60] The episode blew over but not before sharp words from Drukker, accompanied by some coaching on which drugs to prescribe. Later in January 1951, a prisoner presented extremely high blood pressure and suffered a stroke, dying in three hours, despite his efforts to revive him with injections. It was Aleksandrovsky's first patient death and his first time releasing a body from his infirmary to be buried. However, the experience nudged him to immerse himself in his work, and to take it more seriously, 'no, not to forget, but to pacify and calm my sense of my position as a slave of the state and to feel my lack of freedom less keenly'.[61]

Vadim Aleksandrovsky recognised that his study habits in the Academy had been dishonest: he had cut corners, paying most attention to internal diseases since he hoped to specialise in that area. Now his negligence of the remaining curriculum hindered him from grappling with the variety of sickness in his patients. Adrift without mentors, like Mikhail Bulgakov's fictional country doctor marooned in a rural clinic, he had only –

Books. They helped me to really learn. I was allowed to have them in the camp. And I began to order them from 'freedom', from bookshops, with the help of friends and family. Soon I had built up a decent medical library. Particularly helpful were *Surgery for Operations, Methods of Investigating Surgical Patients*, and other manuals. I would read and study a lot, eagerly. And beneath my skin I began to grasp the specifics of camp medicine. The feldshers helped me a lot, of course, because of their long camp experience.[62]

Indeed, Bulgakov's hero often relied on the kindness of his feld-sher and nurses to resolve his medical dilemmas, when he was not running off to look up something in his study, pretending to fetch his cigarettes.[63] If Aleksandrovsky does not give enough information about his textbooks in his memoirs to enable identification, never-theless he asserts repeatedly that access to books was 'not difficult', even praising the KVCh's libraries and free employees for lending to zeks 'despite the official ban'.[64]

A turning point in the young doctor's professional outlook came as a result of a tongue-lashing, one of many he received from Drukker during his time in camp subdivision No. 1. His boss visited on an inspection tour, looking in every nook and cranny, checking medicines, instruments, and the general state of Aleksandrovsky's infirmary.

There was a lot of disorder: and dirt, mess, medicines in a heap and so on. For some reason I remember that episode clearly, and especially my boss's words, 'And you call yourself a doctor! . . .' I was very ashamed, and right away I set about with my lads to tidy up the sanchast. In a couple of days cast-iron order reigned there, and the hygiene was almost ideal. Drukker did not forgive me the slightest bit of negligence, he forced me to do things once and redo them again, making me precise and attentive in my dealings with people, in my work generally, constantly poking his nose in my failings and mistakes. I felt a wild hatred towards him for all this, but gradually I became a more collected, careful, and respon-sible person in all respects. Later I understood that Drukker was being kind to me. He obviously decided to beat the remaining 'prison shock' out of me and make me into a man and a doctor. I think that he felt some kind of weakness for me, a still-green 26-year-old, and he wished me only good things, but his methods of instruction were severe.[65]

Aleksandrovsky owed his recovery from 'prison shock' to the discipline and rigour imposed by a sympathetic and demanding ex-prisoner boss. And yet Drukker is no saint in his account, but a complex figure who straddled the fences between penal power and medical hierarchies. He was not a qualified doctor and had to manage physicians firmly but diplomatically, while burying his kind-heartedness when dealing with the camp authorities. In their presence 'he always spoke in correct and profoundly orthodox speech' – once declaring to dissatisfied prisoners about their morning porridge, that it was 'fine pearl-barley kasha. Comrade Stalin takes care of your nutrition. That is our Soviet humanism.'[66] Was this veiled mockery? 'Read it however you wish. But he really did take care of the prisoners,' Aleksandrovsky comments.

'Standing on my own two feet'

Vadim Aleksandrovsky recognises in his memoir that Drukker's mentorship forged him as a physician. His confidence in his clinical judgement increased with every daily clinic. He began to channel his energy into systematic study of prisoner illnesses, including some conditions that go unmentioned elsewhere in the penal medical memoir literature, such as parasitical threadworm and pinworm infestations. (These were so endemic in the general civilian population that perhaps other medics felt them unremarkable.)[67] Under Drukker's supervision he learned to give vitamin injections to prisoners to combat undernourishment, and his boss also schooled him in setting up his own convalescent station for prisoners in need of refeeding in his camp subdivision.[68] He made house calls to civilians beyond the camp, treating a commandant's wife who suffered from severe tuberculosis so that she could be transferred by rail to Arkhangelsk for hospitalisation.[69] By March 1951 camp subdivision No. 1 was shut down and Aleksandrovsky was convoyed on foot, along with the camp's prisoners, to subdivision No. 5, 10 kilometres from Kodino. His new camp had about 400 prisoners and a substantial sanchast and infirmary, where he took charge, replacing a self-taught 'head of medicine' with only veterinary training. Coming to the end of his sentence, the vet-turned-human doctor had let standards slide in the infirmary. Dr Aleksandrovsky made his first task to raise discipline 'and give our medical barrack a decent appearance'.[70]

He continued to monitor the zeks' blood pressure, conducting an extraordinary 'komissovka' with the camp authorities' approval to detect hypertension and move the worst cases to lighter work categorisations. When the necessary drugs to treat this and other disorders were lacking in the camp's pharmacy, he instructed patients to ask relatives to send these in their periodic food parcels. He began to study, from textbooks, how to conduct minor surgical procedures to remove suspicious growths and drain swellings, and gained experience in performing them on his patients, adhering to the principle of 'doing no harm'. With time he was confident enough to perform amputations of frostbitten fingers without referring these cases onward to the central camp hospital; the penicillin he required to treat amputees came from a supply obtained from prisoner parcels, and he claims there were no complications. Contending with influenza epidemics every winter might lead to a handful of pneumonias, but again prisoners supplied antibiotics to suppress these.[71] Camp No. 5 was closer to Kodino and Dr Aleksandrovsky was able to consult experienced doctors more frequently; zek and free physicians 'would come and help me to figure out a difficult situation'. There were even roving consultants, an ophthalmologist, a dentist, and a neuropathologist, from distant Ertsevo, the administrative centre of Kargopol Camp, and they would leave him in charge of therapies once they diagnosed prisoner conditions. After the isolation of camp subdivision No. 1, he seized on opportunities for learning from mentors and patients. In all of this activity Vadim Aleksandrovsky sought to build a store of knowledge and experience for the future:

> Deep down in my heart I was preparing myself as well for work after prison, in freedom: the more knowledge and experience I acquired here, the easier it would be there. And yet the glimmer of hope was still faint. Wise people then knew well that under the leader of the day, nothing good would come for us, and one had to be ready for the worst.[72]

The stimulus of work and study, combined with mentorship and comradeship among the intelligentsia zeks and free medics, gave

Aleksandrovsky reasons to be cautiously hopeful, even if all were aware that Stalin's grip left little prospect of an easier future.

However his progress might appear, this was not 'a normal, absolutely decent life' in the memoirist's view. His own experience, comparatively comfortable and interesting, was not that of the majority, who suffered 'humiliating unfreedom, the convoy, foul swearing, sometimes physical violence, tough and debilitating labour for 10 or 12 hours ... and if not hunger, then for the majority, a sensation of constant undernourishment'.[73] The knowledge that so many were sentenced for no reason at all, and the 'repugnant yoke' of the hardened criminals who made life in these camps chaotically violent, were inescapable even for those in 'soft' jobs. Indeed, after suffering an attempted stabbing at camp No. 1, Vadim Aleksandrovsky was always on his guard with criminal patients, keeping a knife concealed in his pocket and a truncheon in his reception room desk, with male feldshers ever vigilant. The illusion of normal life was a dangerous one if you forgot where you were.

Early in 1952 Ervin Drukker was released from the Gulag medical service, and although he was not then rehabilitated, with the help of friends he obtained a residency permit for Moscow. Aleksandrovsky reports his mentor's departure drily, and at the time their farewells were probably correct rather than warm: the mentor's tongue-lashings rang long enough in the young doctor's ears and memory. He did not enjoy the paternal embrace Samsonov received from Vittenburg. 'In my years of imprisonment, I acquired great life and medical experience, and finally became a physician. I now see that Drukker played no small part in this, constantly supporting me and pushing me forward. Only later did I realise how much I owed this man.'[74] Aleksandrovsky would quickly get used to a milder boss, ironically, a senior lieutenant of the Gulag Sanotdel, who treated zek and free medical staff with equal respect, even if 'at certain moments the chekist in him' showed itself.[75] Now gaining in experience, Vadim Aleksandrovsky could say 'I felt self-confident and was standing on my own two feet' as a seasoned physician by the time of Stalin's death.[76] Hopes for early release began to press insistently in his heart. He petitioned the Supreme Court and head of state Kliment Voroshilov personally in 1953 and, when his first pleas were rebuffed, again in 1954; he also helped others write petitions for rehabilitation. During this period, 'political' releases were sporadic and the camps he was confined to changed numerous times. Dr Aleksandrovsky continued to work in camp infirmaries, noting the relaxation of the penal regime was worryingly accompanied by an increase in the 'criminal public' among the prisoners. He was now carrying his knife constantly and, with the privilege of 'non-convoyed' status, spending as much time as possible outside the camp away from the criminal element, for safety's sake.[77]

Vadim Aleksandrovsky was summoned to a court near his camp in late March 1955 and given early release without the quashing of his conviction. In June 1955, after much chasing of paperwork through the Supreme Court by a devoted Moscow aunt, Aleksandrovsky heard the court pronounce him innocent and received a rehabilitation certificate. He was restored to naval service. With the help of Boris Aleksandrovich Nakhapetov, he re-entered the Military Medical Academy course in Leningrad. In his 'absence', educational reforms had lengthened the medical course from five to six years, and his final year of study would have included subjects such as hospital therapy and surgical procedures he undoubtedly knew much about from experience.[78] Vadim Aleksandrovsky tells us nothing about his adjustment to military medicine after his Gulag apprenticeship, but the diagnostic and therapeutic skills he acquired in the camps must have affected the way he encountered patients in later life, to judge from his retrospective reflections on what he learned behind barbed wire. Paradoxically, writing a Gulag memoir was also an opportunity to understand who his first teachers were and what he actually learned: the classic medical Bildungsroman.

From an 'ivory tower'

Both Viktor Samsonov and Vadim Aleksandrovsky lived comparatively fortunate lives in the Gulag. They avoided the depredations of general labour, they gained footholds in the refuge of camp medical centres, and they successfully laid the foundations for careers in medicine and in Samsonov's case, academic life, after release.

Aleksandrovsky understood the purpose of his memoir was to describe this place of privilege; 'I consider it my task to show a modest picture of camp medicine and camp confinement from the ivory tower of a camp medic himself.'[79] Both found mentors and allies who made life behind barbed wire bearable and stimulating, who took an interest in their intellectual and moral development, and who protected them from arbitrary penal authority when they could. Within the impoverished prospects of Gulag medicine, they learned how to heal prisoners' illnesses while navigating the bureaucratic and penal restrictions imposed by camp commandants and authorities. They also endeavoured to retain their humanity and to 'do no harm' even when participating in the grim routines of labour categorisation and reception-room triage. They came to understand the moral element that lies behind clinical practice by observing their teachers and by the daily exercise of their own judgement as independent clinicians. They experienced all of this in two different times in Gulag history, and in two very different settings.

The Gulag left its stamp on both men. Samsonov's positive view of the camp medical service was obviously determined by his attachment to a big central camp hospital, and his praise for this special environment and its doctors was evidently why Solzhenitsyn dismissed his perspective. The author of *The Gulag Archipelago* declined to reply to Samsonov's 1995 letter challenging Solzhenitsyn's unrelentingly negative assessment of Gulag hospitals, doctors, and medicine.[80] Samsonov himself knew the limits of penal medicine, and the limits of his own ability to withstand penal life, even if he only reveals them unconsciously in a striking passage of his reminiscences. He could not bear to remain resident in Vetlosian after being given his freedom; he was offered 'luxurious' lodgings there as a free employee but every day after work he 'would have looked out of the window of my fine room at nothing but columns of prisoners, setting off for work or returning to the zone under guard . . .'. Instead, he undertook the daily 3-kilometre commute from a 'kennel' of a room in Ukhta town, where the House of Culture, library, stadium, and friends beckoned.[81] The porosity of the Gulag, the traffic between the camps and 'freedom', has attracted the attention of many scholars, and it certainly mattered to inhabitants on both sides of the barbed wire; but it must not be forgotten that one side of that wire had more freedom and security, even in Stalin's Soviet Union.[82]

Aleksandrovsky's short memoir at first pass would seem to turn its back on the Gulag the moment he was released from confinement. He wasted no time in leaving the zone and even risked several months living illegally in Leningrad while awaiting rehabilitation. He elected to close his memoir with bitter thoughts about the injustice of his imprisonment:

> I often reflected on this position, so absurd, and so humiliating to my human dignity. On the one hand, I was a doctor, worthy of patients' trust. On the other, I was a criminal, who could do harm, and escape, and do all manner of evil. And finally, I was very genuinely a slave, like the slaves of Egypt, of Greece, of Rome. I was obliged to blindly follow the bosses' orders having forgotten that I was still a human being. Yes, I had to forget about that in those days.[83]

Having been deprived of his family and enslaved in the camps, Vadim Aleksandrovsky looks back on a long-silenced part of his life to condemn it. But its stamp was there, in the kind of doctor he became on the foundations laid in the Gulag. The camps, with their unfathomable challenges to the young physician, and with their circles of teachers and mentors, made him 'into a man and a doctor'.

5

SISTERS OF MERCY AND KOMSOMOL GIRLS
Nursing in the Gulag

In 1940, after a year in Kolyma slogging in a succession of back-breaking 'general labour' jobs, Eugenia Solomonovna Ginzburg, a historian and journalist convicted in 1938 of Trotskyist conspiracy, had a piece of good fortune that saved her life. She met a Leningrad surgeon and prisoner-doctor Vasily Ionovich Petukhov, who resolved to 'save' her by taking her on as a nurse. She began her Gulag medical career in a children's home in the harsh Elgen labour camp.

The children's home was as paradoxical as the Gulag world around it. 'Yes, this undoubtedly was a penal camp hut. But it smelled of warm semolina and wet pants. Someone's bizarre imagination had combined the trappings of the prison world with simple, human, and touchingly familiar things now so far out of reach that they seemed no more than a dream.'[1] The paradox flowed from a bureaucratic fact: babies born to prisoners in the camps were 'free' citizens, not prisoners themselves, but the Gulag's Sanitary Department was financially responsible for their care and upbringing until the age of two years, when they were supposed to be transferred to civilian children's homes. The Gulag children's homes were a bubble of civilian life behind barbed wire, a place where the Gulag and the non-Gulag interacted.

Ginzburg, the best-known nurse in Gulag memoir literature, learned children's nursing through direct experience and improvised study. The routines were shown to her by a prisoner-colleague with good sense and compassion: a fourteen-hour day involved bottle feeding, medical treatments, but principally changing babies' nappies, and cleaning 'the enormous pile of soiled diapers'.[2] Knowing that Ginzburg could read Latin, and had 'a bit of education', Petukhov decided to make of her a nurse skilled enough to tend the sickest infants and toddlers. He taught her himself in the prisoners' hospital where he worked. Ginzburg recalled, 'I conscientiously worked through *The Feldsher's Handbook*, I learned to apply cupping glasses and to give injections, even intravenous solutions. I returned to the children's home a full-fledged "member of the medical staff", much encouraged by Dr Petukhov's kind words about me.'[3] Ginzburg would work in this children's home for a year before authorities transferred her through a cycle of minor camps during the war to run small clinics for prisoners. Eventually she became an experienced nurse in larger camp hospitals, including Belichya, where Nina Savoeva gave her a job. Ginzburg left her Gulag medical career in 1947 when as a free employee she took on jobs in civilian kindergartens, which were primarily educational not healthcare facilities. She would not work in medicine again, despite the fact that during her seven years as a penal nurse, and with tutoring from a doctor who became her second husband, she became 'a proper ward nurse. I had learned all the secrets of the art: I could perform with a scalpel and I could give intravenous fluids.'[4] Nursing in the Gulag saved Ginzburg's life, furnished her extraordinary energies with an outlet, and arguably transformed her values and beliefs as the 'naïve young Communist idealist' encountered life's fragility in the cruellest of circumstances.[5]

The realities of nursing in the Gulag for the tens of thousands of medical workers who performed this work behind barbed wire have never been studied. Historians have shown how nursing in Russia's civilian life was an ambiguous profession before and after the revolutions of 1917. Secular and quasi-religious communities of 'sisters of mercy' formed during the tsarist era were an important component of Imperial Russia's medical personnel. Wars transformed nursing from charitable to essential work between 1914 and 1921.[6] However, early Soviet nursing was scarcely a unified profession, and the odour of Christian philanthropy did not endear nursing to revolutionary medicine. The 'virtue script' of the nurse as a 'good, trusting, compassionate figure' in clinics and wards was hard to reconcile with Soviet faith in technocracy, science, and atheism.[7] The more skilled and comparatively prestigious feldshers (military and civilian paramedics) and even biomedically trained midwives challenged the generalist nurse for status in the mid-level 'grey area' of the Soviet medical hierarchy.[8] The health commissariat's bureaucratic term, 'mid-level medical personnel', captured the ambiguity of nursing in the 1920s and 1930s, as just one among many auxiliary medical roles.[9] The lines between the feldsher, nurse, and 'medical assistant' (*lekpom*, a very informal term but widely used in the Gulag) were blurred. Training and certification in nursing was offered by a host of institutions; standards were lax and varied considerably; and the resulting dilution of skills and qualifications meant that in the interwar years many Soviet doctors found nurses 'illiterate' in basic medicine, unreliable, and dangerously overpromoted, especially if they hoped to use nursing as a stepping stone to a physician's training.[10]

Nurses, feldshers, and midwives in the early Soviet years needed only minimal elementary schooling to enter a training course, by the 1930s offered in a 'medical school', that is a college lower in prestige than the Soviet physicians' training ground, the 'medical institute' with its academic ethos. Nurses' subordination to physicians was justified by their usual lack of general secondary education, the practical labour they performed, and the shortness of their training. A nurse in 1930s Soviet civilian courses could qualify in as little as nine months, but two- or three-year courses were the norm.[11] Low educational attainment conspired with gender prejudice to sustain nursing's unattractive reputation. Far from all nurses were female, but the predominantly female occupation of nurse as medical caregiver did not attract many men (males in the role were known as *medbratia*, 'medical brothers', parallel to *medsestry*, medical sisters or nurses). Despite attempts to raise the patriotic status of nursing in the 1930s, men with basic education seeking medical training preferred feldshers' or orderlies' courses.[12] Male nurses were evidently often viewed as unreliable because they were believed to be prone to drunkenness, criminality, or indifference to their patients.[13] Women with feldsher qualifications styled themselves *fel'dsheritsy*, women-feldshers, to assert their superior medical knowledge, and sense of independence. With a paucity of doctors available, Russia's feldshers dominated rural healthcare provision well into the twentieth century, and were trusted, reluctantly, as independent practitioners in a way that nurses seldom were.[14] Yet within the Gulag, nurses like Ginzburg were sometimes given roles of significant medical responsibility, alongside or even in place of feldshers, in remote worksites.

The Gulag's in-house courses for prisoner-nurses mirrored ones in wider society: by the end of the increasingly militarised 1930s, all major factories were meant to offer women workers courses in nursing, and by this time Soviet Red Cross nursing courses were ubiquitous.[15] Gulag nursing courses ran alongside training for feldshers, clinical laboratory, and veterinary assistants in Karaganda camp as early as 1931.[16] In Dmitlag near Moscow in October 1933, eighteen nurses graduated from the first in-house nurse training course and the newly qualified prisoners were assigned to clinics in the camp, with certificates of attestation placed on their personal records.[17] Internal camp newspapers celebrated camp-trained nurses among the many occupational specialities that prisoners acquired.[18] In 1936 a central directive from Moscow, obviously aspirational in tone, ordered all camps to set up six-month training courses for nurses and feldshers from among prisoners. It laid out an extraordinarily ambitious 1,262-hour programme of anatomy, physiology, Latin, biology, chemistry, bacteriology 'with sanitary technique', pathological anatomy, pharmacology, hygiene and fundamentals of healthcare, surgical medicine, infectious diseases, psychiatry, venereal disease, first aid, and gynaecology and obstetrics. There was time in the schedule for political literacy and Russian-language training, too. Gulag doctors (freely hired) were given a 100–150-rouble monthly bonus for running these courses. Students would be selected by camp medical and cultural-enlightenment officials (overseen, undoubtedly, by security chiefs) from among the 'socially friendly' contingent of lesser offenders. The same decree promised these qualifications would be recognised, once the holder had served out their sentence, for military service, and in Gulag medical facilities where they would become freely hired staff. There were to be shorter refresher courses and conferences for prisoners with civilian nursing or feldsher experience.[19] It was through such in-house training that Varlam Shalamov and numerous other memoirists got systematic training as nurses and feldshers. Still others, like Viktor Samsonov and Ginzburg, acquired their training from sympathetic Gulag doctors and by individual study and on-the-job experience.[20]

As with physicians, the Gulag 'recruited' nurses and other mid-level medical staff from the graduating classes of medical schools. The mechanisms for recruitment were ostensibly similar to those for doctors; however, for some 'freely hired' nurses, recruitment was even less 'voluntary' than it was for graduate doctors. For nurses from poor backgrounds a contract in Gulag nursing could represent a step upward in social mobility. The health commissariat paper trails seldom differentiate sufficiently between the various 'mid-level medical workers' to say how many graduating nurses were hired by the Gulag in any given year. In the first quarter of 1944, there were approximately 4,550 nurses working for the Gulag, half of them prisoners and half 'freely hired'.[21] In the post-war years, with numbers of graduate nurse recruits for the Gulag running in the hundreds per year, the camps were able to ensure that at least some politically 'reliable' freely contracted nurses worked alongside prisoner and ex-prisoner nurses and feldshers.[22]

Describing the Gulag nurses' experience is challenging for the historian, principally because mid-level medical personnel usually lacked the advanced education that might encourage them to write their memoirs. If some Gulag doctors took up their pens to record their lives for their children or posterity, nurses apparently seldom did. Historian and lecturer Ginzburg's account of penal nursing is rare for its articulate reflection on the nature of medical care behind barbed wire. Despite its weaknesses, Ginzburg's well-known memoir serves as a useful point of comparison for the accounts on which this chapter is based. To chart nurses' Gulag experience, I have drawn upon a manuscript prisoner memoir, written by Olga Konstantinovna Klimenko, the wife of a Leningrad university professor. Born circa 1900, the daughter of a naval physician, she had trained as a nurse before marriage, very probably during the First World War and then the civil wars that followed. She was from an educated, middle-class background, describing herself as aware of progressive causes but not a radical. Klimenko served in 'ordinary' prison camps in the Vologda region between 1944 and 1954 and wrote her memoir in 1978; it was deposited in the Memorial Society's St Petersburg collection some-time in the 'democratic era'.[23] (No photographs accompany her memoir.) Alongside it I have gathered a handful of similar prisoner-nurse memoirs from the archives of Memorial in Moscow and St Petersburg. To present the experience of freely hired nurses, I will offer a composite portrait of women nurses and feldshers, drawing on interviews, documents, and photographs gathered by local histo-rians in Ukhta and Pechora, cities at the heart of the camps in the Komi Republic. Curators in the Ukhta Museum of the History of Public Health and the Pechora Historical-Regional Museum produced a cache of materials about young women who were sent to work in the Gulag, or who freely chose to work there, in the Stalin era. Many of these are interviews from these women in old age, taken in the 1990s and early 2000s, accompanied in some cases by docu-ments and photographs these women kept into the post-Soviet era about their work record.

'The only place where human dignity was not degraded'

With these warm words Olga Klimenko recalled the sanchast in her memoir, written in the 1970s (and dated 1978), apparently composed for her family's private archive.[24] Her husband, a professor of the Leningrad Polytechnic Institute, was arrested on political charges in February 1942; somehow, Klimenko and her two children survived the next two years in besieged Leningrad. She joined an evacuation convoy with her two children and a nanny, only to be arrested on political charges herself, in July 1944, in a village on the evacuation route. Given a ten-year sentence in a Vologda court in December 1944, she was transported to a series of camps over the next decade, all within Vologda Province. Olga Klimenko's career in the Gulag had a familiar pattern: she seldom 'settled' in one camp but found herself trapped in the 'perpetual motion' of short stays and sudden removals to new places of confinement, perhaps related to the shifting priorities of the Gulag, which had innumerable worksites in the region.[25]

Olga Klimenko knew nothing about survival in the Gulag when she arrived, and yet she landed on her feet by virtue of her nursing qualification. At a farming camp in the village of Sokol, she went before a medical 'commission' examining the new intake of prisoners. A committee of four or five officials sat at a table and without physically approaching the prisoners judged them fit for work. The atmosphere was informal:

> While the commission dragged on, I had the chance to look around. There was a dentist's chair in the corner, and a middle-aged man standing by it. 'Probably a dentist,' I thought, and I went up to him. He began to quiz me very sympathetically – where was I from, what training did I have. Suddenly he exclaimed, 'What is happening out in freedom!? The entire intelligentsia has been put in camps.' Hearing that I had been a nurse, he advised me to write an application to the sanchast to work there. (Yes, there were still sympathetic people.) Then and there I wrote a request and gave it to him to hand to the sanchast director, Vera Ivanovna Fariseeva. I did it all mechanically, understanding nothing, not imagining where fate would send me next.[26]

After two days of hauling and loading work in the camp's sawmill, Klimenko was summoned to the sanchast where Fariseeva interviewed her: where had she studied, when had she last worked in medicine, and then questioning her about medical techniques, 'a little examination on medicine by and by'. It had been 'a long time' since Klimenko had worked in nursing, 'but I remembered my Latin and pharmacology reasonably well and obviously didn't make any major mistakes'. The sanchast director told her:

> Tomorrow you will not go to work [in the sawmill] but come to the sanchast at 12 o'clock, to Dr Levitina. We will take you on in

the sanchast and give you a chance; if you work well, we will keep you. Only, I warn you, do not have any unnecessary conversations with anyone at all. Remember where you are, and that you do not know the people around you. Be careful, and keep quiet.[27]

It was a reduced version of the warnings freely hired doctors received upon entering the Gulag medical service, and by giving this prisoner-nurse this advice Fariseeva recognised that Klimenko was new to the camps and had little understanding of the world she was entering. As the prisoner-nurse recalled, 'I didn't even understand that I had been rescued, without knowing why or how it had come about, and without any expectation or hope.'[28] Other prisoner-nurses recalled similar initial periods of general labour followed by admission to medical work.[29] Klimenko was again 'examined' on her medical knowledge a few years later, when transferred to Sheksna camp hospital; it was a well-ordered facility, she noted, and the examination was part of that thorough approach to its management.[30]

'A few words about medical work in the camps'

Klimenko considered it important to describe her nursing duties and how they varied in the different camps she was assigned to.[31] The freely hired nurses, interviewed decades after their work in the Gulag, had little to say about nursing routines. One suspects that behind this imbalance lay an unequal distribution of the clinical workload: apparently, free nurses supervised prisoners who did most of the work, or perhaps the drudgery itself was unmemorable when they told museum employees about their lives, most of them speaking about their work for the first time to historians.[32] What is beyond doubt is that, regardless of who did it, nursing work in the Gulag was hard work, demanding health, stamina, and physical strength. It was typical Soviet women's work in all-too-familiar Soviet conditions.

As in civilian medicine, the lion's share of clinical care fell to nurses who implemented a doctor's instructions. So often in the Gulag, 'hospitalisation' was the main element of 'therapy' in a resource-deprived medical arsenal. Bed rest, in a ward with clean mattresses, sheets, pillows, and clothing, with clean floors and warm rooms, accompanied by an enhanced 'hospital' diet, was the principal prescription most Gulag doctors could make, assuming beds were free and quotas for work-release were not yet filled. It says something chilling about ordinary living conditions in the Gulag that this minimalist 'hospitalisation' could and did have restorative powers. Such simple luxuries may seem unremarkable but, in fact, their provision in the conditions of the forced-labour camps was anything but easy. Bedding was frequently in short supply; pillows must have been difficult to keep from being stolen, given how lovingly they are mentioned by prisoner-patients; floors and wards were noteworthy in observers' eyes for their filth, exposure to the elements, and lack of cheer; and diets were hardly princely where food was eternally scarce and significant quantities pilfered.[33] Creating an environment free of bedbugs and lice was a key priority, since pests interfered with rest and threatened epidemic disease. In post-war Soviet civilian life, wives ironed their husbands' shirts after work to kill lice they might have picked up from commuting in a crowded bus or train. They sorted through their children's clothes and hair for disease-bearing pests.[34] In the camps, lice were ubiquitous and maternal care absent; it took heroic efforts from nurses and cleaners to eliminate pests from a Gulag clinic or hospital ward. Not for nothing were prisoner-laundresses hailed in the pages of internal Gulag newspapers for their Stakhanovite toil and their record-breaking feats of service, in the face of shortages of wood to heat water, a lack of soap, inadequate ventilation, while fellow laundresses swore and stole the bedlinen.[35]

None of this effort made sense if patients had not washed before entering a clean ward. Klimenko noted that a visit to the banya – the Russian steam bath – was part of the hospitalisation regime, along with opportunities for thorough washing, accompanied by bed rest and the better diet in the infirmary. The Gulag baths for prisoners that she remembered were better than the cold, damp, neglected facilities bitterly condemned by Varlam Shalamov. 'After a few days people revived literally before one's eyes, it was nice to see "the fruits of one's labours" in this way.'[36] Nurses were often drafted in, with

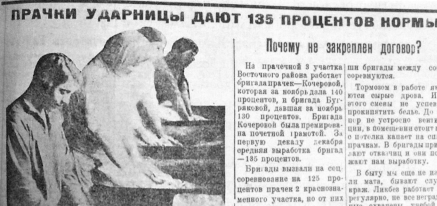

ПРАЧКИ УДАРНИЦЫ ДАЮТ 135 ПРОЦЕНТОВ НОРМЫ

Почему не закреплен договор?

На прачечной 3 участка Восточного района работает бригада прачек—Кочеровой, которая за ноябрь дала 140 процентов, и бригада Бугряковой, давшая за ноябрь 130 процентов. Бригада Кочеровой была премирована почетной грамотой. За первую декаду декабря средняя выработка бригад —135 процентов.

Бригады вызвали на соц соревнование на 125 процентов прачек 2 краснознаменного участка, но от них до сих пор никто не приехал закрепить договор. На

ши бригады между собою соревнуются.

Тормозом в работе являются сырые дрова. Из за этого смены не успевают прокипятить белье. До сих пор не устроено вентиляции, в помещении стоит пар, с потолка капает на спину прачкам. В бригады присылают отказчиц и они понижают нам выработку.

В быту мы еще не изжили мата, бывают случаи краж. Ликбез работает нерегулярно, не все неграмотные охвачены учебой.

Лагкорка

18. 'Shockworker laundresses achieve 135 per cent of the norm; why haven't they all signed up [for socialist competition]?' from the pages of Kanaloarmeika, Dmitlag, 30 December 1934.

orderlies and cleaners, to haul logs from nearby forests, chop wood, and keep stoves burning for heat and bathing; Klimenko actually relished this work – and the ultimate result, revived prisoner patients, was the reason.[37] Similarly, ensuring a clean water supply to create a hygienic environment in the midst of polluted construction or mining sites was often an issue that hospital staff at all levels – inside and outside the Gulag – struggled with. (The country at large had little modern indoor freshwater piping and sewerage.) Medical personnel could get into trouble for taking matters into their own hands on this point, as we have seen with Nina Savoeva. Chekists gave Klimenko a warning for taking prisoners to a distant pond to haul water when nearby supplies were contaminated, despite her repeated reports after epidemics of diarrhoea.[38]

Working days were long. In 1946 at Lnostroi, apparently a camp set up in Vologda's incomplete linen factory suburb, Klimenko's typical day began early:

We had a lot of work to do. I got up at 5 a.m., went to the prisoners' rollcall, then the morning reception of patients, then joined the sanitary inspection of all the camp premises (and in such a slum), then the evening reception of patients. It was good that I was given complete autonomy, and that this contingent of prisoners was healthy, mostly coming from the local Vologda region collective farmers and workers. They got good parcels from home, they did not have political but only minor criminal (*bytovye*) convictions, and so they had relative freedom.[39]

Much of nurse Klimenko's workday was taken up with formal penal-medical rituals: the sanitary inspection of the camp might be a simple matter in midsummer or midwinter, but spring was a particularly muddy period, when low nutrition combined with exposure to the filth that accumulated around barracks in the absence of indoor toilets could lead to outbreaks of intestinal diseases. The daily round of inspections suggests how hard it was to maintain a minimally hygienic environment around the camps. Indeed, Gulag officials routinely sent decrees from Moscow ordering springtime cleaning campaigns.[40] More daily medical rituals for nurses were the morning and evening receptions of prisoner-patients seeking release. These were burdensome, if only because many prisoners would present themselves in the hopes of a day or two of rest. Klimenko's duties in these rituals are unclear but probably included keeping order: fifty prisoners might turn up to an evening clinic, and women zeks laid on 'full-scale hysterics' to get a work-release, Klimenko recalls.[41] Towards the end of her camp sentence, Klimenko was in charge of her own camp subdivision clinic, and responsible for all forms of work-release and treatment: physical examinations, injections, even blood transfusions. She supervised a qualified but inept assistant, 'a dirty, half-literate midwife' who was serving a term for procuring an abortion. 'Aside from my own work I had to correct all this midwife's mistakes, and the patients, who all knew me from my previous work, came to me, so I had double the workload. Yet I was happy to be working in my specialisation and did not ask for anything more.'[42]

A time-consuming task that fell to nurses involved ensuring an adequate diet for the patients. It was not always the case that infirmary kitchens delivered sufficient food to be distributed to patients;

some hospitals were well run and others were hives of pilfering with medical staff eating patients' food or cooks and orderlies purloining it for barter transactions. Klimenko herself struck deals to feed her patients. This illegal 'food-trafficking' evidently grew out of her own experiences of survival of prison after arrest: she smuggled a note with gold valuables to a trusted friend outside the prison, who then sent her money at regular intervals for food and necessities.[43] When assigned to the sanchast of the Vologda Transit Prison for four months in 1946, Klimenko sympathised with prisoners, some of them mothers with infants, and accepted small sums of cash from them 'that would be stolen by the criminals anyway' to buy bread, sugar, and food in a prison-colony shop. 'I did it gladly, trying to help these famished people somehow, and then I would summon the poor patient to the sanchast to see me, on the pretext of giving an injection, and gave him the food I'd obtained for him.'[44] Klimenko played cat-and-mouse with the authorities, hiding food for prisoners from guards as she entered the prison: she risked discovery and punishment to feed prisoners she sympathised with. Later, in camps with high rates of mortality, nurse Klimenko befriended cooks in the infirmary kitchens, who let her send emaciated patients in small groups to 'work' peeling potatoes and washing floors. It was understood by all that cooks would feed these emaciated prisoners in return.[45]

'A real sister of mercy, a real Christian'

Olga Klimenko passed through so many camps in the dense Vologda archipelago that she had the opportunity to serve in 'fortunate' camps where mortality was almost non-existent (such as Lnostroi in 1946) and to witness those where death was ubiquitous, very likely the result of the wider Soviet famine of 1946–47.[46] In January 1947 in Sheksna camp, she begged for a new assignment to escape 'the insults and abuse' of a children's 'barracks' where criminal nurses and a corrupted doctor neglected their duties, treated the children cruelly, and made her life as a staff nurse 'hell'.[47] She was assigned to a 'tuberculosis town', four barracks barricaded from the rest of the camp, where she was horrified by the conditions, but embraced the work willingly: 'I entered the ward. My heart contracted: it was a dreadful sight. A long barrack with a ramshackle ceiling. One flickering lamp for the entire barrack. It stank of sour cabbage and creosote. Half-dead patients lay on the bunks covered in dirty and torn bedclothes.'[48]

The 'town' was feared by most of officialdom because of the threat of infection; but even with its demoralised zek-doctor, the fact that authorities seldom visited made it a more harmonious workplace.[49] Many prisoners died here: they had been front-line soldiers, later arrested and worked to exhaustion in swampy forests cutting down trees and hauling logs. (Their situation resembles that reported by Eugenia Ginzburg in the 'tuberculosis block' at Belichya under Dr Nina Savoeva.) Klimenko says that she 'kept watch over the dying and many times got up in the middle of the night to be by the side of the severely ill.' She tried to lift their spirits by reading aloud to patients, telling stories, and encouraging prisoner singers to visit the wards. Recovering patients worked in the 'town' gardens in fair weather; 'labour therapy' was a typical treatment for tubercular patients everywhere in the early to mid-twentieth century.[50] Tuberculosis patients could not be sent to 'work' in the kitchens for extra food but Klimenko enlisted free employees to buy and bring them berries, milk, and potatoes from outside of the camp. To treat TB, she had only glucose, vitamin C, fish oil 'with vitamins', 'endless' injections of calcium chloride, and 'some kind of home-made device for pneumothorax' (collapsed lung).[51]

However, 'TB patients rarely left the hospital: their path led primarily to the morgue.' Klimenko found herself tending to the dying with particular care. At the bedside of an old Belarusian peasant, on the eve of his death, she recalled his last requests:

'Sit by me, Olga Konstantinovna, I want to speak to you. Tomorrow I will die, please write down my last requests.'

'Maybe you should ask the doctor,' I said.

'No, I'm asking you, please stay,' and suddenly he added, 'The spark of God is not yet extinguished in you.' Then he fell silent. He started to dictate: '1. Please inform my wife at this address. 2.

Dress me in my best clothes; there is a shirt and underwear under my pillow. 3. Here is some money, give it please to the men who carry me and place me in my grave.'

He died the following day at exactly two o'clock. His surname was Skurat. Of course, I carried out his wishes.[52]

Recalling the death of another patient, who asked her to his bedside to kiss her hand, Olga Klimenko reflects on the kind of nurse she became in the camp. 'Looking back now and taking stock of that period of my life, it seems to me that I truly was then a real sister of mercy, a real Christian.'[53]

Just as Ginzburg's encounter with Gulag medicine and prisoner deaths unsettled the confident communist's ideals and ultimately led her to adopt semi-religious, humanitarian, values associated with the pre-revolutionary era, Olga Klimenko, a Soviet Leningrad professor's wife, turned to religious values in the Gulag clinics.[54] For Klimenko, Christian sympathy and forgiveness animated medical care for prisoners, and contrasted with doing medicine 'the labour-camp way' (po-lagernomu).[55] Behind that phrase seemingly lay the shadow of doing medicine as 'sisters of mercy' had during the pre-Soviet era. Giving water to an arriving transport of severely weakened German prisoners of war, she promised them food and rest, 'and life will not seem so terrible'. One of the POWs turned to his comrades and said this was 'the first humane word' they had heard in captivity.[56] Klimenko in her memoirs reserved her strongest condemnation for doctors who allowed criminal prisoners to commit murder in their infirmaries, for demoralised physicians who failed to perform their duties conscientiously, and for female nurses, work colleagues, who allowed sexual intrigues and romantic jealousies to consume their minds and poison relations among medical workers. Looking back at her Gulag nursing career Olga Klimenko had no doubt (like free doctor Nina Savoeva) that the sanchast was the only positive feature of camp life: 'Only the sanchast comes to the aid of those who commit mistakes or misdemeanours.'[57] However we assess Klimenko's attempts to memorialise her values in the late Soviet era, her detailed description of nurses' work routines and her foregrounding of the prisoner-nurse's experience remains a valuable addition to this small body of Gulag nursing memoirs. Comparison in the next sections with the recollections of 'freely hired' nurses highlights some important contrasts.

'Komsomol girls whose hearts had bid them come . . . and help develop the Far North'

Eugenia Ginzburg's ironic characterisation of freely hired nurses who worked with her in Kolyma children's homes sums them up as naive at best.[58] Later speaking of these young women contractors for the Gulag, she observed that they had grown up immersed in Soviet propaganda and believed it wholesale, regardless of the reality around them. She understood that propaganda well, having at one time sympathised with it, propagated it as an educator, and admired its products, her students from disadvantaged backgrounds.[59] In her jaundiced retrospective view, many 'Komsomol girls' came to the camps simply to find a husband among the geologists, bosses, and guards. For Ginzburg the 'Komsomol girls' were not thoughtful or perceptive, in contrast to the deprived but woefully experienced prisoners' children they cared for as nurses and daycare staff.[60] She remained wary of 'contractors' during her time in nursing as a prisoner.

The experience of 'Komsomol girls' journeying to the remote corners of the Soviet Union 'to build socialism' has attracted some scholarly interest.[61] However, as with Gulag freely hired doctors, little has been said about nurses who 'chose' to work for the camps. In this section I examine the fates of seven nurses, their 'choices', and their medical values, as traced in interviews with local historians in Ukhta and Pechora. Their fragmented reminiscences limit access to any single individual's life course, but as a group they paint a portrait of the free-contract Gulag nurse that is worth considering alongside Ginzburg's dismissive glimpses and Klimenko's reflections about doing her job as 'a real sister of mercy'.

The Gulag recruited five of the seven women in this sample straight from graduating classes of nurses in small-town Russia. In 1940 Liubov Mikhailovna Deriabina graduated from Yoshkar-Ola's medical college and was assigned a job in the Pechora Railway Construction camps of the NKVD. She sought to resist the posting, making enquiries with the Yoshkar-Ola NKVD office, where she was told, 'If you don't go, we'll take you there.' After hearing this, her father told her, 'You have to go.'[62] In 1940 Maria Ivanovna Komleva finished training as a feldsher in Kharkiv, 'and they sent us Komsomol conscripts to the colonisation of the North, to Arkhangelsk'; she in fact ended up in Pechora.[63] A graduate of the Kovrov Feldsher-Midwife School, collective-farm girl Serafima Stepanovna Davydenko came on assignment to Pechora as well, in 1946.[64] A group of nurses was sent from Ivanovo Feldsher School in 1947: 'we were sent "to railway construction" in Abez' and onward to Pechora, recalled Yulia Grigorievna Sokolova, interviewed in 2001.[65] One other nurse whose account is in the Pechora archives did not mention her school by name, but had similar experiences.[66]

It is striking that none of these women recalled a sincerely romantic desire to 'colonise the North', unlike freely hired doctor Sofia Guzikova. Still less do they remember 'choosing' the Gulag out of selfless professionalism, like Nina Savoeva. The Komsomol 'draft' clearly smelled of compulsion and contending with the NKVD about an undesirable assignment suggests that, for some mid-level medical personnel, a Gulag assignment was involuntary.[67] Maria Komleva remembered a ruse the NKVD employed not infrequently to tie these new 'free employees' to their jobs: 'We were only allowed to receive our diplomas after two years of work in the North, so you could not call our arrival voluntary.'[68] Still, there were nurses who seem to have exercised a degree of choice about working for the labour camps. Post-war collective farms were sufficiently miserable and unremunerative to make the Gulag seem an attractive proposition. Even if the chekists withheld her diploma, collective-farm girl Serafima Davydenko signed her contract with them in September 1946, jumping at this escape route from badly paid rural toil for the camps' monthly salary of 637 roubles. She kept her crumbling contract for over half a century before donating it to the Pechora regional museum.[69]

Other routes to nursing in the Gulag made sense in Soviet terms. Raisa Ivanovna Akolzina, a student in a pedagogic institute at the

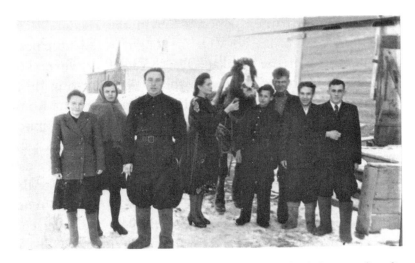

19. *Collective farm girl to Gulag medical worker: far left, nurse Serafima Davydenko with colleagues in Salekhard, 1953.*

20. *Serafima Davydenko's first contract in 1946 with the Gulag, treasured for half a century.*

time of arrest in 1937, was a prisoner working as a self-taught nurse in Pechora's camp hospitals until release in August 1942. She married another ex-prisoner, physician Aleksei Ivanovich Akolzin, upon his release in 1943; the pair decided to work as freely hired employees of the local Gulag medical system until rehabilitation in the mid-1950s.[70] Akolzina's salary in 1946 compared poorly to Davydenko's: nominally it was just 425 roubles per month (but with a 50 per cent 'bonus', a symbolic equalisation of pay with 'voluntary' free employees but one that authorities could revoke).[71] Another path to nursing in the camps is demonstrated by Elena Ivanovna Kharkova, who qualified as a nurse in Sarapul during the Civil War. She worked in a series of civilian hospitals and clinics near Ukhta, including a stint from 1933 to 1938 in an outpatients' clinic in Vodnyi Promysl, where radium waters were being developed by Gulag scientists. It is unclear whether she had any role in radium-water therapy, described in chapter 8, but she certainly attracted the attention of Gulag medical authorities in this small settlement. She had urban hospital experience; probably, work in the larger facilities of the adjacent Gulag offered more scope for professional advancement. In 1939 she voluntarily transferred into the labour-camp system, where she worked in Vetlosian Central Camp Hospital, the training ground of prisoner-feldsher Viktor Samsonov.[72]

The freely hired nurse in the clinic

The 'Komsomol girls' traced by historians in Pechora and Ukhta said little to describe their nursing duties in their interviews, giving the impression that the work was unremarkable. In fact, their comments on their jobs are rare but revealing. 'Free' nurses evidently expected prisoners to scrub floors, wash linen, and keep wards spotless. Maria Petrovna Kolinenko, a graduate of an unspecified feldsher college, was assigned in late 1941 or early 1942 to run a medical station in Kochmes camp. In an interview she recalled that it was demanding and heavy work since there was no 'sanitary and epidemiological service' (prisoners to clean and do laundry) and 'we did everything ourselves'.[73] Prisoners were normally tapped to provide the labour needed to keep wards clean and supplied with fresh bedlinen. Arriving in Abez in 1946, Serafima Davydenko found she had a surprisingly light workload: her boss, a prisoner-doctor, insisted she keep her uniform in exemplary starched condition but otherwise relied, one infers, on prisoners to perform most duties.[74] For the post-war years, Yulia Sokolova observed that the Central Transit camp infirmary in Pechorlag was always in an ideal condition. 'Well and why wouldn't there be cleanliness, they used unpaid labour: the prisoners themselves put everything in order.' No cockroaches or bedbugs plagued prisoners there because sheets were regularly boiled and all linen checked by the sanitary brigades.[75]

Certain kinds of nursing work seem to have been better suited to 'free' hands, at least in the eyes of Gulag bosses. Escorting prisoner transports was recalled by one freely hired nurse; such trips made for awkward reminiscences, because the journeys were arduous for sick prisoners some of whom surely died en route. Yulia Sokolova accompanied a group of tuberculosis patients from Pechora to a nearby specialised TB prisoner-hospital in Mishayag in 1948. In an elliptical passage in her 2001 interview she said it was a big facility where prisoners from the entire railway camp network with infectious tuberculosis were concentrated. She must have been aware of the grotesquely high death rate at this hospital, which may be the reason why she remembered taking prisoners on this relatively trivial journey, only 6 kilometres from Pechora town. Studies of the hospital precinct by local historians have revealed a complex of mass graves, where thousands of prisoner-patients were buried in the 1940s.[76] Other tasks which reliable free nurses undertook included fetching drug supplies from remote pharmacies in district centres (Sokolova did this routinely); and accepting special assignments in infirmaries for free employees, to suppress epidemics in the 'free' population (Davydenko took part in an anti-scarlet fever campaign in 1946).[77] Free mid-level medical employees were likely also preferred for compiling medical statistics. Klavdia Petrovna Belova worked as a statistician in Pechora's main Gulag hospital from 1948.[78]

In the extreme conditions of some Gulag camps, where facilities were not yet built or wartime emergency required all hands to the pump, free nurses were drafted in to perform heavy labour alongside prisoners. Some free nurses recalled these episodes of hard labour with notes of resentment about the loss of status they entailed. Maria Komleva told a historian:

> We, the lowest of the freely hired employees, were similar in many ways to the prisoners: they sent us to the construction sites and fed us nothing but turnips three times a day. You worked your day shift [in the infirmary] and then you had to go to the earthworks and drag a wheelbarrow to the tipping point along the railway embankment. The only people who lived well were the '*blatnye*' among the criminals. For them places of confinement were home sweet home. Sometimes they even gave us food to eat.[79]

Liubov Deriabina, the nurse who questioned the NKVD's decision to assign her to the Gulag, remembered 1940 to 1943 as a time when distinctions between prisoners and the lowliest of freely contracted workers seemed to collapse. 'They fed us, the freely hired workers, with oats,' she marvelled. After a day of looking after patients the bosses would send them out to clear snow from roads or haul logs to fuel locomotives. 'The prisoners prepared the logs and we free workers carried them out of the forest. They scraped your shoulders so that you couldn't wear a dress. That's how I remember 1940 to 1943.'[80] The famine year of 1947 was also remembered ruefully. At one new camp near Pechora Maria Kolinenko recalled the lack of facilities, shortages of basic goods, no cafeterias, not even ration coupons: 'at first there were tents, then barracks. We starved . . .'[81]

Authorities recognised free nurses' labour in ritual praise, and the fact of recognition resonates in free nurses' testimony, and in their archives donated to local museums. These routines of praise did not dispel freely hired nurses' resentment at their low status, and yet praise from above mattered to them. Such recognition showed that contract-nurses were 'insiders' in the system, like the freely contracted doctors and their medical administrator bosses. Rituals of reward coincided with the annual October Revolution holiday (7 November) and, significantly for female nurses, with the 8 March observance of

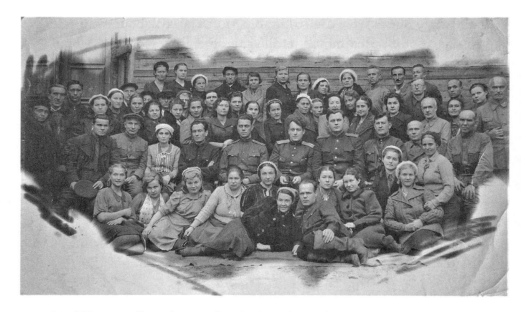

21. 'We starved': conference of medical workers, Abez, 1944. Maria Kolinenko
is seated on the ground, third from the left.

International Women's Day. While she was working in Vodnyi
Promysl for civilian healthcare, Elena Kharkova was designated
a shockworker (March 1935) and awarded cloth for dressmaking
(November 1935), and a further bolt of silk for a blouse in 1936 on
the women's day holiday. Her labour book records that she got no
material gifts when she transferred to her Gulag employer; but in the
post-war years, camp officials did award her at least three citations of
merit (*pochetnye gramoty*) for participation in 'socialist competitions'.[82] Higher salaries and regular access to scarce consumer goods
through closed distribution networks incentivised Gulag employees.
The symbolic gift of cloth Kharkova got as a civilian nurse was but a
scrap compared to the privileges available to employees of the camp
system.[83] Other Gulag nurses got prizes during the war. Liubov
Deriabina, the nurse who ate oats and hauled logs in the early war
years, received a dress, 5 metres of cloth, and slippers in 1943 in
recognition of her shockwork, and was twice cited in the Pechora
Railway camp newspaper for her successes in socialist competitions,
according to clippings and printed decrees she saved for half a

century.[84] Rituals of recognition made the status differential between prisoner and free nurses visible and contributed to the ideologised atmosphere that alienated prisoner-nurse Eugenia Ginzburg.

'Honourable' women or Ginzburg's 'Komsomol girls'?

What did freely contracted nurses make of the Gulag's harsh treatment of prisoners? What was their attitude towards the Gulag authorities and the security police in the camps? How did they respond to mass emaciation and death in the infirmaries they worked in? Were they frivolous 'Komsomol girls' keen to marry a Gulag boss, as Eugenia Ginzburg tartly observed? In the brief interviews and employment records in this sample, direct answers to these questions are rare, and it is impossible to say how typical these women were. Instead, what emerges is a spectrum of attitudes towards the Stalinist Gulag running from reflection on the injustice suffered by prisoners to an unwillingness or reluctance to recall such traumas. Most of this evidence was gathered in the years after the Soviet Union's collapse and reflects the reassessments typical of the early post-Soviet era.

Yulia Sokolova, nurse in Pechora's transit camp hospital (who escorted prisoner-patients to the TB hospital in Mishayag), reflected carefully on some of these issues in her early twenty-first-century interviews. Sokolova had read Alexander Solzhenitsyn – presumably, his *Gulag Archipelago* – and her thoughts about her past seem to reflect his influence. She does not evade acknowledging that diseases of starvation ('dystrophy' and scurvy) prevailed in the late 1940s in the facilities where she worked, and she adds that mortality was always high. Unusually among the free nurses, she specifically mentions two incidents when she intervened to enforce regulations protecting prisoner health. In the late 1940s during a morning roll-call she sent four Moldovan inmates back to barracks as unfit to work, because they lacked shoes. Sokolova caught a reprimand from the foreman in charge, but she appealed to the camp director who forced the foreman to apologise. In another confrontation she protested that prisoners were being sent out to work in minus 40-degree weather; again, the camp director supported her against

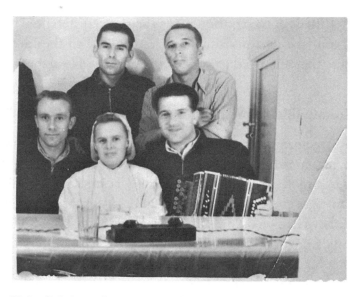

22. Yulia Sokolova, free nurse, with prisoner-orderlies, Pechora transit hospital, psychiatric ward, 1949.

the engineer who had mustered the work party.[85] Other injustices and acts of disobedience remained vividly on her mind after fifty years. She recalled how Pechora camp authorities curbed innocent conversations between free female and male prisoner-nurses by having the prisoners transported to distant outposts. This experience made her wary of unguarded speech with any prisoner-medic; she also recalled cases where Party members were expelled for marrying ex-prisoners, similar to Dr Nina Savoeva's ejection in 1949. She participated, with other free employees, in food-trafficking across the camp boundary to feed starving prisoners, not unlike prisoner-nurse Olga Klimenko. The most daring act of disobedience she recalled was breaking open personal prisoner files and reading them 'all night long'. Along with other free nurses, she had been entrusted with transporting files from Pechora to Abez: the folders were sewn shut and the women unpicked the stitching and read the details of crimes supposedly committed by 'enemies of the people'. Sokolova remembered that she doubted that political prisoners known to her could be genuine traitors.[86] It is impossible to gauge whether such doubts arose at that time, or during the de-Stalinisation era, or as a result of her re-evaluation of her life under Solzhenitsyn's influence.[87]

Elena Kharkova, the nurse awarded bolts of cloth for her shock-work in the civilian clinic at Vodnyi Promysl, was warmly remembered as a trustworthy freely hired colleague by prisoner Viktor Samsonov. This testimony about her actions more reliably accounts for her attitudes at the time. In 1942, while Viktor was still a prisoner, free employee Elena shared a whispered secret with him in her bandaging station at Vetlosian Hospital: '"Viktor, there was a revolt in Vorkuta."' Samsonov reflects, 'I was struck then by the exceptional trust of this freely hired woman, for what she said was not only terrible to say, but to hear as well.' In 1943, after his release, Viktor and Elena met again during a medical conference. Elena confided that when Viktor's sentence finished, she had 'been called in' to

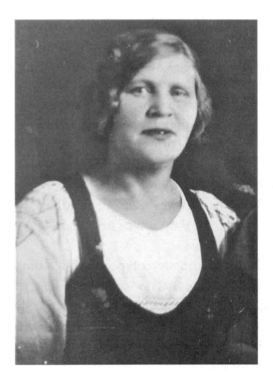

23. 'This honourable woman': Elena Kharkova, the freely hired nurse who did not betray Viktor Samsonov, Ukhta, 1939.

answer questions about him. 'Without explanations I guessed where exactly she had been called and what they asked about, and I was sure that this honourable woman told them nothing bad about me, she did not "squeal" on me.'[88]

Maria Komleva, the nurse who recalled being sent to the Pechora railway embankments to haul wheelbarrows of earth after her daily shift in the infirmary, was painfully conscious of the terrible death rates in the railway-construction camps. She remembered her first assignment, to infirmary No. 1 of the Pechora main camp where, in the summer of 1940, she panicked when confronted with a ward full of dying prisoners. She recounts:

> I was on my first night shift. I went into the ward and recoiled in horror: the patients were side by side in their clothing, half-alive, hardly able to look at you, and you could hear them, 'Help me, help me!' But help them how? There were no medicines at all. I stumbled out and howled with fear until morning, terrified to go back inside to the patients. At dawn, the orderly reported: 25 corpses. Who died? Go and check. Later the patients them-selves made a 'rationalisation suggestion': they started to tie a wooden tag to their big toe with their name and criminal-code article written on it. In the summer the dead were buried imme-diately; in the winter the corpses were stacked up like posts. They were buried in bast sacks, like dried fish. They would put six or seven people in sacks and lower them into common graves. On the site of these mass graves near our infirmary there is now a monumental tablet 'To the Victims of Pechorlag'.[89]

Komleva hardly fitted the stereotype of the 'Komsomol girl' who married a Gulag boss. She married an ex-prisoner, the Gulag physi-cian Boris Vasilyevich Komlev. They both began testifying about the Gulag origins of Pechora and its terrible human cost in the 1980s, when local historians began to interview them.[90]

In the testimonies of two other free nurses, Davydenko and Kolinenko, little is said to answer our questions about their attitudes towards Gulag authorities and their understanding of the injustices

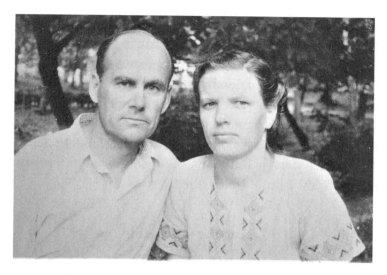

24. Witnesses to Gulag mortality: the Komlevs, Boris and Maria, in the 1950s, Pechora.

they confronted in the infirmaries of the camps. Serafima Davydenko had escaped the collective farm and taken a nurse's job in the Gulag; her interview dwells on the arduous toil expected of kolkhoz peasants in the 1930s and 1940s. In her short passage reminiscing about life in Abez as a Gulag nurse, she discussed her ineptness at bartering for food and her enjoyment of the cultural and social activities organised for free employees. In a similar vein, Maria Kolinenko, who remembered free workers 'starving' in 1947, said nothing about the condition of prisoners or how she viewed authority. Their brief interviews might give an impression of indifference to the fate of their prisoner-patients. One critical detail suggests rather that their attitudes were more nuanced than interviews given late in life, with little evident preparation on their part, might allow. In the late 1940s, both free nurses married ex-prisoners. This was an ideologically suspect choice for 'Komsomol girls'. Serafima Davydenko married a veteran of the Soviet–Finnish War, a soldier taken prisoner by the Finns and then imprisoned by the NKVD upon repatriation. Maria Kolinenko's husband was a Lithuanian physician, arrested in the wartime Soviet occupation of his homeland and deported to the camps.[91] Both women took risks in marrying ex-inmates, and both chose men under clouds of political suspicion. In the predominantly male Gulag towns, they were women in a buyers' marriage market; they could have chosen from free Gulag guards or bureaucrats, or indeed ex-cons from among the 'socially friendly' common criminals. Like Dr Nina Savoeva and other Gulag free medical staff, they doubtless encountered hostile attention from authorities for this choice, and they understood that not everyone who was a Gulag inmate deserved to be there. In such details, hints of a more complicated assessment of the Gulag world by these freely hired nurses arise.

Doing the impossible

Caring in the Gulag was a task full of dissonance and ambiguity. Kind words and generous deeds have long been an element of medical therapy, but providing these acts of mercy to prisoners jarred with the ideologically amplified rhetoric of prisoners' punishment and alienation from the community in the Soviet camps. Nurses perhaps came closer to violating the ideology that said 'this patient is an implacable enemy of the people' than even doctors. Physicians on their daily rounds or in clinics quickly examined patients and prescribed treatments, but it was nurses who had to dispense the medicines, inject the drugs, keep watch over the hospitalised, and perform many of the innumerable tasks that constituted 'therapy'. Their proximity to the prisoner-patients made their work in the camps' hospitals, infirmaries, and clinics a delicate balancing act of professional and political values. The Gulag nurse struggled with an already ambivalent 'virtue script' since Soviet nursing as a whole wrestled with how to reconcile tenderness and caring with militant patriotism and proletarian vigilance.[92]

Within the Gulag, much of the work performed by nurses was 'impossible'. Keeping wards clean, bedlinen fresh, vermin away, and patients bathed were not simple tasks, but enormously burdensome and challenging feats where primitive or semi-industrialised conditions made hot water and soap luxuries procured through sweat and toil. It is hardly surprising that nurses were drafted into chopping wood, stoking furnaces, boiling linen, and scrubbing floors, to maintain hygiene and make 'hospitalisation' in the Gulag into a regime resembling something approaching twentieth-century sanitary norms. It is equally unsurprising that prisoners in 'sanitary and epidemiological services', and prisoner-nurses too, were given the lion's share of this work. Clearly, there were divisions of labour based on prisoner or freely hired status, with a lighter load for the freely hired. At moments when the boundaries between the two groups dwindled or threatened to disappear, markers of status took on enhanced significance. Free nurses cherished their contracts, citations, medals, and perquisites of the job, and they remembered times when they were fed or put to work 'like prisoners' with some alarm. Ultimately, freely hired nurses enjoyed opportunities for professional advancement and had choices prisoner-nurses could not dream of.

If Eugenia Ginzburg viewed freely hired nurses as frivolous 'Komsomol girls' immersed in Soviet propaganda and lacking the desire or intellect to question Soviet reality, it would be an injustice to think of all nurses who 'chose' to work for the Gulag in these terms. If young graduates of Soviet nursing schools lacked the memory of pre-revolutionary nursing's ethos, the mindset of the 'sisters of mercy', they nonetheless had to show professional concern for prisoner-patients and practise medical care according to basic standards. They were low on the medical ladder, and most had limited educational attainments. Many came from deprived or disadvantaged backgrounds: a salaried job in a semi-skilled profession was a palpable advance in prospects. They worked in institutions that were themselves immersed in Soviet ideology and values, and if they spoke and acted in alignment with those values, they were hardly alone in the Sanotdel world or the wider Gulag administration. The moments when free nurses strayed from Soviet orthodoxies therefore suggest we need to think more carefully about their place and predicament.

6

THE PLACE WHERE DEATH DELIGHTS IN HELPING LIFE
A prisoner in the morgue

Winter above the Arctic Circle, early in 1946. Impulsive and principled, Eufrosinia Antonovna Kersnovskaya, a prisoner-nurse in the Central Camp Hospital in Norilsk, ejects herself from yet another posting in this large and complex penal medical facility. A job in the infectious-diseases department had seemed an opportunity to learn about another side of medical care, after her first job in the surgical department went sour. In fact, most jobs prisoner-nurse Kersnovskaya took up in the hospital were efforts to put distance between herself and oppressive managers. She had reached a point of no return with her immediate superior in infectious diseases, the freely hired 'sister without mercy' Aleksandra Mikhailovna Fliss, and the corrupt doctor who ran the unit. Kersnovskaya's mentor and ally Dr Leonard Bernardovich Mardna, an Estonian prisoner, who had been to Paris in 1936 and visited the Sorbonne's famous medical school, persuaded her to take a new post in the hospital morgue. He tried to inspire her by explaining how the motto engraved over the entrance to the Sorbonne's morgue celebrated its role as 'the place where Death delights in helping Life'. And Kersnovskaya let herself be convinced, reluctantly:

> There it is – the city's most welcoming institution: the morgue [...] Its doors are always open to everyone! Day and night, winter and summer [...] Maybe at the Sorbonne, the morgue's inscription in golden letters is impressive: 'Hic locus est ubi Mors gaudet

180

succurrere Vitae'. But here? Just in front is the Medvezhy Brook; behind, the stables; and next door, the pigsty of the Engineering and Technical Workers' cafeteria and the Central Camp Hospital refectory. Say what you like! It wasn't the Sorbonne . . .[1]

Norilsk's morgue was, by any means of transport available to a prisoner in the 1940s, not less than 9,000 kilometres from Paris and its analogue at the Sorbonne. The puzzle of the existence of the morgue in Gulag hospitals and Kersnovskaya's work in one is the subject of this chapter.

Eufrosinia Kersnovskaya was an unusual Gulag prisoner, headstrong, blessed with an iron constitution and a fierce love of work for its own sake: one editor of her memoirs says labour was for her a 'shield' against the humiliation and dehumanisation of prisoner existence.[2] If the Soviet ideological logic of 'reforging' promised redemption through labour, Kersnovskaya's values, formed in an upper-class family that escaped the crumbling Russian Empire in 1919 and settled in Bessarabia, were very different. She was not a 'Soviet-minded' person; like the many thousands of inhabitants of the borderlands annexed by the USSR in 1939–40 who ended up in the Gulag, she brought a leaven of something freer. Kersnovskaya in the camps submerged herself in work and preserved her individuality and her freedom of spirit by throwing herself into every task she thought worthy of her efforts. Her compass in the Gulag when confronted with moral dilemmas, according to her own testimony, was not 'what will I gain from this?' but 'would I be ashamed before the memory of my father?'[3]

Born in 1908 in the Ukrainian port city of Odesa, Eufrosinia was the child of a well-born jurist father and a mother who taught foreign languages. In the revolutionary civil wars the family was dispossessed and the father arrested by the Cheka. They escaped to Bessarabia where they had connections and Eufrosinia completed schooling and a veterinary course. She spoke several European languages and showed talent as an artist. She rejected her father's proposal to send her to university in Paris, and instead chose to become a modernising farmer on a smallholding of 40 hectares. In 1941, after the Soviet annexation of Bessarabia, Eufrosinia Kersnovskaya lost her farm when she was deported as an enemy of Soviet power and exiled to Siberia as a 'special settler'. After escape and rearrest in 1942, she was held in Siberian camps; in 1944 she was given a Gulag sentence of ten years and transported to the far northern mining camp at Norilsk. She was not released until August 1952. Like many prisoners, she was frequently moved between work assignments. After a period in hard labour on construction projects, Kersnovskaya, weak from emaciation and feverish, fell and injured her knee.[4] Taken to the Central Camp Hospital, doctors considered amputating her leg, but a prisoner-surgeon managed to restore her to health without the loss of the limb. Her remarkable recovery, and her lively personality, attracted the sympathy of prisoner and free doctors alike. The hospital's director, contract-physician Vera Ivanovna Griazneva, spotted her medical know-how and hired her as a nurse, sending her to the surgical department under former prisoner Viktor Alekseevich Kuznetsov. In her spare time, Kersnovskaya illustrated his medical treatises in proctology. Kersnovskaya worked in the Central Camp Hospital of Norilsk for two-and-a-half years. In 1947, at her own request, she was reassigned to the nickel mine at Nagorny camp; she worked underground as a miner in various capacities. Except for one further unsatisfactory interlude in hospital jobs, Kersnovskaya toiled as a miner, underground, virtually until the end of her sentence.[5]

If Kersnovskaya was an unusual prisoner, Norilsk was in many ways a unique outpost of the Gulag. Remote and forbidding, Norilsk largely remains a puzzle for historians, unlike other major Gulag centres which have been studied extensively. Founded in 1935 as a nickel-mining camp, Norilsk tapped a massive deposit holding 22 per cent of the world's reserves of this metal. Prisoners built refineries, processing plants, and service industries alongside the mines. The camp complex also became an important Soviet source of cobalt, copper, and platinum.[6] As in Kolyma, Norilsk had no railway connection with 'the mainland'. Prisoners were transported the 1,900 kilometres to Norilsk by barge down the Yenisei River, north from Krasnoyarsk, the regional capital on the Trans-Siberian Railway. Only the hardiest Gulag prisoners were selected for Norilsk; given the harsh conditions above the Arctic Circle, orders from Moscow dictated that

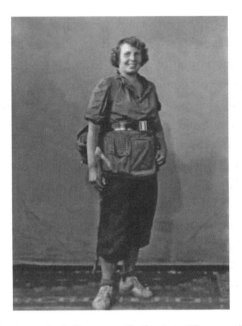

25. *Not a 'Soviet-minded' person: Eufrosinia Kersnovskaya in 1957.*

weaker prisoners were not to be sent there.[7] Prisoners were supposedly fed more generously, and mortality rates were reportedly lower than in other Gulag camps, although during the war Norilsk suffered the same privations as others, and food deliveries were interrupted and reduced, worsening prisoners' health and 'labour capacity'.[8] The Norilsk deputy camp commandant Vasily Petrovich Eremeev was remembered, however, as a leader who respected medical prisoner-experts and encouraged their research and plans for development. One report from Norilsk on sixty scientific papers presented at medical conferences held there between 1940 and 1947 mentions free and prisoner-speakers without distinction, including Kersnovskaya's mentor Dr Mardna.[9] The intellectual climate in the medical facilities of Norilsk was exceptional, but this impression has to be balanced against the episodic bursts of arbitrary rule, and abusive medical practice recalled by Kersnovskaya and other prisoner-personnel.[10]

The puzzle for Eufrosinia Kersnovskaya in moving from helping living prisoner-patients, to 'serving medicine' after their deaths as an anatomist (*prozektor*) in the morgue, was that the work seemed pointless to her. Caring for the sick was self-evidently a chance to do good. Cutting up the dead was horrifying, apparently meaningless in conditions of constant undernourishment, and perhaps even sacrilegious. What purpose could it possibly serve?

To understand the requirement for anatomists in the Gulag it is essential to ask why Soviet – and European – civilian hospitals valued the autopsy of deceased patients in the early twentieth century. Autopsy had long served medical scientists to understand human anatomy and physiology, and students of medicine were taught in their courses how to dissect human corpses. In the nineteenth century, practitioners of pathological anatomy depended on a steady supply of corpses from hospitals (and bodies procured by less salubrious means) to investigate the forms which disease took inside the human body. In an era long before the computerised tomography scanner, when X-ray machines were far more primitive, identifying and tracking a disease process inside the living human body was a tricky business, and frequently a doctor's careful inferences led to misdiagnosis. Often patients presented a picture complicated by more than one clearly defined illness: comorbidities could obscure the principal condition bringing the patient to seek medical care or leading to death. The autopsy of patients who died in hospital was a routine means of establishing a cause of death and detecting medical errors. Autopsy, and the practices and perspectives around it, transformed the dead patient into a teaching tool, an audit trail, a scientific curiosity, and finally a corpse to be buried.[11]

Soviet medical planners of the 1930s and 1940s deemed that autopsies should follow virtually every hospital death. A comparison of the patient's case history with the results of post-mortem was supposed to confirm the cause of death or reveal its cause where medicine's inadequacies or doctors' failures had led to erroneous conclusions. Autopsy would also reveal cases where treatment was mishandled, or untimely.[12] Soviet ideological sensibilities dictated that doctors should enter into the spirit of 'self-criticism' where such flaws or misperceptions and misdiagnoses were uncovered. 'The review of mistakes is a very important school for the doctor,' wrote one optimistic expert.[13] Collectively, 'epicrises' or patient case histories compared with their autopsy results formed a monthly audit trail that hospital directors and staff were intended to study and discuss, looking for local trends, lessons in diagnostics, and ways to improve therapy. Such audit trails went all the way to the top, in digested form, and affected health policy. The post-war civilian health minister, Efim Ivanovich Smirnov, was so convinced that Soviet physicians needed better skills and training that he launched a campaign against misdiagnosis in a May 1947 speech. There was too much variance in diagnosis between specialists treating the living patient and the pathological anatomist's reckoning after death.[14] A February 1948 decree required post-mortems on all deceased patients and discussions of epicrises at periodic hospital conferences.[15] The freely hired doctor Anna Kliashko reported routinely attending conferences in the Dalstroi and Magadan hospitals, where she worked in the 1950s, to review autopsy data and discuss causes of death.[16] The morgue in the Gulag was a mirror of its analogues in civilian medicine: it was part of a modernising medical system of science-led verification of physicians' decisions and treatments.

Soviet values deprived the human body of traditional sacred meaning, and this was evident in expert discussion of pathological anatomy. It was 'thanks to the disappearance of all sorts of religious and popular prejudices' that the routinisation of the hospital autopsy had come so far in Soviet medicine.[17] In 1951 Stalin's *Great Soviet Encyclopedia* dispassionately described for the man in the street the process of opening up a corpse for study. A long, straight incision from throat to pubes gave access to the internal organs which should be examined in situ then any pathologies investigated by removal of organs for closer inspection and sampling for laboratory analysis. Perhaps aware that armchair anatomists might find this passage distressing, the anonymous author reassured readers that autopsy restored the wholeness of the body: 'When the autopsy is completed the organs are put back inside the corpse, and all sections are sewn up again. No noticeable injuries or traces remain on the corpse, save for the stitching at the place of incision.'[18]

Such dignities were hardly routine in the Gulag after death. Corpses were frequently treated with as much brutality as the human beings previously inhabiting them. In Alexander Solzhenitsyn's view,

the autopsy behind barbed wire lost all pretence of a medical function; it became part of the punitive penal regime.

> Corpses withered from pellagra (no buttocks, and women with no
> breasts), or rotting from scurvy, were verified in the morgue lean-to
> or in the open air. The act rarely resembled a medical autopsy – a
> long vertical slash from neck to crotch, smashing legs, pulling the
> skull apart at its seam. Usually it was not an anatomist but a convoy
> guard who verified the corpse – to be certain the zek was really
> dead and not pretending. And for this they ran the corpse through
> with a bayonet or smashed the skull with a big mallet.[19]

This 'literary' description of 'autopsy', a composite from survivors'
testimony, comes after an account of extremely high prisoner
mortality in the worst years of the war, when camps were over-
whelmed with death. The atrocious treatment of prisoners drained of
life was by all accounts widespread in the Gulag, and the lack of
dignity accorded the dead was surely the norm in the 'worst' years
and the camps with highest mortality. Medical autopsy such as
Viktor Samsonov or Eufrosinia Kersnovskaya witnessed could only
have been conducted where a prisoner-patient expired in a major
camp hospital.[20] And yet it was far from a rarity there. In her relatively brief service as a Gulag anatomist, Kersnovskaya conducted
1,640 autopsies in just over a year from 1946 to 1947, a plausible
number according to archival sources.[21]

A closer examination of this period of Kersnovskaya's penal servitude can help in understanding the environment of the Gulag
morgue. Eufrosinia Kersnovskaya recorded her experience in the
camps in an extraordinary illustrated memoir, parts of which were
composed in preliminary fashion inside the camp, but she only fully
completed it in 1963–64, revising it in the two decades that followed.[22]
They are compared with survivor-memoirists' accounts of working
with Kersnovskaya in the camp hospital. The richest of these is the
transcript of 1989 reminiscences of another Gulag prisoner and
medical worker, Zigurd Genrikhovich Liudvig, a student in the final
year at the Moscow Medical Institute when the war broke out. Before

getting his doctor's diploma, he was detained as an ethnic German and in 1943 sent to Norilsk.[23] Kersnovskaya taught him French by helping him read a medical textbook in the language, and Liudvig worked with many of the same prisoner and free doctors Kersnovskaya mentions. Kersnovskaya's assignment to serve in the morgue; her duties; her disputes with doctors over their medical mistakes and falsifications; and the end of her Gulag medical career – these all reveal the paradoxes and challenges of work in a place where death was supposed to delight in helping life.

The Central Camp Hospital, Norilsk

Eufrosinia Kersnovskaya's memoir describes the day-to-day world of the Norilsk camp central hospital in the late 1940s, but accessible archival information about its origins and development is scant. An ideologically conformist essay about healthcare in Norilsk, penned in 1948 by its Sanotdel director, captain of the medical service, Dr Sergei Mikhailovich Smirnov, tells a familiar story.[24] As in Ukhta, where the Vetlosian and Sangorodok hospitals grew with rising prisoner numbers, Norilsk Gulag medical services evolved rapidly. From clinics in barracks at the outset in 1935 to an 18-bed infirmary in 1938, the Norilsk camp complex finally opened a 250-bed Central Camp Hospital in 1941. The new facility had all the attributes of a modern 'scientific' hospital: an X-ray facility, clinical laboratories, a 'functional diagnostics cabinet with an electrocardiograph', and finally 'a patho-logical anatomy department with a histological laboratory and a large medical library'. The pathological anatomists had facilities enabling the study of 'the pathology and the clinical course of disease in the conditions of the Far North'.[25] If, in 1938–39, there were just four physicians in Norilsk, by 1948, sixty-four doctors of varied specialisa-tions worked for the Sanotdel system (the camp complex clinics, infirmaries, and the central hospital), and they were served by 296 mid-level medical staff.[26] Smirnov neglected to tell his readers (Moscow Sanotdel officials) what proportion of these medical workers were prisoners, but the usual hierarchy of prisoner-staff supervised by freely hired managing physicians and senior nurses applied.[27]

Kersnovskaya's career as a nurse in the hospital started sometime in 1944 after her recovery from her leg injury. Vera Griazneva, the director of the Central Camp Hospital, the only doctor there who had arrived as a free employee, spotted her skills. She was attentive and focused on details across the hospital, constantly appearing to inspect wards, to check patient records, to instil confidence in her prisoner staff. Kersnovskaya praises her for not becoming a hardened Gulag careerist. 'All honour and glory to Vera Ivanovna – the director who did not lose her human feelings, a person who saw the human even in us!'[28] Griazneva assigned her to work in the surgical ward under the zek surgeon Viktor Kuznetsov. 'He was our "God",' notes Kersnovskaya. Imperious at the bedside and in the operating theatre, Kuznetsov's malign professional and personal values became obvious to Kersnovskaya over time, although she admits she worked so closely with him that a dispassionate assessment is impossible.[29] Indeed, her colleague Zigurd Liudvig thought him a memorable teacher, and a skilled surgeon who performed 'virtuoso complex operations'; their evaluations diverge enough to arouse the suspicion that nurse Kersnovskaya's critical perspective, and very probably some of her medical opinions, are flawed.[30] In the mining camps, industrial accidents required surgical attention and the department was busy, with nine hours per day of 'planned' operations and seven further hours of reception for emergencies. Kuznetsov dutifully kept up this schedule but Kersnovskaya thought 'instead of knowledge he relied upon intuition' in his medical decision-making. It was his study of rectal surgery, conducted on emaciated prisoners, illustrated by Kersnovskaya, that alerted her to the voluntarism of his medical ethics: he was 'a man lacking all human morality' because he took unwarranted chances in operations on prisoners already victimised by a cruel regime. Kuznetsov was also bitterly envious of any other doctor's successes, offloading hopeless patients on colleagues and denying them the tools or permission to cure them effectively, at least in Kersnovskaya's estimation and experience.[31]

An important guide to Gulag hospital ways for prisoner-nurse Kersnovskaya was Leonard Mardna, the Estonian physician who had been to Paris; he ran the hospital's therapeutic department. He developed a strong professional bond with Kersnovskaya, who also illustrated his ill-fated scientific studies (they were destroyed by Griazneva, who decided they made it 'too obvious that the camp system crippled people').[32] Mardna encouraged Kersnovskaya's skills as a diagnostician; in one 1945 episode, she was challenged by a group of doctors to rethink her treatment of a patient forwarded from a camp outpost clinic where a Dr Bachulis had diagnosed croupous (lobar) pneumonia. Mardna lent her his stethoscope and Kersnovskaya checked his chest, rapidly establishing through examination and deduction that the patient had pericarditis (heart inflammation, detected from changes to the heartbeat), not pneumonia in the lungs. Leaving the room, Kersnovskaya overheard Mardna comment not without pride, 'I have mid-level medical staff who know how to conduct a diagnosis, but Bachulis, a doctor, doesn't even know what croupous pneumonia is!'[33]

Kersnovskaya is imprecise about how much time she spent working in each department of the hospital, but she appears to have served for several months in the surgical department under Kuznetsov before being transferred, involuntarily, after conflicts with her senior nurse, to the infectious disease 'branch' (*filial*) of the central camp hospital. It was a place of revulsion that even punctilious Griazneva seemed to ignore. The department consisted of at least three divisions. The largest barrack held 80 to 100 patients suffering from starvation diseases (dysentery was the official diagnosis) and tuberculosis; a second held up to 50 patients with syphilis, some combined with tuberculosis, and these patients died in large numbers. A third barrack housed female prisoner-syphilitics. Additionally, box-rooms on the site were used to accommodate free patients with syphilis, since there was no venereal ward in Norilsk's hospital for civilians, and the only VD specialist in the region was a prisoner.[34] Civilian syphilitics paid handsome bribes to get sulphapyridine (an antibacterial drug), and penicillin, rare enough in 1945, leaving prisoners without adequate medication. The staff, many serially infected with venereal disease themselves, purloined what was left. Kersnovskaya was dismayed by the staff attitude to prisoner-patient mortality:

Everyone was firmly convinced that the main thing was not to look after the patients. They should lie there quietly and die without complaining. After all, they were being well treated: they could die in a hospital bed and not on the bare bunks in the camp barracks. It was pointless for them to cling to life! What was available for their treatment was too insignificant to help them, so best to hold it back and use it for the staff's needs: some glucose with your tea, a bit of ascorbic acid to season the soup, eat vitamins like sweets, and as for sulphapyridine and penicillin, they could be procured on the black market.[35]

Working alongside such colleagues, Kersnovskaya fell into constant conflicts with them over the neglect of patients, the bribe-taking, and the diversion of resources formally destined to prisoner-patients. The senior nurse Fliss accused her of wasting bandages on patients whose sores needed rebinding; she chided her about threatening to expose the bribe-taking for washing the branch's dirty linen in public. Ultimately, a dispute between Fliss and Kersnovskaya, requiring her to sign a pledge not to let the ward's only pair of scissors out of her sight (they were stolen frequently by women hospital staff for their private needlework sidelines), exasperated the prisoner-nurse. 'You must sign,' Fliss screamed, 'or we'll be parting company!' 'Then goodbye!' answered Kersnovskaya. She realised that she might lose her place in the hospital 'oasis' and be sent to the mines.[36]

Hic locus est ubi Mors gaudet succurrere Vitae

In retrospect, Kersnovskaya realised that her assignment to the morgue saved her from becoming a prisoner-miner, which she regarded, at the time, as a death sentence. Hospital director Griazneva had caught her 'on a harpoon' after she jumped overboard from Fliss's ship of fools, and her ally Dr Mardna 'had helped to reel her in' by persuading her that anatomising corpses would in fact be 'helping life'.[37] Paradoxically, Kersnovskaya found that 'the year and a bit' that she spent in the morgue was 'a happy time' because of the intense learning and work that went relatively undisturbed by camp authorities.[38] The pathological-anatomy department of the Central Camp Hospital evidently repulsed the average commandant and was, rather like the venereal wards, seldom willingly visited by authorities. 'Death helped Life' in unintended ways, as the Gulag morgue served living prisoners as a place of refuge and relative freedom. Kersnovskaya's Norilsk fellow prisoner Zigurd Liudvig recalled the Norilsk morgue as a sociable spot. Three 'leading medics', Mardna, Kuznetsov, and morgue director Pavel Evdokimovich Nikishin – all prisoners – shared quarters in a room there. 'The morgue was a scientific centre with its own anatomical museum. After work everyone gathered in the morgue to read, play chess, or to talk while knitting caps for sale.'[39] Kersnovskaya recalls how the entire morgue staff from director Nikishin to the lowest orderly pooled rations and ate from a common pot. In his documentary fiction, Varlam Shalamov depicts a similar atmosphere of liberty and opportunities to study in a main camp hospital morgue in Kolyma at this time.[40]

Dr Nikishin, who ran courses for mid-level medical staff, taught Kersnovskaya how to open a corpse for autopsy, how to isolate the organs needed for examination, and how to recognise pathological states in the body and diagnose retrospectively. She had time after the day's work to study anatomy textbooks in its library and to continue her medical illustrations for Kuznetsov. Kersnovskaya recalled her teacher and boss Nikishin with sorrow and affection. A 'genuine' Communist, his convictions broken after the Great Terror, Nikishin was loved by all but respected by none for his cowardice in the face of authority. He was an informant for the security police, but Kersnovskaya insists he made every effort to know nothing incriminating about the people around him, such was his awareness of his fearful, craven nature.[41]

As the morgue anatomist, Kersnovskaya's first task was to carry corpses into the autopsy theatre. They were often so light from emaciation that she could manage two at a time, one under each arm – a feat she commemorated in an illustration. The lightest corpses came from two penal camps: Kalagron and Alevrolitov.[42] Her keenness meant she often began the dissection alone, while Nikishin was still finishing his breakfast.

And even so from time to time it was strange to see Nikishin, still breakfasting in the next room, suddenly dash into the autopsy theatre with his bowl of kasha in his hand and start to explain things, very nearly touching the giblets of the open corpse with his spoon, 'Look, Frosinka, at the hyperaemia of the large intestine! Colitis, the result of chronic dysentery. Here's the haemorrhaging, here! And here!'[43]

'Dysentery' was a euphemism for starvation disease. Kersnovskaya recalls the 'skeletons' of the emaciated prisoners as the most tragic bodies she encountered, 'bundled in loose grey skin, with dulled, deeply sunken eyes, all resembling each other and all with the same singular look of surprise in their blank eyes, as though to ask in puzzlement, "Why?" They were all like that. It was tragic, but understandable. Or typical, at any rate. But here...'[44] Despite supposedly receiving better rations, not every Norilsk prisoner was able to resist the draining exhaustion of hard labour underground; and Kersnovskaya knew that conditions worsened during the war and after, when officials' attitudes towards new contingents of prisoners hardened.[45] The broken bodies of prisoners came into the morgue after industrial accidents, too. Kersnovskaya recalls the 'terrifying' remains of miners caught in the collapse of an underground tunnel, and the formless horror of a body mangled under a locomotive. 'Accidents of daily life' (a bureaucratic classification) including shootings of prisoners by guards in attempted escapes and wanton murder furnished more memorable incidents requiring post-mortems. Kersnovskaya attended a post-mortem by an unnamed doctor of seven corpses brought to the morgue by guards who said they were shot while trying to escape; the bullet entry wounds were, however, deemed by this courageous doctor to be evidence of deliberate killing.[46] The hundreds of bodies that Eufrosinia Kersnovskaya anatomised taught her, paradoxically, to fear death less.

After autopsy, the corpses needed to be buried. Burial was not part of Kersnovskaya's job but her observations about them generally align with those of other Gulag memoirists and show how official procedures in the treatment of the prisoner-dead were disregarded. She helped load naked corpses on what she drily termed their 'catafalque', a horse-drawn cart that took them to trenches for interment. Prisoners were buried at Norilsk on 'Shmidtikha', a bleak plateau overlooking the town.[47] Kersnovskaya says that the rising mortality of the wartime years led to the end of individual burials at Norilsk. Indeed, the rule of individual graves was frequently disregarded in remote camps before the war, and common graves were formally permitted across the Gulag by at least 1943. From November 1941 the dead prisoners' gold teeth were to be extracted in the presence of officials and transferred to state coffers (an order not mentioned by Kersnovskaya, who surely witnessed this desecration).[48] By September 1946 Moscow Gulag commanders had ordered a return to individual graves for bodies clothed at least in 'underwear', although Kersnovskaya shows these rules were violated in Norilsk.[49] Evidently speaking of late 1946 and 1947, Kersnovskaya recalls that in summer gravediggers cut trenches on Shmidtikha for communal graves that held 200; in the winter (average low temperature: −33 degrees Celsius) trenches were cut in the snow and corpses buried in them until they could be interred in the summer months.[50]

In contemplating her work and the flow of corpses to Shmidtikha, it is unsurprising that Kersnovskaya turned in her memoirs to reflect on the tragedy she witnessed and, from this indelible experience, to her purpose in writing and illustrating her memoirs. Gulag literature often turns to philosophising in the depiction of the lifeless corpse and its interment. 'From the deft hand of Shakespeare, we have long been accustomed to thinking of gravediggers as semi-professional philosophers,' mused Georgy Demidov's gravedigging prisoner-hero in his documentary short story, 'The Stiff'.[51] And yet his hero claims the burial-brigades of the Gulag were not populated by amateur philosophisers out of *Hamlet*, but ordinary sloggers who thought of nothing but 'the camp ration, the soup, and sleep on barrack shelves'.[52] In her illustrated memoir, Kersnovskaya declares her fear that the passage of time distorts memory and history, and that Soviet education and propaganda finish the job of distortion by 'hiding or perverting the lessons of history'. She is resolved to '"photograph" that which I witnessed' with her notebooks and drawings. 'People should know the truth, so that such times will never be repeated.'[53]

'A dog in a game of skittles'

'Let's cut to the chase,' Kersnovskaya says. 'Does any doctor want to see their mistakes? Frankly speaking, rarely. Does the doctor have the opportunity to apply a different treatment? Almost never. Do the other morgue staff feel like showing their zeal or at least spending their time on this revolting work? You can answer without a shadow of a hesitation – no! So it was that I wrought havoc in the calm, peaceable lives of the morgue personnel! I was about as useful as a dog in a game of skittles, as the French say.'[54]

Kersnovskaya's habit of truth-seeking, and her keen interest in pathological anatomy, led to conflicts and a few triumphs in the autopsy theatre for the memoirist. In her recollection, her colleagues apparently did wish to be elsewhere: Dr Nikishin supposedly trimmed his medical opinions to match the ante-mortem diagnosis in the patient case history, so that he could rush off to the library, or participate in Party meetings. In confirming doctors' diagnoses he was allegedly abetted by the morgue's secretary, who just copied their diagnoses from the case histories straight to the post-mortem paperwork; he preferred wandering the tundra in the summer months. The orderlies looked forward to the moment they could disappear in pursuit of their black-market trade in dead prisoners' clothing and other contraband.[55] 'They shouldn't bother with the motto from the Sorbonne, "Here Death delights in helping Life",' observes Kersnovskaya of this morgue, 'but just stick up a sign saying "Right this way, please!"'[56]

Her manner in the autopsy theatre was far from diplomatic with senior doctors, upsetting hierarchies of expertise and gender. In her blunt assertiveness she differed from other prisoner-anatomists who found subtler ways to expose the cruelty evident on the mortuary slab.[57] When on one occasion she was charged with anatomising the corpse of a prisoner diagnosed with 'dysentery' and evidently starved, Kersnovskaya's attention was caught by the long patient history, 'not a case-history but a whole book' detailing tests, X-rays, and the patient's status as a political prisoner of the 1937 intake. For three years he had complained of difficulty swallowing and breathing; despite various medical consultations the indifferent local camp medics had put off investigating until he was near death when they sent him to the Central Camp Hospital (to save their infirmary statistics from including his death). In the autopsy, Kersnovskaya, having suspected cancer, demonstrated the extensive growth and put her hypothesis bluntly to Dr Andrei Vitalevich Miller, her one-time boss in the infectious diseases ward ('he was coarse, cruel, and cynical' and a perpetual adversary); he was the doctor responsible for the patient's diagnosis and treatment. The haemorrhaging characteristic of starvation diseases was absent, she pointed out.

> Here Miller's voice rang out. 'Haemorrhage of the large intestine. Write: dysentery and alimentary dystrophy of the third stage.'
> 'No! Cancer. Cachexia, caused by carcinogenic intoxication.'
> 'Silence! This is none of your business!'
> 'I know my business – which is impossible to say about you . . .'
> Not quite apoplectic, he turned as purple as an incensed turkey and leaned across a chair, waving his fist to strike. I raised my arm pointing my knife blade at him. Miller dropped back. Knocking over the chair, Vladimir Nikolaevich [Dmokhovsky, the morgue secretary] jumped up. I don't remember what he said . . . Joking as was his habit, he led Dr Miller to the office in the next room. I finished the autopsy alone.
> Death might delight that it was able to help Life, but I did not feel like laughing.[58]

In another autopsy, attended by hospital director Griazneva, and doctors Mardna and Miller, Kersnovskaya demonstrated that in this patient, the original diagnosis of tuberculosis had been incorrect, first explaining that an X-ray had shown a shadow in the wrong part of the lung. Miller, 'my constant opponent', let out a noise that 'might have been a guffaw or an oath', and mocked her as a 'fantasist'. A sympathetic Griazneva invited Kersnovskaya to continue. As she worked, the anatomist showed that the patient's pain in the lower chest had been caused by septic thrombophlebitis – infectious blood clotting with a lethal outcome; it was the result of an untreated frost-bitten toe. Griazneva thanked Kersnovskaya for her skilled detective work, but the prisoner-anatomist felt her knowledge was becoming a source of 'annoyance' instead of a service to Life.[59] If the review of mistakes was 'a very important school for the doctor', as the Soviet textbook said, Kersnovskaya's male doctors were reluctant to be taught by a female veterinarian-turned-dissector.[60]

Kersnovskaya's thirst for perfection in her understanding of pathological anatomy led her to make 'yet another enemy' over the dissection table: Aleksandr Aleksandrovich Baev, physician and biochemist, one of the most illustrious ex-prisoners in Norilsk at the time, soon to defend his delayed dissertation in Leningrad, and a future member of the Academy of Sciences.[61] The deceased had been an engineer, an ex-prisoner, hospitalised with chest pain, enlarged liver and spleen, declining heart function, and increasing debilitation. Baev had diagnosed miliary tuberculosis, a deadly generalised form of the disease spread throughout the body. He considered the case hopeless, according to Kersnovskaya, prescribing morphine and codeine; the patient died within ten days. At the autopsy, Baev said, 'An uninteresting case. There's no doubt here. Nothing could be done . . .' However, writes Kersnovskaya, '[d]uring the autopsy I observed no tuberculosis of any sort, still less miliary TB.' Instead, the anatomist declared the case one of croupous (lobar) pneumonia 'in the stage of grey hepatisation, with an unresolved lesion that had suppurated in the lower left lobe. Myocardial dystrophy. Liver congestion.' The morgue secretary refused to record her opinion. 'Let it be "miliary TB" . . . There's no help for him now . . .' Kersnovskaya's reaction was a bitter commentary aimed not at the secretary, but at Baev:

No, he can't be helped now. But ten days ago he could have been. And should have! Was he given sulphapyridine . . .? No! Not even camphor and caffeine to support the heart, and we know from Laënnec that croupous pneumonia 'is one of the most perilous illnesses for the heart'. So just how did you treat his heart?

How the physician responded, Kersnovskaya neglects to record. The secretary wrote down her version – but morgue director Nikishin was appalled to learn what had happened. 'Frosinka, what have you

done? It's Baev we're talking about! He writes scientific papers ...'
'All the more reason why such a gross mistake is impermissible', was
her reply. Fearing Baev's displeasure, Nikishin ripped her conclusion
out of the morgue's protocols and rewrote it with Baev's diagnosis.
Indeed, recent editions of Kersnovskaya's memoir exclude this
episode.[62]

'To burn my bridges'

Eufrosinia Kersnovskaya's time in the morgue as anatomist under
Nikishin ended sometime in 1947. A change of management in the
Central Camp Hospital that year, related to a general strengthening
of the penal regime, saw the demotion of Vera Griazneva from
hospital director to staff doctor: she had married an ex-prisoner, a
hydrologist, and she faced the same Party displeasure that freely
hired Nina Savoeva did after marrying ex-prisoner Boris Lesniak.
'Vera Ivanovna had the courage to tell them, "I found in him my
soulmate!"' and this 'heroism' cost her a managerial job and her Party
card.[63] A cascade of personnel changes brought new management to
the hospital and morgue. Nikishin was now supervised by one 'doctor'
Liandres, an ex-prisoner by this time, and Kernovskaya's 'enemy No.
1 in the Central Camp Hospital'.[64] It was not long before the
prisoner-anatomist and the new morgue director fell out. He forbade
her to stay in the morgue, which lay beyond barbed wire, after work
to complete her illustrations and read in its library: guards escorted
her back to barracks every day once her autopsy duties were done.
Nikishin did nothing to soften the loss of privileges, and more
humiliations followed. Soon after, Kersnovskaya characteristically
challenged Liandres over his purloining of hospital chemicals to
repaint his new quarters, and the new director fired her.

As Kersnovskaya tells it, she was now determined 'to burn my
bridges' and leave the hospital, so demoralised was she by the succession of repressive and corrupt bosses to whom she had refused to
submit. Typically bold, she refused the offer of another post in the
hospital from its new director, a Sanotdel major who did not want to
transfer her to the mines. She spent a week refusing to eat (she says)

to convince him that she would only take a job underground. Thoughts of suicide loomed. She recalled the words of the morgue secretary Dmokhovsky when she first arrived there: 'Remember, Eufrosinia Antonovna, there are only two ways out of the morgue, the path to freedom and the path to the grave!' Secretly, she prepared to kill herself, but her plan to slash her wrists in a bath was foiled by Dmokhovsky, perhaps inadvertently, when he buttonholed her as she was approaching the bathroom with a concealed scalpel. He asked her not to forget that 'you belong to us!' and that when she got fed up with mining, she should write to him to get another medical job 'and we will have you back here right away'.[65] The moment for self-destruction passed, softened by this human kindness. Kersnovskaya realised that she knew very little about how prisoners worked in the mines and what life was like there. Through the corpses of miners that she had anatomised, the mines had come to symbolise death. She was sent to Nagorny camp, where some 800 women worked in the underground mines.

Her apprenticeship underground ensued, and her appetite for hard work and fearlessness impressed foremen and fellow miners. Despite the usual conflicts with bosses, she recalls that everyone underground, free and prisoner-miners, were 'equals before death' in this exceptionally dangerous environment and that, whatever their status, 'a miner, above all else, is a comrade'. Kersnovskaya experienced an epiphany soon after her adoption by a shift with a respected foreman and crew:

> I understood that the mine, in my imagination a thing so repulsive that it only eased my decision to die, turned out, on the contrary, to be a bright lighthouse that lit up the pitch darkness, calling to me 'You are not alone! Take hold of my light, and it will guide you through the storm and darkness to safety.'[66]

Paradoxically, Eufrosinia Kersnovskaya's search for humanity and solidarity in the Gulag led not to the camp hospital, where many other prisoners found refuge, but to the forbidding nickel mines of Norilsk.

'The morgue for prisoners is a special morgue'

Varlam Shalamov, in his short story 'The Geneticist', comments that the camp morgue differed from civilian ones in many ways, but chiefly in the content of a prisoner's medical case history, with the tales it told or concealed that were specific to Gulag life.[67] His hero, Professor Umansky (based on the pathological anatomist Yakov Mikhailovich Umansky, a zek in Kolyma) walked the line between serving as a 'judge' of the medical facts and as an 'accomplice' to medical mythologising. The prisoner-anatomist encountered doctors' diagnoses he considered pusillanimous, conforming to bureaucratic instruction, especially the florid collection of euphemisms for starvation disease, 'avitaminosis, polyavitaminosis, scurvy stage III, pellagra, their names were legion'. He felt contempt for the physician applying wildly inaccurate cancer diagnoses when no tumour was present inside the starvation-wasted corpse. For such doctors he performed elaborate demonstrations of the underlying cause of death: malnourishment and withering of the organism, implicitly mocking the fabrications they spun. But he forgave the prisoners who in desperation sought frostbite (and the loss of a limb), or who infected themselves deliberately with tuberculosis, to escape hard labour – especially those who ended up on his morgue dissection table. Umansky's medical degree from 'Brussels' (the real Umansky studied at the Sorbonne), and his pre-revolutionary practice, Shalamov says, gave him a troubled conscience that was only assuaged in the Gulag by working with corpses rather than suffering prisoner-patients.[68] Perhaps for the same reason Eufrosinia Kersnovskaya found working with the dead consoling – at least until her persistent thirst for truth got the better of her, and she could no longer put up with 'the tufta, the deception' and the corruption, which she suspected reigned in the morgue before Mardna persuaded her to take the assignment.[69]

Medical tufta was a critical part of the Gulag morgue's special character. The lofty aspiration that Death should delight in helping Life ran up against the challenge of letting Death speak truth to power. 'Death' was not capable of speaking, however: the Latin motto personifies abstract forces. The medical facts of a death were fashioned by human beings in a penal system that shaped – and routinely warped – the form of those facts. That prisoner-doctors with consciences like Nikishin and Umansky were sometimes selected to run Gulag morgues reminds us that some administrators like Vera Griazneva wanted to be able to tap the facts about the medical practice in their facilities. They knew they could not always trust their staff physicians. At the same time, the educational function of autopsy, closely associated with the morgue, required authentic knowledge about medicine. The Gulag's pathological anatomists, among the principal teachers on courses for mid-level medical staff trained up inside barbed wire, were custodians of precious lore, of what prisoners and medics alike called 'medical literacy'. Literacy and illiteracy, medical truth and deception, worked side by side in the Gulag hospital. The penal setting made imposture more possible and, for the qualified doctors, lies easier to offer than truth.

PART III
RESEARCHERS AND DREAMERS

7

'I DO NOT ASSIST SIMULATORS'
A prisoner-psychiatrist challenges
Gulag conventions

In a forest somewhere near Ukhta in November 1943, L.F.S., a 36-year-old woman from China, a prisoner in a deadly timber-felling camp, had a nervous breakdown. Her situation must have been desperate. On the day of her crisis, she threw aside her work, broke into sobs and shouts, hurling words in her native Chinese. (She knew very little Russian and had been arrested on charges of spying.) Grabbing at those around her, raving and refusing to let go, she was removed from the worksite. For weeks before the breakdown she had seen 'visions' of her parents, who supposedly had come from China to visit her in the prison camp. Forced to cut logs, she justifiably believed that her physical strength was draining away. Before being sent to the forest camp she had worked in a Gulag sewing workshop for several years – much lighter indoor work. At the logging camp she was terrified of failing to fulfil her norm, of losing her pitiful ration of bread, of being sent to the punishment block. Those near her reported that she had spoken to them about committing suicide, and often talked in gibberish. She constantly addressed herself to an imaginary 'big boss' – apparently pleading for an end to her suffering. Inconsolable, disruptive, and agitated, L.F.S., by a stroke of luck unrecorded in her file, was soon taken to the psychiatric department of Ukhta's Vetlosian Central Camp Hospital. On admission, she threw herself at an unidentified male hospital employee, believing him to be the 'big boss'. It was perhaps the psychiatric department's head doctor, Lev Grigorevich Sokolovsky, himself a prisoner.[1]

L.F.S. spent approximately three-and-a-half months in Vetlosian Hospital under Sokolovsky's observation and treatment. For the first six weeks the patient was agitated day and night, slept nervously, reacted fearfully to her surroundings, and ate with a poor appetite, often retching, rejecting nourishment. Her suicidal thoughts continued. She was anaemic, and evidently undernourished. In the mornings in the hospital she often rose, dressed, and expected to be led off to work. Her hallucinations about her parents continued for weeks. An X-ray scan revealed she had tuberculosis of the lungs, a typical cause of death among Gulag prisoners in 1943, and particularly common in camps where the zeks slogged outdoors in timber-cutting and logging operations. In mid-January 1944, L.F.S. was transferred to a tubercular ward, where her condition was described as 'good, quiet, reserved, hard-working, yet not very physically strong'. She was discharged from the camp hospital on 2 March 1944 – to an unknown fate. Looking back on his case notes later that year, psychiatrist Sokolovsky came to a conclusion at once stark, and dangerously truthful: her mental disturbance was not a fabrication, an attempt at malingering; it was genuine, produced by her own mind, 'the direct result of prolonged mental traumatisation without the participation of her consciousness, nor of the deeper spheres of the psyche – the so-called "subconscious"'. 'She felt that her strength was failing, and she sought a way out, even considering suicide. Pathological fits were the only means of escape from an unbearable situation.' The 'unbearable situation' was, of course, the life of a Gulag prisoner.

Sokolovsky presented this case history in an unpublished scientific paper, a manuscript 'for service use' only, painstakingly handwritten in block letters, a study of the simulation of psychoses and neuroses by Gulag prisoners. He wrote the study in summer 1944 and read it out to a scientific medical conference held in Vetlosian Central Camp Hospital on 15 September that year. No indication of how it was received remains in the written record, and yet its survival hints at the regard – or concern – it commanded. The manuscript sits in the central archives of the Gulag Sanitary Department in Moscow, a curiosity among a collection of labour-camp medical 'research

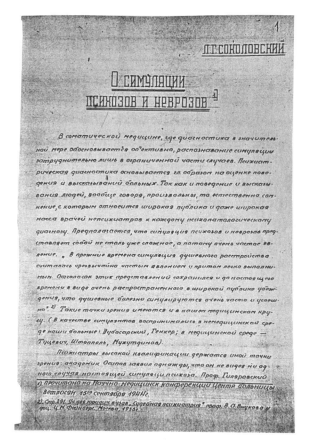

26. *For service use only: Sokolovsky's handwritten research paper on the simulation of psychiatric illnesses by Gulag prisoners.*

papers', mostly on nutrition, or on occupational disease among prisoners, produced by doctors working for the Gulag in camps scattered across the country. The tone and approach of the vast majority of these research papers is ideologically conformist, production-focused, aiming to boost prisoner output while overlooking the desperate conditions of Gulag life.[2] The Sokolovsky study, by contrast, is a rare investigation into the mental health of labour-camp prisoners, and even more intriguing is the humanity and truthfulness of this work. How was this candour possible – from a prisoner-doctor no less? What forces drove him to pen an investigation into prisoners who faked mental illness? How did the zek-psychiatrist regard and treat his prisoner-patients? What tools and ideas did Lev Sokolovsky bring with him to the Gulag and how did he interpret the 'unbearable situation' of the Gulag prisoner that generated madness? To answer these questions, we look first at how Soviet healthcare reckoned with the problem of malingering and simulated illness, before considering how Gulag officials and doctors translated this reckoning to the penal setting. The specific role of the psychiatrist in the Stalin-era Gulag needs to be explained. We then turn to Lev Grigorevich Sokolovsky's career and his work in the Gulag, to build a context for his extraordinary investigation of cases like that of the Chinese convict L.F.S., prisoner-patients who seemed to be faking mental illness but who were in fact often driven to genuine insanity by the inhumanity of labour-camp life.

Malingering in civilian and Gulag eyes

From ancient physicians to modern healthcare professionals, doctors have struggled with the problem of malingering, the feigning of illness to escape obligations of work or military service.[3] The patient simulating illness in the modern era troubled the conscience of some physicians, exposing a conflict of interest between the doctor's role as a healer of the individual patient, and his or her duty to powerful employers or state authority. Other doctors viewed the malingerer as a professional challenge, a contest of wits to be won. The army, industrial, and company doctor all served two competing imperatives: to treat the individual's medical condition, and to do so within the constraints and priorities of the institutional setting. Few medical issues brought the tension between the medical professional's Hippocratic duties, and their obligations to real-world masters, so vividly to light.

Soviet military doctors and psychiatrists admitted little about simulation of illness in print, but they were keenly aware of attempts to evade conscription via symptom-faking and self-mutilation. Their civilian counterparts in industry were equally alive to the problem of workers demanding medical certificates excusing the bearer from work to escape penalties for illegal absence, to search for scarce consumer goods or conduct illegal trade, to care for family, or indeed to reap the privileges of the ill or disabled citizen. A 'malingering folklore' circulated in the Soviet backstreet, with a semi-criminal coterie of 'experts' giving advice on how to simulate credible perform-ances of specific illnesses. Professional self-esteem and institutional quotas and monitoring prevented the soft-hearted doctor from excusing every case with a dubious claim from work or military service. Medicine in the Stalinist era walked a tightrope between the state's demands for labour and the physician's duty to attend to and heal the individual patient.

Within the Gulag, camp bosses and production managers believed that prisoners in the forced-labour system had a strong incentive to shirk work via the camp's clinic or hospital. While they seldom tried to quantify simulation and self-mutilation, Gulag statisticians in Moscow did track the number of workdays lost to sickness, the frequency of visits to camp infirmaries, and rates of hospitalisation, in the major camp complexes. Such indicators reveal concern not only for losses of productivity due to illness, but also for coping with prisoner demand for medical care.[4] The malingerer blocked beds, consumed staff time, and prevented genuinely ill prisoners from getting treatment. Another set of routines designed to monitor prisoner physical condition also opened routes to escape from work via illness. The Gulag's twice-yearly medical inspection of all prisoners is another indirect indication of the central authorities' anxiety about malingering.[5] Each May and November medical commissions examined and classified all prisoners according to their 'labour capacity', as fit for heavy, medium, or light labour; completely disabled prisoners were also identified or rechecked. The labour classification system allowed work-shy prisoners to find refuge in a lighter work category than the rules dictated; malingering was thus possible by degrees and not merely in absolute terms. Regular admonitions from inspectors and central Moscow bureaucrats indi-cate officials were alive to this possibility.

Malingering in the Gulag is a major theme in the archives of the camp administration and the materials produced by the labour-camp Cultural-Education Department. In official camp decrees and in documents for internal use, malingering was often rhetorically linked to loafing and refusal to work. Surprisingly soft-hearted attitudes circulated in the early 1930s but, by the time of the Great Terror and the late 1930s, camp commandants and Gulag bosses in Moscow dropped the sympathetic language and adopted a much tougher stance against faking sickness, deeming it a criminal act of sabotage.[6]

In the early 1930s, when the secret police promoted their forced-labour camps as the ideal vehicle for reforging the 'socially close' criminal while contributing to socialist construction, paternalistic encouragement backed by threats of penalties was tried on malingerers. Reforging through pep-talks and rousing lectures would transform the prisoner's attitude towards work and persuade him that honest labour was the route back to the family of Soviet toilers. Camp guards and bosses who neglected the 'human' needs of the prisoner were said to undermine the reforging of inmates, as a series of administration decrees from the early 1930s show.[7] Paternalistic reforging through labour figured as well in Cultural-Education Department propaganda aimed at Gulag inmates, with dramatisations of work-refusal and malingering in plays, newspaper stories, and posters. An entire page of stories about malingering appeared in 1933 in *Reforging*, the newspaper of the Moscow–Volga Canal Construction Camp. 'Unmask malingerer-loafers, hold them up to shame! [...] The best and the worst: brigadiers report; We taught them how to work', headed up stories calling for more pep-talks and redemptive toil.[8] *The Dream of a Work-Refuser*, a play published in 1936 in the newspaper of the White Sea–Baltic Canal camp, for performance by prisoners in propaganda work, offered a sentimental tale of the reforging of Tsyganov, a young thief who rejects gentle chivvying by a solicitous commandant. Feigning a long list of illnesses, his examining doctor diagnoses him 'a simulator and a shirker' who should be 'thrown out on his ear – then he'll stop moping and find life is cheerier!' Tsyganov mends his ways after dreaming of Moscow only to find that all the beerhalls have been closed, and the thieving and pimping fraternity all now have honest factory jobs.[9] More skits, stories, as well as posters for barracks and dining halls, some made by prisoner-artists, relayed similar messages of reforging the malingerer.[10]

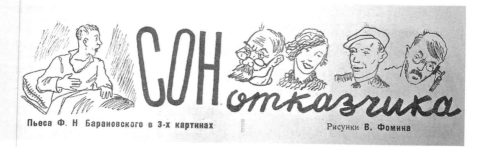

Пьеса Ф. Н Барановского в 3-х картинах   Рисунки В. Фомина

27. The Dream of a Work-Refuser, *a play by F. N. Baranovsky in three acts,* *from* Pod znamenem Belomorstroia.

With the Great Terror the tone of official Gulag treatment of the 'simulator' darkened. The Terror brought an influx of hundreds of thousands into the Gulag, and many sought refuge in the camp infirmary from overcrowded barracks, criminality, and exhausting labour. Pressure on the medical system was overwhelming. An inspection of Gulag hospitals in spring 1938 revealed many 'simulators' occupying beds with the presumed connivance of medical staff. Moscow ordered twice-monthly patient inspections by Sanotdel managers in camp hospitals to shake out fakers. New rules limiting hospitalisation and marking malingerers' files with their offence were set.[11] The same Moscow bureaucrats issued a sterner set of orders about malingering in February 1939. Simulators of illness and their 'instigators and accomplices' must receive well-publicised punishments; a meeting of medical staff and camp administrators should come up with measures to prevent malingering tailored to the individual camp. Doctors signing off prisoners should have armed guards to prevent bullying from patients, and the paperwork to release prisoners on medical grounds would require more detailed entries and cross-checking. The deputy chief of the Gulag Sanitary Department in Moscow supplied a four-page list describing the most notorious methods of simulation, and self-inflicted wounds, and called on camp doctors to report any new ruses they observed.[12]

Such orders cemented the Gulag medical system's official view of the malingerer as a cheat to be detected and punished. The significant expansion of Gulag hospital beds during and after the war, enormous fluctuations in morbidity and mortality, onerous war work and post-war reconstruction under reduced rations, and the huge influx of battlefield-hardened, less docile, prisoners in the 1940s, led to an increase in systematic malingering. With more women as a proportion of the inmate population during and after the war, officials noted more cases of female malingering.[13] The scale and variety of malingering in the camps and prison system was incalculable but undermined the camps' profitability. It is striking that just six days after Stalin's death, prison officials issued for internal use an 'orientation note' cataloguing in excruciating detail twenty-six general categories of simulated diseases, and eight major types of self-inflicted harm observed in Soviet jails.[14] In the immediate post-Stalin years, with successive amnesties and camp closures, the population of the camps slumped, but the Gulag prisoners who remained continued to fake tuberculosis, sexually transmitted diseases, and mental illness, often hoping to secure early release.[15]

Psychiatry for the Gulag?

What role did psychiatry play in this grim cat-and-mouse game where inmates played sick, and doctors played detective? We may begin by asking why have psychiatrists at all in Stalin's forced-labour penal system. To be sure, prisoner mental health, battered by arrest, detention, deportation – and then ground down by hard labour on meagre rations – was the least of the camp system's concerns. Prisoners struggled to keep their mental balance in the face of separation from loved ones and exhausting forced labour.[16] It seems odd, even exceptional, that psychiatrists like Lev Sokolovsky were working in their specialist field in the Gulag's medical system. The answers to these puzzles can be found in the broader story of labour-camp organisation and medical services.

The call for psychiatric medicine in the Gulag mirrored the modernisation of Soviet medicine in civilian life, but it also reflected the perverse logic of Stalin's penal-medical system. The Soviet regime granted civilian psychiatry enhanced status as a recognised specialist branch of scientific medicine. Building on a significant, if modest, platform of pre-revolutionary psychiatric clinics, asylums, colonies, and research centres, the Bolshevik leaders of the first health commissariat sought to give Soviet psychiatry parity of esteem with somatic branches of medicine.[17] They saw its potential as a science-based tool for improving humanity's capacity for healthy labour and they even overestimated this relatively young discipline's ability to deliver cures for severe mental illness and minor psychiatric complaints. An experimental, 'utopian' phase of psychiatric and mental health research in the 1920s licensed explorations of a host of questions geared to capacity-boosting and labour-enhancing the human machine: 'genius' studies, 'mental hygiene' initiatives to prevent workplace mental illness, expansion of outpatient psychotherapy, and experiments in new forms of drug and labour therapy for mental illness.[18] Until a shift of policy in 1936, considerable resources in a relatively underfunded healthcare system were devoted to 'mental hygiene' services designed to address psychological problems via medical means.

In that year Stalinists intervened to shut down 'paedology', child-focused, educational mental health support; and 'psychotechnics' – 'mental hygiene' services for industrial workers. The state denied that minor mental-health issues required medical care, and compelled Soviet psychiatrists to turn attention to major psychiatric illness, and to new curative procedures, like insulin-shock and electroshock therapy, that promised an ideologically orthodox material basis for explaining and curing mental illness.[19] During the 1930s, as Soviet medical education and infrastructure expanded, so too did specialist psychiatric training and therapeutic institutions, although the scale of provision trailed behind Western psychiatric services. Military psychiatry expanded and flourished during the war. In 1946 the director of the new civilian Institute of Psychiatry in Moscow, Vasily Alekseevich Giliarovsky, noted that in all of the USSR there were just 1,900 psychiatrists (1 per 90,000 in the population), while the USA had at least 3,500 (1 for 40,000). His ambition was to expand numbers of psychiatrically trained physicians to the point where every major hospital would have a staff psychiatrist able to diagnose mental illnesses competently.[20] Pavlovian dogma and Party ideology interfered with the evolution of psychiatric research and treatment, and an unknown degree of secret police intervention led to the abuse of forensic psychiatry for political purposes before Stalin's death.[21] Despite these considerable faults, Soviet psychiatry came of age as a modern science during the Stalin years.

A Gulag version of this psychiatry also matured in these years. Its history has not been written, but the outlines can be sketched from archival sources. The camps offloaded many severely mentally ill prisoners on the nearest civilian facilities, a habit that persisted into the 1950s. The earliest decrees by labour-camp medical bureaucrats in 1931 and 1935 directed that 'incurably mentally ill' prisoners should be removed from valuable camp hospital beds and transferred to civilian asylums. Their presence in the camps disrupted production and barrack life, demoralised prisoners, and wasted medical resources.[22] The Great Terror, with the mass influx of traumatised and unjustly detained victims, greatly increased the numbers of mentally ill prisoners. Now, however, these 'spies', 'anti-Soviet terrorists', and 'enemies of the people' with psychiatric illnesses could not easily be released to civilian institutions, and an in-house alternative was needed. The number of dedicated 'psychiatric hospitals' within the Gulag jumped from four in 1937 to seventy-six in 1938.[23] The 793 general Gulag hospitals in 1938 also had a limited number of psychiatric wards and beds. The number of psychiatrists in the system grew too, from 19 in 1936 to 34.5 (*sic*) in 1938. The puzzle of their distribution and their ability to run so many facilities is unanswered in the statistical data, but 15 per cent of Gulag doctors held more than one post in 1938, and specialists were likely to be among those managing wards or departments in general Gulag hospitals and special psychiatric facilities too. The system probably deployed prisoner-physicians like Sokolovsky without recording them in this data and sent doctors without psychiatric knowledge to cover for shortages. By the end of the 1930s, an experienced and learned psychiatrist like Sokolovsky could be a valuable asset in the Gulag. Offloading inmate psychiatric cases to civilian facilities continued in the 1940s, despite the growing internal network of psychiatric hospitals, and decrees from Moscow forbidding the practice. As late as January 1952 the Gulag's top medical official admitted there were still not enough psychiatric beds to handle prisoner-patient need.[24] The regular amnesties of prisoners with incurable health problems included those with severe mental illnesses, but only if these inmates were not among the categories of criminals regarded as politically dangerous. An unknown number of mentally ill prisoners who could not be released before the end of their sentences crowded Gulag mental hospitals.

The Gulag medical system needed mental hospitals and doctors of the mind, and its psychiatric branches expanded inexorably in the late 1930s and into the 1940s to accommodate some fraction of the total need presented by its inmates. Its expansion held a cracked mirror up to the Soviet Union's growing civilian psychiatric provision. The Gulag's focus of resources on severe mental illness was dictated not merely by the general ideological and planning priorities of Soviet psychiatric medicine, but by the logic of state terror. An accumulation of mentally ill prisoners who could not be released because of the severity of their so-called crimes needed to be confined. If possible, the Sanotdel hoped to cure prisoners and restore them to the unfree labour force, if not then psychiatric confinement at least saved them from disrupting camp production.

Lev Grigorevich Sokolovsky – Gulag psychiatrist and prisoner

Sokolovsky was the 'big boss' of the Vetlosian Central Camp Hospital's psychiatric department during the early 1940s. His pathway to serving as the principal psychiatric practitioner in the Ukhta camp region was a bitter one, only hinted at in contemporary histories and reminiscences. At the same time, we encounter in his biography the marks of revolution and Five-Year-Plan development that moulded him in ways that served him well in the Gulag.[25]

Born in 1907 in Kazan, the sophisticated provincial capital of one of Russia's major Tatar regions, Sokolovsky was a member of the pre-revolutionary Jewish intelligentsia, from a relatively secular and urban background.[26] His family seems to have navigated the Revolution successfully, placing him in an experimental secondary school run by the Eastern Pedagogical Institute of Kazan. He graduated in 1925 and entered the medical faculty of Kazan State

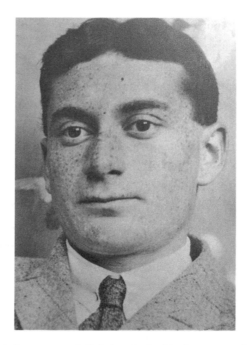

28. Bright prospects? Sokolovsky in his first year of medical school, Kazan, 1926.

University. At a time when Soviet medical education was still academically oriented, he received a strong education while he taught biology part-time, back in the experimental school that formed him. His exposure to revolutionary teaching methods and 'utopian' Soviet ideas of reshaping the human mind, as well as to a broad range of Russian and international literary and cultural influences, came from this period in his life. In 1930 he graduated as a physician-psychoneurologist and was called up for naval service.

Sokolovsky served seven years in the Baltic Fleet, based in Leningrad, in a 'military-medical expert psychoneurological laboratory' as a physician-psychophysiologist. Although little is known about his experience of this first appointment, it evidently gave him the experience and the mental skills to weather the coming storms. Military discipline and an assured sense of emotional reserve were qualities that observers of his Gulag work ascribed to him. As in the case of other Gulag prisoner-doctors, a background in military

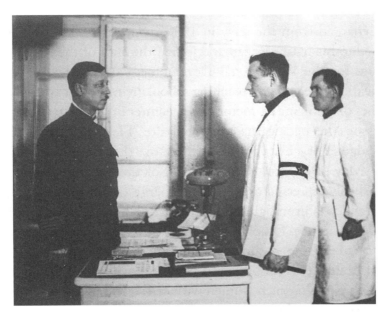

29. *Advancing career: Sokolovsky (second from right) in naval service at Kronshtadt near Leningrad, c. 1935.*

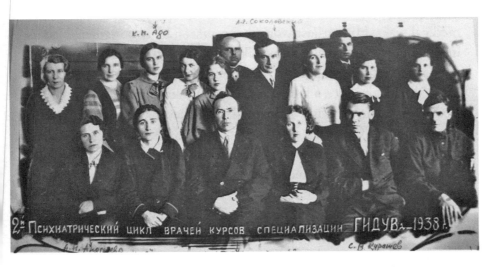

30. *Sokolovsky (top row, fifth from right) among doctors during his course on psychiatry in Kazan, 1938.*

medicine assisted the physician behind barbed wire in his adaptation to labour-camp medical service.

Discharged from the navy in 1937, at the age of 30 Sokolovsky returned to his native Kazan and joined the staff of the Kazan State Institute for the Professional Development of Physicians, a post-qualification research and teaching school giving courses on specialist branches of medicine to doctors. As a lecturer in psychiatry, he applied the lessons he had learned in the Baltic Fleet and deepened his knowledge of psychiatric medicine. He married. Seven months later, on 20 May 1940, Lev Grigorevich Sokolovsky was arrested and 'groundlessly repressed on a political charge' (as his brief biographies put it) and was eventually transported to Ukhta's camp complex to serve his sentence. Quickly after his arrest, his wife divorced him; such acts of self-protection were commonplace and had a bitter logic. One of Stalin's decrees outlawed being the wife of an enemy of the people, threatening such women with arrest, and a Gulag sentence.[27] An observer from the camps commented that Sokolovsky 'suffered in his hours of loneliness' as a result of his wife's reaction to his arrest.[28]

The record of Sokolovsky's early days in Ukhta camp in 1940–41 is scant; we do not know if he was first sent to general labour in the usual pattern, nor do we know how he was spotted and assigned to medical tasks. His earliest work was overseen by two medical leaders in this book: Nikolai Viktorov, Ukhta's very first prisoner-physician, now a free employee, and by this time chief of the camp's Sanotdel; and Yakov Kaminsky, a fellow prisoner-physician and director of the Vetlosian Central Camp Hospital. (Viktorov was introduced in chapter 1, and Kaminsky appears in chapter 8.) Kaminsky recognised in Sokolovsky a like-minded professional, educated in the old school and with a talent for medical organisation. They traded language lessons, conversing in French and German and correcting each other's mistakes. Sokolovsky's psychiatric specialisation was a major asset for this central camp hospital, so remote from civilian psychiatric facilities. In March or early April 1941, and with Viktorov's approval, Kaminsky assigned Sokolovsky to establish a psychiatric department in Vetlosian's expanding camp hospital.[29] The department was allocated a separate building on the edge of this complex, next to barbed-

216

wire fences and a watchtower staffed with armed guards. Close by were buildings housing the infectious diseases wards, a house devoted to *dokhodiagi* (prisoners so exhausted they were near death), a maternity hospital, and the radiology department.[30] It seemed a world away from the lecture theatres of Kazan's medical schools, and yet not entirely unlike the militarised milieu of navy psychiatry where Sokolovsky served his apprenticeship. Lev Sokolovsky embarked on his third career, this time as a Gulag psychiatrist.

Studying the Gulag 'simulator'

By the summer of 1944, when Sokolovsky wrote his study 'On the simulation of psychoses and neuroses', he had treated over 400 patients in his psychiatric department. What motivated Sokolovsky's turn to the question of faking mental illnesses is unknown; he could easily have chosen to write about other, less controversial issues, or indeed to remain silent. However, the Gulag hospital he worked in was an environment where experts were given a significant degree of latitude. Vetlosian had a well-developed research culture with frequent medical conferences and an atmosphere created by ex-prisoner physician-managers that encouraged zek-doctors to develop professionally and to mentor colleagues.[31] Golfo Alexopoulos has rightly called Lev Sokolovsky's study 'a bold challenge to Gulag dogma regarding the ubiquitous threat of malingerers'.[32] To appreciate his audacity, this section delves more deeply into this research.

Sokolovsky had clearly spent some time thinking about simulators, displaying knowledge of what leading authorities in Soviet psychiatry had to say about them, and showing he had access to a broad medical library in Vetlosian camp hospital. It is also fair to surmise that he had encountered suspected cases of malingering in the navy and discussed them in his professional development lectures in Kazan. His research paper begins with the apparently mundane observation that 'the broad public and even a broad mass of physicians'believe that faking mental illness 'is even less complicated [than faking somatic illness], and therefore it must be a common phenomenon'. He doubles down on this axiom by citing the leaders of Soviet forensic medicine for a similar view: to the present day, a 'holdover' of this attitude is found in the commonplace public view that 'mental illnesses are often and easily imitated'.³³ The ticklish issue for a zek-psychiatrist writing in a Gulag hospital is that the 'broad public' feeling sceptical about psychiatric illnesses were not simply comrades in the street, but commandants in the camp. The research paper begins, in other words, by discreetly announcing its intention to refute a viewpoint that Sokolovsky had undoubtedly heard from work-assignment officials, camp managers, and internal security officers. Indeed, if 'even a broad mass of physicians' might be guilty of the same prejudice, the paper also implicitly takes a swipe at the NKVD's young and green contract-hired medical staff whose loyalties were first to the penal regime rather than Hippocratic ideals.

Continuing his theme, Sokolovsky points out that '[h]ighly qualified academic psychiatrists think differently: [V. P.] Osipov claimed he never observed even a single case of genuine simulation of a psychosis; Giliarovsky distinguished between the recognition of crude mimicry and simulation in the specific meaning of the presentation of a [. . .] mental illness.' Perhaps that is why they devoted so little attention to it in their textbooks. 'Specialists rarely suspect simulation while laypersons often do, and this is understandable if we recall the methodology of medical and especially neuropsychiatric diagnosis' in which experts readily see when the 'picture of illness presented' fails to match what they know from scientific literature and clinical experience. The prisoner-doctor does not mince his words: the more 'professional competence' one has, the less likely one is to suspect simulation of mental illness. And yet, Sokolovsky admits that faking mental illness 'is a form of crime, and therefore the task is to forbid the criminal from hiding under the mask of illness'.³⁴ This phrase, justifying the research paper, is the most ideologically orthodox passage in the entire work, and a necessary bid to 'satisfy his captors' under these circumstances.³⁵ Yet much of what follows refutes the notion that Sokolovsky relished tearing off the masks of these 'criminals', unlike other medical practitioners in the Gulag.³⁶

Sokolovsky reviewed the case histories of his prisoner-patients: in 34 months he had treated 400 for psychiatric illnesses; he sifted their records to focus on 23 cases where the suspicion of malingering was significant, a part of the process of diagnostics. Perhaps mindful of the priorities of commandants, he divided malingerers into groups according to the length of hospital time they received. Noteworthy were the few successful prisoners who faked a mental illness for a long period of time, getting several days or weeks of hospitalisation in the bargain. Less impressive were the ones who let their perform- ance drop once they had arrived in hospital, displaying their lack of illness on the ward; and those who did not make it as far as the ward, having been recognised as simulators at the threshold. In all, Sokolovsky found only eighteen obvious or probable malingerers, out of the 400 (4.5 per cent) who managed to achieve a significant hospital stay, and on average these were only a month or less. He argued that statistically only perhaps two or three out of 100 mental patients could be simulators. By implication, the administration's suspicion that each psychiatric patient must be a deliberate work- refuser was wide of the mark, and the loss to Gulag production via this especially refined ruse, minuscule.[37]

Medical competence, deliberate changes to the hospital food ration, and careful examination of the patient's past exposed this small group of simulators sooner or later. Sokolovsky begins by presenting the most clear-cut cases, showing his medical detective skills and a forthright approach to malingering, evidently to give 'his captors' the story they expect, but possibly as well to distract them from his Aesopian arguments about Gulag mistreatment of pris- oners. Two of the clear-cut cases, both thieves who managed to spend two months in Sokolovsky's wards, presented mismatched combina- tions of symptoms and were found out partly on this basis, and partly after apparently admitting their deception to hospital staff. The other four malingerers managed to confuse the doctor with psychosis-like fits and howling or struggling against the ward regime, mutism or deafness, lack of concentration when addressed, and talking to them- selves or refusing to respond to questions. Yet they slept well and generally ate 'with a big appetite'. In these cases, Sokolovsky had provoked responses that exposed the malingerer by deliberately altering their hospital rations: in one case omitting the butter portion caused a malingerer to complain; in another case, the greatly reduced portion aroused overt dissatisfaction. Both reactions were clues to the prisoner-patients' motivation and will. When another young patient presenting mutism and complex symptoms over several weeks was told he would only get liquid food he refused these meals and became hysterical; he had to be tied down to his bed for twenty-four hours until he calmed down, was fed, and began to speak to Sokolovsky. The psychiatrist retrospectively thought his case was more ambiguous than the others, but concluded the mutism was feigned.[38] Other supposed psychotic cases with brief hospitalisation quickly exposed themselves in examination by the doctor: these might be thieves, with violations against camp discipline in their histories as 'work-refusers', self-harmers, or inmates coming from the Gulag's internal punishment-camp subdivisions.[39] A further collection of cases in Sokolovsky's sample, he realised, had been simulators of mental illness who managed to avoid being detected; he only recognised their deception as he reread their notes in preparing this article.[40] Sokolovsky's forensic and factual presentation, and measured self-criticism of his diagnostic and detective practice in these relatively unambiguous cases, all presented in the first few pages of this article, establish his credentials as a psychiatrist not easily deceived and alert to the requirements of Gulag medicine. A busy censor might have waved the rest of the article through on this basis.

Like messages in a bottle, the prisoner-psychiatrist finds subtle ways to expose Gulag abuse of prisoners in his brief summaries of each patient case history. Hunger and anxiety about food, physical malnourishment, and somatic and mental diseases of starvation are observed and explicitly mentioned in seventeen out of twenty-three cases. The period when Sokolovsky encountered these patients was the worst for mortality and starvation diseases in the entire life of the Gulag, the years of the Second World War when Gulag official statistics registered one million prisoner deaths. The camps were desperately undersupplied at the bottom of national priorities during the wartime emergency. Diseases of malnourishment such as tuberculosis and vitamin deficiencies stalked the camps and resonate in these cases. The Chinese woman L.F.S. was found to have tuberculosis and remained 'not very physically strong' even at the point of discharge from Sokolovsky's department; another prisoner, male, Russian, whose mental derangement brought him to the psychiatrist had died in December 1941 from advanced tuberculosis. Sokolovsky could not rule out 'psychogenic reactions' (in other words, genuine mental illness triggered by his life circumstances) as the cause of this patient's derangement, but his physical demise was due to TB.[41]

Sokolovsky describes numerous patients in passing as 'in poor physical condition' and in two cases he goes farther, using terminology that risked at very least a caution from medical managers. One describes a 34-year-old male Russian with heart disease and 'alimentary dystrophy' – the Soviet wartime term for starvation disease.[42] This man spent nine months in Vetlosian Hospital evidently being treated for his physical depletion and heart condition; he had a week's stay during that time in Sokolovsky's department after a psychotic episode four months into his hospitalisation. Had he presented with psychosis in a smaller camp clinic, or not been surrounded by medical staff who understood his full diagnosis, Sokolovsky comments that 'suspicion of simulation' would doubtless have been ascribed to this hapless prisoner.[43] The psychiatrist's description of another case as 'severely emaciated with polyavitaminosis' (a 21-year-old Russian man) used a term, 'emaciation', which had by this time long been restricted for internal use only in the Gulag.[44] The young patient had arrived in Sokolovsky's care in January 1942, directly from the NKVD's holding cells where he had spent at least three months awaiting a death sentence, in conditions that amounted to starvation. The supreme punishment was commuted to a ten-year sentence; the young prisoner suffered from paralysis caused by the vitamin deficiencies he experienced and displayed complex mental-health problems. Sokolovsky assessed his mental and physical debilities as simultaneously unconsciously induced by his trauma, and consciously exploited in his statements and behaviour.[45] The extremes of hunger, physical depletion by hard labour, and traumatic stress brought on by arrest, interrogation, transportation, and camp existence all contributed to the appearance of mental illnesses, and in some, an 'escape into illness'.[46]

Literary diagnosis behind barbed wire

The puzzle of the simulating psychiatric patient, and the doctors who suspect them, clearly captivated Lev Sokolovsky as he reviewed his case notes in the summer of 1944. Reflecting on his flawed professional practice, he asked whether doctors tended to minimise or avoid the accusation of malingering because they were afraid to call an ill person a faker by mistake. Ruefully he writes that 'looking retrospectively at the catamnestic data of our diagnoses over the past two years of our work, awkwardly we feel that we have become convinced of the opposite.'[47] Medical scholarship suggested to him that schizophrenics were frequently taken initially for simulators. He also recognised that the problem of discerning 'schizophrenia or simulation' was well explored in Russian and European literature. Like many Russian psychiatrists with academic training, Sokolovsky referred to literary and cultural works to explain psychological states.[48] To engage in 'literary diagnosis' at length in a Gulag research paper was unusual, to say the least.

Sokolovsky opens his literary approach to his research question by pointing tersely to a novella by the radical, decadent, and notoriously neurasthenic writer Leonid Andreev: 'The Thought' (1902).[49] This work luridly dramatised the borderline between schizophrenia and fabricated mental illness. Its hero, Anton Kerzhentsev, a physician, kills a boyhood friend on an apparently Nietzschean impulse to assert his will and his distance from ordinary human emotions. Suspected of mental derangement, Kerzhentsev is confined to an asylum and observed by doctors. In his first-person narrative, Kerzhentsev explains to them how he intends to simulate insanity and escape punishment for his crime, but as his internal monologue advances, he comes to doubt his mental balance, and the novella ends inconclusively: is Kerzhentsev genuinely mad, or merely simulating an illness? Sokolovsky makes no allusion to the author Andreev's own travails with neurasthenia, depression, and alcoholism. Still less does he mention the psychiatric profession's intrusive, gossipy, and negative response to 'The Thought' and its author's health problems, a low point in the ethical probity of Imperial Russian psychiatric medicine.

Nevertheless, the well-informed Gulag psychiatrist was very likely aware of the backdrop to this story that attracted so much attention from the press and Russian medical experts, including a 1903 lecture by a psychiatrist at Sokolovsky's own Kazan university.[50] With Andreev under a cloud of ideological disapproval and confusion in the Stalin era, Sokolovsky's foregrounding of his novella in this research paper takes on added piquancy. The Gulag psychiatrist clearly esteemed Andreev's fiction as illuminating; in the analytical section of his article 'The Thought' is the first literary depiction of the psychology of simulation Sokolovsky refers to. He immediately turns to observe that in real life as in art, Soviet psychiatric authorities such as Vnukov and Feinberg found distinguishing the boundary between simulation and 'hysteria and reactive conditions' nearly impossible in some cases.[51]

Sokolovsky then reached for an analogy from the stage to pinpoint the border between simulation and hysteria. At this border lay the heart of his critique of the official Gulag attitude towards mental illness, and indeed the camp system's neglect of prisoner well-being. Having suggested up to this point through Aesopian language that the extremes of daily life drove prisoners to extreme responses, he now argued overtly that genuinely pathological hysteria, produced by the patient's response to his stressful environment, generated an impulse 'to escape through illness'. The pathological mimicry of illness resembled the deliberate faking by a malingerer, because both were performances.

Sokolovsky continues,

Speaking schematically, simulation is the conscious deception of those around the subject; hysteria presents itself as the same kind of deception of others, but it is involuntary, because at the same time it is a self-deception. In both cases, the illness is performed by the patient like an actor. In the first case, this is rational play, playing in the words of [Konstantin] Stanislavsky 'in the art of performance', while in the second it is emotional play, the actor totally inhabits the role, Stanislavsky's 'art of experience'. The simulator knowingly presents himself as a sick person, while the hysteric, who presents himself as a sick person, also imagines himself to be ill. In our professional terminology we say simulation is *ideogenic*, while hysteria is *timogenic* [i.e. generated by emotions]. It is difficult to explain the difference between genuine, non-pathological and therefore criminal simulation, and that simulation which we regard as a sickness in itself, as a peculiar kind of reactive condition.[52]

To drive the point home Sokolovsky adds, 'There are times when the subject's position seems so hopeless that he views simulation as the only escape hatch, and once he has started, he simulates blindly, heedlessly, and he cannot stop himself regardless of changing circumstances that he does not even notice.' The Gulag psychiatrist draws on the authority of Konstantin Stanislavsky's physical and psychological method for stage actors (enunciated in his 1938 *An Actor Works upon Himself*) to delineate the line between simulation and hysteria, malingering and blameless derangement.[53] By adapting the language of fiction and stage drama, Lev Sokolovsky made explicit his argument that his psychiatric prisoner-patients became sick because of their environment. The Gulag made some prisoners so desperate to be ill that they literally became mentally ill.

'I do not assist simulators'

What did Lev Sokolovsky actually think about prisoners who simulated mental illness? His careful research paper pays due attention to the conventional 'crime' of malingering, while offering clues to something more humane than this standard Gulag approach. His repeated observations about prisoner malnutrition and his old-school 'literary diagnosis' suggest this labour-camp prisoner-psychiatrist was painfully aware of the reasons why his patients might wish to be ill. A late-Soviet memoir written by a Gulag survivor and deposited in Memorial's St Petersburg archive intimates that Sokolovsky was equally careful with patients, but capable of taking great risks to help them.

Three years after the Gulag psychiatrist had written and delivered his paper on simulators, he encountered a 25-year-old prisoner,

Oskar Yosifovich Gurvich. Arrested on a political charge in 1945 in Leningrad, the young zek had been through a series of mining camps and was deeply depressed. He had resolved to kill himself by refusing food. He was 'in a state of utter apathy to everyone and everything, including [his] own life'.[54] Sokolovsky hospitalised Gurvich. After a few days he called Gurvich to his office,

> ... and closed the door tightly. 'You're not mentally ill,' he said to me softly and assuredly. 'You are in a reactive condition tied to extraordinary psychic burdening. Do not make anything up: there's no need to play at being mad. I do not intend to send you back. Act naturally and do not do anything stupid.'
>
> I looked at Sokolovsky with mistrust. When you have seen so much evil from people it is hard to believe in the benevolence and noble intentions of a stranger.
>
> Even though the future seemed ephemeral, an inner voice was contradictory – sometimes calling for death, other times for life. I was 25 years old.
>
> I remained silent. Lev Grigorevich told me sympathetically, speaking like a friend, 'Politicals do not get amnestied. Even if your simulation were successful (and I doubt it would be!), then you would face a life confined to an insane asylum. There, with time you really would go out of your mind. Even in life's most difficult circumstances there is some good. I will try to help you to survive.'
>
> I burst into tears, and sobbing asked, 'How can you help me?'
>
> Sokolovsky looked at me, then away, thinking, and after a pause replied, 'You have landed in a good camp. It's difficult to stay here. But there is one way ... I will not rush to discharge you and I will try to fix up something ... But remember: I do not assist simulators. Maybe you started off with simulation, but right now you are genuinely unwell.'[55]

The prisoner-psychiatrist coaxed Gurvich to eat after three weeks of 'delirium' and, when he had recovered sufficiently, enrolled the young man in a nursing course for prisoners. Oskar Gurvich qualified as a male nurse and worked for three-and-a-half years in Vetlosian Central Camp Hospital, before being transferred to another camp. Under Sokolovsky's mentorship Gurvich adapted to Gulag life and 'became a camp veteran. I believe that Lev Grigorevich saved my life.'[56] Writing in the late 1970s and early 1980s, Gurvich describes how Sokolovsky assisted other 'political' labour-camp prisoners to escape emaciation and hard labour using his privileged position to hospitalise them, and perhaps coaching them to simulate illness. 'I knew several people whom Sokolovsky helped to survive. He never spoke of his good actions himself.'[57]

Did Lev Sokolovsky routinely 'assist simulators' to escape hard labour and criminalisation as work-refusers? It hardly seems likely that he was able to do so in the majority of cases that passed through his care. He certainly argued robustly that there were fewer malingerers in his psychiatric department than his bosses thought. In his research paper he sought to reduce the number of genuine fakers of mental illness in his case notes to the tiniest number possible, through his retrospective review of his patients' illnesses, his professional erudition, and his literary and dramatic analogies. In this written argument there are flashes of the inspirational Kazan medical school lecturer. Sokolovsky was a brave man who took risks: in his words and actions he teased the boundaries between mental illness and health. He took advantage of the good fortune that he 'landed in a good camp' and in a Gulag hospital that indulged his expertise. In Gurvich's words, Vetlosian Central Camp Hospital was both 'cherished, and puzzling' to its staff, its patients, and perhaps to the zeks of Ukhta who heard of its existence.[58] Lev Sokolovsky was a piece of the puzzle to be cherished.

8

'YOU WILL BE SINGING THESE SONGS'

The radium-water spa of the zeks

Dear comrade descendants. When, having arrived at the luxurious sanatoria of Ukhta, you stroll along the shore of this once-legendary river, by the mouth of the Yarega creek, you will see the derrick for bore-hole No. 3.

By then it will be old, very old . . .

You should know that you must address this tower with respect.

Moroz managed to get here trudging through snow up to his neck; Romanenko sank this bore; and its bitter-salty waters yielded so very, very much – yielded, in fact, the result that you are walking here in Ukhta and getting medical treatment.

Its waters, and the selfless devotion of Ukhta's first inhabitants, made of this place one of the most remarkable in the world . . .

As you pass you will recall Ukhta's first inhabitants . . .

They are worthy not only of recollection, but of legends and songs . . .

And you will be singing these songs.[1]

Ostap Vyshnia, the author of these lines, was one of the best-known writers to be imprisoned in the Gulag camps of the Ukhta region, or Ukhtpechlag, as this complex was known in the mid-1930s. The Ukrainian prisoner edited a grand chronicle of the history of Ukhtpechlag, described in the Introduction.[2] This passage addressing the imagined future visitor to Ukhta's 'luxurious sanatoria' concludes a chapter entitled 'Ukhta's Healing Water. OGPU Factory No. 2', written by Vyshnia himself. In it he describes an improbable story worthy of the looking-glass world of the Gulag. At a settlement 20 kilometres from Ukhta called simply 'Water' (Vodny), a unique source of radium waters rich in radioactivity was discovered, developed, and exploited by prisoner geologists, doctors, labourers, and their Gulag overseers. Gulag physicians and scientists experimented on humans and animals with these waters for medical purposes in a programme of research into radioactive substances. Between 1932 and 1941, a 'physiotherapy laboratory' operated at the site, staffed by prisoner-doctors who sought to devise medical treatments based on 'Ukhta's healing water'.

Hailing the future spa visitor, Vyshnia manages to compress allusions to a host of themes pertinent to this chapter. In his fast-forwarding to a bright future of luxury and song, he taps the tomorrow-facing currents of socialist realism which were only then being dogmatised in Soviet art. By alluding to this remote corner as one of the most remarkable in the world, he writes the story of the prospective spa into the Marxist-Leninist 'world-historical' narrative of socialist construction.[3] Ukhta's spa proponents, conscious that a multi-day rail journey to a northern Gulag town was not a selling point, argued tenaciously that the unique properties of the region's therapeutic resources merited the trip. The waters at Vodny were truly of global significance: Gulag scientists would claim that their radium content was ten times that of the famed springs of Czechoslovakia's Jáchimov, a spa town where the grand Radium Palace Hotel and many lesser hostelries served a bourgeoisie eager for the latest therapeutic rituals offered by scientific medicine.

In Vyshnia's hymn to Ukhta's healing waters it is axiomatic that this Soviet spa will be socialist, intended to benefit not capitalist parasites, but the working class, like all Soviet spas, be they run by civilian authorities as most were, or by the more shadowy organs of state security. The imagined Ukhta spa would take its place within a growing national network of resorts run on strictly scientific and non-commercial, non-capitalist lines, to serve the workers and their representatives in the Communist Party. The Soviet passion for spas grew from the long-standing influence of German medicine in Ukrainian and Russian medical science: the German 'cult of water cures' had long taken root in Imperial Russia where spas operated in the empire's southern fringes, in the Caucasus and Georgia.[4] Pioneering prisoner-doctors working in Ukhta brought with them an existing Soviet template of resort medicine and research (known in Russian as *kurortologiia*), one that was evolving rapidly in Stalin's Five-Year-Plan economy. Gulag commandants and freely hired employees brought an expectation that as deserving Soviet workers they would (eventually) earn paid sojourns in resorts with the kind of 'luxury' promised by Ostap Vyshnia despite their remote posting to the Soviet empire's farthest regions. The Gulag's contract workforce did not check its thirst for the abundance promised by socialism at the labour-camp gates.[5]

The improbable image of Vyshnia's 'luxurious sanatoria' emerging from Ukhta's camps of forced labour and high mortality is only explicable if we recall that the colonisation of the remote spaces of the USSR was a seriously held objective set by NKVD top leaders and Gulag managers. These resorts were integral offshoots of the geological expeditions from which all the major Gulag camp complexes began in the late 1920s and early 1930s. Gulag geologists and cartographers noted mineral and hot springs, healing muds, and other therapeutic resources and added them to the inventory of natural wealth they compiled as plans were drawn up for the expansion of the camps. Talaya, a hot-water spring north of Magadan, the capital of the Kolyma gold fields, was a model for these Gulag free worker resorts. The spring was discovered in 1933, and by 1940 the first twenty patients got treatment in rough-and-ready reindeer sheds. By the late 1940s the resort had its own dormitories, and by 1954 it had physiotherapy, X-ray, and dental clinics, as well as a gymnasium, pharmacy, library, and auditorium with a dancehall and billiards room. To be sure, all these luxuries in the wilderness were built by prisoners. By 1959 it had served 30,000 visitors, supposedly the cream of Kolyma's 'deserving' workers.[6] Freely hired physician Nina Savoeva was sent there in the summer of 1942 to relax for two weeks after an apparent emotional crisis in her adjustment to the

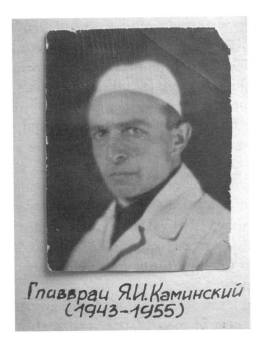

Главврач Я.И.Каминский
(1943-1955)

31. Chief doctor of Vetlosian Central Camp Hospital,
Yakov Kaminsky, c. 1950.

'specific conditions' of the Gulag camps. Following this short break, she assumed command of Belichya Central Camp Hospital, and seemingly her stay at the spa ensured that the young contract doctor returned to work refreshed and recommitted to socialist labour. Contract physician for Dalstroi's civilian medical service Anna Kliashko recalled that her husband, a freely hired geologist, had joint problems, and had a series of treatments at Talaya in winter in 1950. It was easier to get passes to go there in the winter because in summertime the top management of the Dalstroi camps and industries crowded its comfortable lodgings.[7]

In 1944 an ambitious Gulag prisoner-doctor, Yakov Iosifovich Kaminsky, wrote a proposal to establish a 'Northern Resort', a facility of 'all-Union significance' at the Vodny radium water source.[8] Kaminsky hoped it would be built on the basis of more than a decade's experimentation in the radium-springs physiotherapy laboratory established in Vodny. The Ukrainian prisoner-doctor from

Odesa had an unusual background that fired his enthusiasm for the radium spa. He had long specialised in radiology, studying and teaching the therapeutic uses of X-rays from the 1920s until his arrest as a supposed 'Trotskyite' in July 1937. Additionally, he had devoted a significant part of his early career to the study of physiotherapy and the curative effects of physical exercise in resorts and sanatoria around Odesa. The twin tracks of his career fused in the prospect of a resort that promised cures using the beneficial effects of radiation alongside physical exercise calibrated to the individual patient. At the time he wrote his proposal, Kaminsky was the new chief doctor of Vetlosian Central Camp Hospital. He was a close friend, and boss, of prisoner-psychiatrist Lev Sokolovsky, who, at about the same time, was writing his research paper on simulators of mental illness. A physician from Ukraine's urban and proudly Jewish community who had tasted many forms of anti-Semitism before and after the collapse of the Russian Empire, Kaminsky had also experienced his share of professional setbacks under Soviet rule. His early attempts to parlay his scattered research interests in Odesa into an accredited doctoral dissertation were scooped by a powerful rival in Kyiv. Later in the 1930s Kaminsky was robbed of the chance to defend his doctoral thesis because of his arrest just weeks after it was submitted. The 1944 'Northern Resort' proposal was an eye-catching bid to broaden his reputation in the Ukhta scientific community, where he was known principally as an expert on tuberculosis; and perhaps even to catch the attention of Gulag leaders in Moscow.

The puzzle of Kaminsky's decision to immerse himself in the dream of a radium-water resort for the Gulag is the focal question of this chapter. Like his Vetlosian colleague the psychiatrist Sokolovsky, captivated by a research question that enabled him to escape and even contest the bounds of the forced-labour camp, Kaminsky seems to have been gripped by a fascination with an enterprise that offered glimmers of a future after confinement. How did his early career prepare him for this unlikely enthusiasm? What actually went on in the 'physiological laboratory' attached to OGPU Factory No. 2, and for what ends? At what point did the 'dream' of radium therapy turn into a nightmare of radioactive poisoning? As a man of science, how did Yakov Kaminsky respond as he observed and studied the harmful effects of radiation unleashed by Gulag experimentation and industrialisation on the inhabitants of Vodny? Kaminsky left an unusual 'documentary memoir' that enables us to explore these questions.[9] Published in 1995, his memoir was a joint creation of the aged doctor, then in his nineties, and members of Odesa's Memorial Society, who interviewed Kaminsky and interspersed his words with official documents from his personal archive, and testimony by colleagues from the Gulag. When compared with the documentary record of Ukhta's museums, a rich picture of the man, the radium-water factory, and the 'dream of a Northern Resort' emerges.

Kaminsky's path to Vetlosian Central Camp Hospital

Yakov Kaminsky was born in 1897 in Kropyvnytskyi, a market town in the heart of central Ukraine, where his father was a prosperous ear, nose, and throat doctor with a thriving prosthetic dental practice. The family holidayed in Germany and Austria, in Františkovy Lázně with its middle-class spas, and in Berlin and Vienna where young Kaminsky picked up a lifelong facility for the German language. The boy flourished in his local gymnasium where he excelled in the sciences and took a deep interest in physical fitness. In 1915 Kaminsky graduated with a 'silver medal' for his excellent results and aspired to get a studentship in the city of Dnipro's Mining Institute to study engineering. However, the tsarist quota of Jewish higher-education admissions blocked entry, and his father persuaded him to try medicine instead. Yet even here the quota stood in young Kaminsky's way, and his father took the matter into his own hands, asking a favour of an old patient in a demonstrative gesture that must have become a family legend:

Then my father acted decisively. He put on his dress uniform with his three medals, and we went with him to Petersburg to the reception room of his patient, a comrade chairman of the State Duma Mr [Sergei Timofeevich] Varun-Sekret. My father asked him, in view of his services, if the medical faculty of Odesa

232

University would admit me outside the quota. The request was granted. With my father glowing in happiness, we returned to Odesa.[10]

Yakov Kaminsky entered the medical faculty to train as a physician in 1915.

Physiology and biomechanics were the young student's favourite subjects, building on his love of physical fitness, his active participation in the Maccabi Society for Jewish Fitness, and a passion for fencing.[11] He supported himself through teaching in another institute. In his account, the First World War does not seem to have affected him, but he notes how the Revolution threw life out of its normal groove, and he briefly joined an improvised student militia keeping order in the streets in 1917; he left Odesa for Kropyvnytskyi at some point that year. The fall of the Provisional Government barely mattered there, where successive regimes flashed past with lightning speed. Kaminsky remembers from a diary he kept at the time that power changed hands thirteen times in the town where he sought refuge, and courted his wife, Vera. They were betrothed in a Jewish family ceremony in January 1918 and married in religious then civil rituals in May 1919.[12] In his memoirs Kaminsky cultivates a studied distance from politics. 'Party political discord never interested me [...] I did not wish to join the ruling party of communists. In principle I shared the ideas of socialism.'[13] Sympathetic to the Bolsheviks' apparent respect for national diversity and religious toleration, at the same time he observed how they persecuted 'innocent' Christians, and made arbitrary use of arrest, terror, and violence. Like Dr Yuri Zhivago in Boris Pasternak's eponymous novel, his first loyalty was to 'the feeling of medical duty. To assist the patient regardless of his estate or nationality, or personal qualities – I followed that principle my entire life, whatever the circumstances.'[14] And rather like Zhivago's fate, politics came looking for Kaminsky regardless of the would-be doctor's indifference and sent him on a three-year odyssey.

In the flux of regimes Kaminsky witnessed two pogroms against Kropyvnytskyi's Jews: the first inflicted by Ukrainian nationalist leader Symon Petliura's forces in January 1918 and a second, devastating, wave of violence under a Bolshevik Ukrainian warlord, Nykyfor Hryhoriv, in February 1919. The pogrom under the Bolsheviks left more than 2,000 Jews dead and destroyed the homes and property of 85 per cent of the town's Jewish community.[15] Kaminsky's now impoverished family returned to Odesa, where Yakov worked as a feldsher while resuming his studies, and Vera made and sold pies to hungry students. In autumn 1919 General Anton Denikin's White forces occupied Odesa and Kaminsky, now in the fifth year of a six-year medical course, was among forty students deemed 'qualified' to practise and drafted into military-medical service for the anti-Bolshevik force. He found himself in Novorossiisk in Russia, ill from typhus, when the Whites disintegrated, and Bolsheviks took over; the Reds assigned the recuperating 'doctor' to serve their army. Finally, in May 1920 the Bolsheviks released him to resume studies and he made his way through anarchist-held territory to Odesa and the medical faculty. Yakov Kaminsky finally graduated as a qualified doctor in Odesa in 1921.

With Ukraine now under Soviet rule, Kaminsky began a career in medicine that followed several paths in practice and research. He was drawn into famine relief work in 1921–22 and served as an agent for the American Relief Agency and the American Jewish Joint Distribution Committee (the 'Joint'), both operating at the invitation of Bolshevik Moscow to alleviate mass starvation in the wake of the civil wars on Soviet territory. It was thanks to Kaminsky's work for the 'Joint' that he first engaged in radiological treatments, which became a lifelong interest. Using X-rays to cure fungal infections in orphaned children in Odesa, he studied the therapy, participated in courses on X-ray technology, and eventually in 1925 formed a radiology section in Odesa's medical trade union. One of his first reports for the union was a call for better safety measures for workers in X-ray clinics.[16] Regardless of the dangers of this technology that were by now increasingly apparent, the benefits of X-rays were confidently explored in the 1920s across Europe, and Odesa's medical scientists followed the trend.[17] Under the mentorship of Professor Yakov Moiseevich Rozenblat, a leading Ukrainian radiologist,

Kaminsky authored a manual on radiological therapy, and conducted studies of treatment for tuberculosis using X-ray radiation, reporting his findings at the All-Union conference on tuberculosis in Tbilisi, Georgia, in 1928. By this time, Yakov Kaminsky had become personally aware of the harmful effects of radiation. When in 1927 Rozenblat fell ill to X-ray-induced cancer, Kaminsky took over his private practice, but not long thereafter doctors diagnosed Kaminsky himself as having had excess exposure to the rays and he was banned from working in radiological clinics for three years. Rozenblat died in 1928, and his name would later be inscribed on a monument to 'X-ray and Radium Martyrs' in Hamburg, Germany.[18] Kaminsky was forced to seek another specialisation and he looked to his fascination with sport and physiotherapy, which he had pursued simultaneously during the 1920s.

Like many Soviet physicians, Kaminsky worked in two or three posts in order to put together a viable income. For a time in the early 1920s he held a clinical post in a war invalids' sanatorium in Odesa, where he used physiotherapy in his practice; the experience encouraged him to seek out mentorship and more work in sanatoria, including a stint in a mud-bathing spa, Kuyalnyk, near the city. He wrote a paper on the impact of physical therapies on patients in this sanatorium which he presented in 1925 at a conference on resort studies in Pyatigorsk, Russia, and a daring pamphlet (not mentioned in his memoir, but clearly a profitable venture) on 'sex life and physical culture' in 1927.[19] Soviet physical education ('physical culture') was an increasingly important arena for medical, industrial, and military sponsorship, and Kaminsky found a key mentor in the local secretary of the region's Physical Culture Council, L. L. Sakhnovsky, who steered him towards work in military and factory sanatoria and sport-related physiotherapy. Kaminsky's life took a glamorous turn: the charismatic Sakhnovsky got him placements studying horseback riding as a training method for military servicemen, and in 1931 made him the ship's doctor on a yachting tour from Odesa across the Black Sea to Istanbul with a Soviet football team.[20] By the early 1930s Kaminsky was directing a section of a new Institute of Physical Culture in Odesa and held a researcher's academic post; colleagues encouraged him to seek a first-level doctoral degree in the field. Collecting a series of research papers into a manuscript, 'Physical culture as a therapeutic method', he sent it to Kyiv's physical education institute requesting that it be published. After a long wait, Kaminsky was stunned to learn that the Kyiv institute's director insisted on his name on the book as 'co-author'. Between 1934 and 1935 Kaminsky quarrelled with the Kyiv institute director trying to retain control over the book and get the doctoral degree from his physiotherapy research. Ultimately, in 1936 Kaminsky abandoned physiotherapy and wrote a dissertation on radiology, submitting it to the Odesa Medical Institute in May 1937. The defence was set for October – but on 30 July 1937 Yakov Kaminsky was arrested on charges of 'counterrevolutionary Trotskyite activity' and sentenced to eight years' imprisonment. A colleague in the Medical Institute had denounced him, and his NKVD inquisitor twisted his early activity for the Maccabi Jewish fitness society as 'anti-Soviet' and Trotskyite political agitation.[21] Instead of rising on the academic ladder, he found himself in a railway carriage headed for the Russian Far North.

Kaminsky does not say how he first came to practise medicine while being transported to the Gulag; however, his commitment to medical service undoubtedly propelled him to make himself known when prisoners fell ill. By train he travelled to the railhead at Kotlas, some 900 kilometres northeast of Moscow, after which his prisoner group went by a river barge holding hundreds of prisoners for the next stage of the journey. On board Kaminsky was one of twelve doctors working in an improvised clinic to deal with prisoner illness. At Kniazh-Pogost, a river station 120 kilometres from Ukhta, the prisoners were unloaded for distribution to the region's camp divisions; some were being sent as far north as Vorkuta, beyond the Arctic Circle. Here, Yakov Kaminsky was interviewed by Nikolai Viktorov, the Ukhta camps' Sanotdel director who 'was courteous and in general made a good impression on us'. Luckily, the camp's chief radiologist was about to finish his sentence, and Kaminsky was assigned to work in the radiology cabinet and run a tuberculosis department at Vetlosian Central Camp Hospital.[22] Within months Kaminsky was directing the radiology cabinet, and his reform of the

TB wards reduced mortality and gained him a reputation as the best expert on the disease in the region. Viktorov sent him on short assignments beyond Vetlosian, to clinics for free employees and other camp subdivisions to give advice on TB therapies. Kaminsky organised medical conferences at Vetlosian (recalled warmly by Viktor Samsonov); he presented papers on the problems of tuberculosis in the camp.

Yakov Kaminsky tells the story of how in 1943 he was appointed chief doctor of Vetlosian with characteristic panache. The director of the entire Gulag Sanotdel, Dr David Maximovich Loidin, made an inspection visit to Ukhta, and Vetlosian Hospital in 1943.[23] At this stage in the war, with supplies exhausted and labour demands unchecked, prisoner mortality was enormous – in these years as much as one-quarter of the camp inmate population perished, according to official statistics.[24] Real death counts were even higher. According to Kaminsky, the Sanotdel director convened a meeting of Vetlosian's medical staff, free and prisoner alike, berating them for the high mortality rate in the 600-bed hospital, threatening them with charges of sabotage; he demanded explanations. After a long silence, Kaminsky says that he spoke up:

'I will explain the mortality!' I spoke these words harshly and confidently, but in my throat, I was choking with anxiety. 'Who are you, state your identity,' Loidin sharply replied. I reeled off the words I'd used for five years: 'Kaminsky Yakov Iosifovich, born 1897, sentence eight years for counterrevolutionary Trotskyite activity, commencing July 1937 ...' And then a hot, decisive monologue: 'Citizen director, you are simply incorrect! You do not know the crux of the matter ... You do not see the people who are brought to the hospital, they come to us in a state of extreme emaciation, unconscious ... The reason for the high mortality is that the prisoners are so very poorly fed. They become emaciated and perish from it. And you say that we don't treat them ... If you would like to see how we treat them, I invite you to come to my department right now. There we are using everything we have today to care for tubercular patients. And there you will certainly see patients who are doomed …' Behind me someone started, 'That's enough, sit down!' But I had the bit between my teeth and went on at length. I told him what I thought needed to be done to keep people in the camp from dying. Loidin listened attentively, not interrupting. He left without speaking, and without saying goodbye.[25]

Within days, after a shake-up of Ukhta's local Sanotdel leadership, Kaminsky was appointed chief doctor of Vetlosian Central Camp Hospital.

Whether the prisoner-physician actually dared to speak so boldly to the Gulag's top medical bureaucrat is impossible to verify. Loidin was a Moscow-educated doctor who had seen some of the best and worst Soviet medicine had to offer. He earned his spurs in the Soviet railway's embedded medical service, only to move in 1932 into Gulag hospital work for railway-construction camps. Nevertheless, Loidin's harangue as recalled by Kaminsky conforms to the top Sanotdel director's 'aggressive and accusatory style' as seen in lengthy September 1945 conference transcripts that do survive.[26] At this gathering of Gulag medical managers, he took a similar approach, cynically blending harsh accusations of his doctors' 'criminality' and negligence with honeyed advice to be more resourceful medics, and more collaborative with camp commandants (a dubious pathway to prisoner well-being). Loidin the Sanotdel chief seems gifted with selective hearing in this meeting, too, giving Kaminsky's account a degree of authenticity. Another confirmation that Kaminsky was not simply embellishing his recollections comes from contemporary commandant testimonials not solicited for his memoirs, but held in Ukhta's museum collections: he was genuinely respected for his 'conscientious attitude towards his work', for the high demands he made of himself and his team, his 'modesty and self-criticism' in his assessment of his performance.[27] His enthusiasm for establishing a radium-water resort in Ukhta would be of a piece with this profile of restless medical service. By turning to examine the background to the Ukhta radium-water factory, we can guess what Kaminsky could have known and understood about its operation by this time.

Ukhta's radium-water factory and
the physiotherapy laboratory

Awareness of the natural riches of this remote corner dawned before the 1917 revolutions, and yet it was only in 1926 that the first expedition mapped and discovered the radium-salt waters of the district. Their exploitation did not begin until the 1930s when the Gulag started to develop the Ukhtpechlag complex of oil, gas, and coal-mining camps in the region. Scientific testing of the waters found at Vodny began in summer 1930 and established that they had an exceptionally high concentration of radium – eight to ten times the concentration found at comparable sources in central Europe. In November 1931 construction began on a factory to distil radium bromide crystals from the water. It was fully operational by 1934 and secretly produced significant quantities of the radioactive crystals. The factory grew in size and complexity: by 1936 almost 4,000 prisoners and 500 freely hired workers lived in nearby barracks and worked on a site with seven 'factories' and dozens of huge distillery vats connected by several kilometres of wooden pipes (no more serviceable materials were available). Radium was an extremely rare element in the first half of the twentieth century. By 1952 the entire global stocks of radium consisted of 2.5 kilograms; the Vodny factory complex had by then produced 271 grams. Over one-tenth of the world's supply of radium came from this secret Gulag installation.[28]

In September 1932 the director of the entire Gulag camp system, Matvei Davydovich Berman, visited Ukhtpechlag and, in a meeting with local commandants, decreed that a resort should be established at Vodny to exploit the radium waters. Experts of the Institute of Resort Studies in Moscow made a rushed visit to the site and, despite the difficulties of access, agreed it should be developed as a 'resort of all-Union significance', in other words, a major spa with investment from the centre, and elite access protocols. Such all-Union resorts were distinguished from resorts of 'local' significance, where access was easier to gain for middling and lower officialdom and workers. At Vodny, the Ukhtpechlag Sanotdel chief, a career NKVD medical bureaucrat, Yakov Petrovich Sokolov, conducted tests on twenty-eight people suffering various ailments; all but two experienced some improvement, and on this basis the medical value of the waters was considered proven to Gulag officials and the Institute's experts.[29] In autumn 1932, following Gulag director Berman's decree, a 'hydrotherapy hospital' (*balneolechebnitsa*) also called a 'physiotherapy laboratory' (*fizlaboratoriia*) was constructed in Vodny. A prisoner-doctor, A. A. Titaev, began treating more patients and studying the effects of his treatments. The resort institute in Moscow also made a hurried analysis of the water and its healing properties, publishing a study of their findings for Ukhtpechlag in 1933.[30] This study appeared in Russian with French and German summaries that suggest early uncertainty about the secrecy of the physiotherapy experiments; the report remains classified in the State Archives of the Russian Federation to this day.[31]

The principles of radioactive water therapy were well established by the early 1930s, but internationally and in the Soviet Union, experts were also aware of the dangers of excess exposure. The 1933 report of the Institute of Resort Studies on the effects of Ukhta water acknowledged that its findings were merely preliminary, but presented

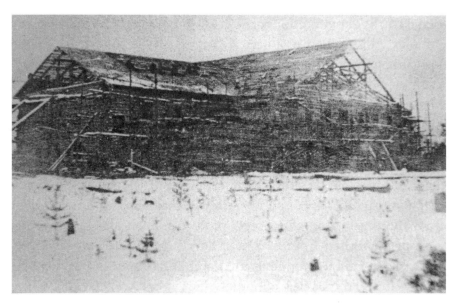

32. Ukhta's radium-water factory under construction, early 1930s.

an optimistic view of prospects for therapies, including drinking and inhalation, but especially in baths. Immersion produced a stimulating effect on muscles, joints, and other tissues, and such treatment was held to be effective in relieving the symptoms of or even curing arthritis and defects of the organs of movement, and of the peripheral nervous system. For the Institute's scientists and doctors, an exciting feature of the Ukhta water was that its radium could be distilled into crystals, transported with apparent ease around the country, and the healing water reconstituted by dissolving the crystals when and where it was needed, although it would prove that the wherewithal to achieve this advantage taxed the available human and physical resources beyond reasonable limits.[32]

At this time, scientists had an incomplete, and disputed, understanding of the dangers of excess exposure to radioactivity. Soviet experts were well aware of international precautions, debates, and tragedies (an American steel magnate died in 1932 having drunk radium-salt water every day for a year, noted a Moscow resort studies institute professor); and yet, Soviet radiation hygiene protocols were comparatively primitive.[33] Well into the 1940s, the Vodny Radium Factory official who personally conveyed refined radium to the Leningrad Radium Institute slept on an ordinary sleeper train with the vial of radioactive material under his pillow. When arriving at the institute, its director received him by hiding in the farthest possible corner of a large room, directing him to remove and store the vials securely.[34] A 1935 secret manual for a Moscow factory handling 'rare elements' – an early uranium-processing facility – recommended safety measures to reduce workers' exposure to radiation. These measures, judged rudimentary by today's standards, might have been implemented with civilian workers in the capital, but very little was done for prisoners or even free workers who distilled radium in Vodny, or handled the highly concentrated waters in the physiotherapy laboratory.[35]

Who were the subjects of the Vodny physiotherapy laboratory, and what were their treatments like? The first human 'patients' (a word to use advisedly) were both prisoners and free members of the camp staff: commandants, bureaucrats, guards, and their families.

The proportion of prisoners to free patients is unknown, but if we consider that for every free worker there were eight prisoners in 1936 in Vodny, and that they were less healthy than their free counterparts, then prisoners probably constituted a large share.[36] According to one source, in its nine years of operation, the physiotherapy laboratory treated 1,500 individuals.[37] They presented a wide range of illnesses: rheumatism, sciatica, gout, 'various chronic illnesses of the female sexual sphere', scurvy, nephritis, and neurasthenia.[38] Bathing was the chief technique employed: typically, patients bathed once a day for ten to fourteen days in succession in the radioactive waters, carried in wooden buckets to open-air bathtubs. Following a German medical researcher's 1931 report that the benefits of radium-bathing were extended if the bather did not towel off the healing waters, the Ukhta bathers also refrained from doing so. In Moscow, at the Institute of Resort Studies, patients given experimental Ukhta-water baths were allowed an hour's rest after bathing and were then subjected to a battery of blood and urine tests. The Ukhta physiotherapy laboratory conducted similar tests, albeit in the more primitive Gulag setting and using less sophisticated equipment.[39] One prisoner-doctor, A. A. Lyubushin, nevertheless managed to invent a special radioactive toothpaste to cure dental ailments using the radium waters, an attempt to develop a substitute for an expensive German imported brand. Research papers on the effects of the 'healing waters' on various illnesses were written, but not published, by Lyubushin and his colleagues. They were evidently assisted in this work by free nurses and technicians.[40]

A significant body of subjects came from the prisoners working in the radium distillation factory itself. Titaev and his successors as director of the laboratory (all prisoners themselves) were responsible for monitoring the health of this unfree workforce through the typical Soviet system of 'dispensarisation', or periodic outpatient examination, tests, and treatment.[41] Prisoner-workers suffered sharply declining health in the factory, and were effectively guinea pigs, studied for the effects of radiation in humans. Alongside them, rabbits were kept in the factory workshops and regularly slaughtered and examined for anomalies due to radioactivity. Monthly and annual reports of the human dispensary observations were fed back to the Gulag headquarters in Moscow. The physiological laboratory paid special attention to blood and urine anomalies, female reproductive disturbances, and motor disorders. The overall loss of 'labour capacity' was such that by 1937 the Gulag's management finally directed the doctors in this laboratory to investigate Vodny's workplace conditions and recommend safety precautions. The physiotherapy laboratory's director Lyubushin presented a stiff report calling for special protective clothing, protective shields in the distilleries, supplements to the prisoner-worker diet, and a shortening of their total work time in the facility. Some of these recommendations were acted upon since prisoners reportedly regarded Vodny as 'a resort' because of the reduced workday and extra rations. And yet they continued to reject wearing heavy rubber gloves and aprons, ate their lunches next to radioactive vats, and smoked while exposed to high radioactivity.[42]

Kaminsky's dream of a 'Northern Resort'

For reasons that remain unexplained, the physiotherapy laboratory at Vodny closed in 1941. One local historian suggests that the laboratory declined after its chief sponsor, Ukhtpechlag chief commandant Yakov Moroz, was arrested and shot in 1938.[43] Nevertheless, a new director of the laboratory, Oskar Avgustovich Stepun (a prisoner and physiologist) was appointed that same year and served until it closed, generating more research papers on radium-water therapies. Two authoritative local historians of the radiation facility indicate that the archives say very little about the Vodny factory at all for the 1940s and point out that secrecy about it intensified in these years.[44] In 1941 the prisoner-doctor Stepun was transferred to work in Ukhta's hospitals. With the rise of attention paid to the development of nuclear weaponry and radioactive materials during the war, the top Gulag hierarchy clearly began to see Vodny as highly strategic and wanted fewer, not more, unmonitored visitors to the site. In March 1940 in frigid conditions, a large, multidisciplinary commission from the Academy of Sciences in Moscow visited Vodny and spoke to local doctors and geologists. It received a report from the

Vodny radium factory's exasperated chief geologist Kulevsky explaining how critical information 'was buried in the secret archives and not made available' to experts who were trying to do their jobs efficiently. The visitors from the Academy of Sciences apparently concluded that, as regrettable as this secrecy might be for local scientists, Vodny and its radium source should remain cloaked in secrecy.[45]

As the war was drawing to a close, and not long after his appointment as chief physician of Vetlosian Hospital, Yakov Kaminsky became a staunch advocate of reopening the physiology laboratory and expanding it as a radium waters treatment centre. He learned about Ukhta's 'healing waters' from his colleagues in Vetlosian, including the poet and feldsher Ostap Vyshnia who had been so captivated by the radium-water story that he outlined an entire novel (never published) based on its discovery.[46] Moreover, the 'famous pathophysiologist Professor Stepun' persuaded an initially disbelieving Kaminsky of the efficacy of radioactive bathing. Stepun shared copies of the laboratory's research works with him.[47] In 1944, in a handwritten, self-published pamphlet with a striking watercolour cover, Kaminsky assembled the scientific data about the resources available for a 'Northern Resort', and arguments for urgent investment in a resort of all-Union significance.[48] Given the geologist Kulevsky's complaints in 1940 about information hidden in 'secret archives', it is striking that Kaminsky had access to the detailed Moscow Institute of Resort Studies 1933 report assessing the radium-water therapy's potential, as well as to eight years of the Vodny physiology laboratory's reports and observations. According to Kaminsky, of the hundreds of patients treated at Vodny, the vast majority reportedly experienced some degree of improvement in their conditions, with 10 per cent making full recoveries. 'Many cases have been observed where one can speak of a "miracle cure",' he wrote.[49] Kaminsky's conversion to curative radium bathing was evidently rooted in his experience, early in his career, in therapeutic radiology, the subject of his ill-fated second dissertation, and still more in his enthusiasm for sanatorium healthcare and physical culture. He imagined a facility that would offer not just radium-water bathing, but sulphur and mud baths using natural resources in

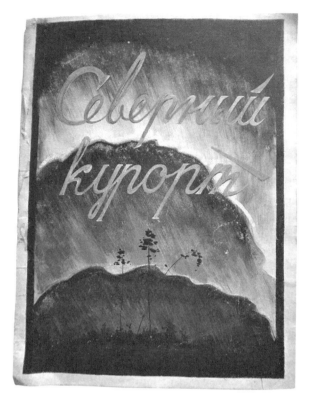

33. Kaminsky's pamphlet, 'Northern Resort', with a cover illustrated by Lithuanian prisoner-artist Boleslav Motuza-Matuziavichius, 1944.

the vicinity of Ukhta, previously studied by geologists but never fully exploited.[50]

Kaminsky offered a lyrical vision of the new resort, which he proposed to site not at Vodny, but on a lakeside near the principally civilian hospital complex outside Ukhta, at the Sangorodok. A programme of exercise and physical activity would round out the daily regimen of the Northern Resort. He wrote,

The long, windless, snowy winter creates conditions for healthy recreation, for the organisation of many forms of winter sports for patients, that, in conjunction with therapeutic physical culture, will enhance the effect of the resort treatment. The large quantity of birdlife in the virgin forests would attract hunters here, and in the summer months delicious fish (grayling) would reward the labours of amateur anglers. There are many wild berries (cranberries, blackberries, raspberries) and mushrooms in the forest. The resort-visitors' free time can thus be put to use productively and with interest.[51]

Kaminsky also devoted several pages to making a business case for the Northern Resort that would attract state planners' attention. Wounded soldiers would require specialist treatment for trauma and nerve disorders, and the Ukhta waters with their unique healing potential constituted a resource of not merely Soviet, but international medical significance, justifying the investment. He also argued that local workers merited a high-grade resort on their doorstep, since before the war the Soviet health commissariat had already made the localisation of resort therapies a goal (ostensibly, to relieve the strain on the national railway network).[52]

Yakov Kaminsky sent copies of the pamphlet to the Komi Republic's branch of the Soviet health commissariat, and a summary to Moscow's Institute of Resort Studies, and also tried to get articles promoting the scheme published in the local press. The silence that greeted Kaminsky's proposal was total, apparently another indication that the secret police wanted no curious hunters, anglers, or mushroom-pickers roaming in the vicinity of the classified radium distillery. The reason for all this secrecy was only revealed by local historians after the collapse of Soviet rule. They explain how the Vodny radium-water distillery expanded dramatically during and after the Second World War. At the height of its operation in the 1940s, it had 150 wells producing radium water, and twelve factories distilling about 17 grams of the radioactive element each year.[53] What is more, beginning in 1946, Moscow sent waste products from uranium-processing conducted at the Moscow Uranium Factory No. 12, for refinement at the Vodny factory site. In the Cold War nuclear arms race, curated for Stalin on the Soviet side by the secret police, it became an outpost, far from Moscow, where materials more suitable for weaponisation than radium, a comparatively weak element, could be processed.[54]

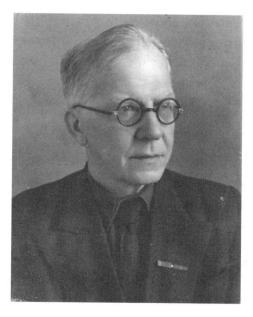

34. Fyodor Toropov, ex-prisoner and future Stalin Prize laureate, early 1940s.

The Vodny factory's archives explain what was then happening. Vodny's chief chemical engineer, Fyodor Aleksandrovich Toropov, a long-serving ex-prisoner 'free' employee of the facility, had developed the process for distilling radium bromide from Ukhta's water. In a 1939 report to state planners, he too proposed that the radium waters should be in a bathing-therapy resort. Like Kaminsky's proposal it was ignored. In the 1940s his star was on the rise, becoming one of the first Ukhta scientists to receive the Order of Lenin in 1943. In 1947 he was awarded a Stalin Prize for his radium-waters formula. Now his expertise would turn towards uranium as the vital ingredient for a bomb. In 1948 the Vodny commandant praised the Stalin laureate for developing 'a completely new technology for [. . .] extraction of uranium from the by-products of production' from the Moscow uranium plant. A 'politically literate person able to keep state secrets', Toropov remained at the heart of Vodny's shifting Cold-War mission until his sudden death, from natural causes, while on a family visit to Kazan in December 1953.[55] Fyodor Toropov's career, commemorated by the 'Progress' factory that still operates in Vodny today, illustrates why Ukhta's radium-water spa was never launched: the secret police were determined to keep it a 'state secret'.

'The water was not to blame – it was human carelessness and ignorance'

At some point during the war, Yakov Kaminsky began to suspect that the workers of Vodny were suffering from excess exposure to radiation. Perhaps this was even at the same time as the Vetlosian chief doctor was writing his upbeat pamphlet about Ukhta's 'healing waters'. Kaminsky's memoirs distinguish carefully between the therapeutic value of the radium water, as he then understood it, and the consequences of radioactive contamination around the Vodny factory for human health, which he came to investigate later in the 1950s–1960s. (It is also clear that Kaminsky and his Odesa memoir editors were unaware of the uranium-processing at Vodny.) Kaminsky's account suggests that, as he looked back in the 1990s, he recognised his own ignorance of the dangers, in the wider context of the Gulag's 'workplace negligence' that considered the medical monitoring and protection of Vodny's prisoner and free workforce a low priority.

> In Vetlosian I didn't know anything about this, even though there were prisoners working in the factory. Yet even before the war I was struck by the large number of patients presenting symptoms without an explicable cause. The symptoms reminded me of something very familiar! In the course of a year, I carefully conducted up to 2,000 blood tests and came to the conclusion: radiation sickness. Of course, I myself had suffered from it in 1924!
>
> But what should I do? Who can a zek turn to? Who to write to? The only accepted route was via a written report to the Sanitary administration of the Gulag. But who would be interested in some kind of radiation sickness, still only hypothetical, in wartime when the country demanded radium? People would get infected and die for many more years . . .[56]

As a prisoner, then ex-prisoner 'exile' confined to live in Ukhta after release in 1945, Kaminsky the hospital doctor lacked the authority and the scientific knowledge, he says, to challenge the secret police bosses at Vodny.[57] Maybe he could have spoken up, but in retrospect the problem was far larger and more complex than he imagined. Many sources point to the 1949 reconstruction of the factory, until then consisting of wooden sheds, vats and even pipes, as a factor in extending local radiation exposure. Vodny's inhabitants, resourceful Soviet survivors that they were, spontaneously repurposed the heavily irradiated building materials from the factory, using them in schools, homes, and street furniture.[58] Kaminsky describes the contamination of the settlement in his memoir, but he may not have become aware of it until the later 1950s. Even in the 1990s, he was clearly unaware of the uranium-processing at the factory, and he may in fact have encountered patients with more than just exposure to radium.

Whatever he knew about failures of industrial hygiene at Vodny, Kaminsky used the changing political context of Khrushchev's de-Stalinisation to learn more. Receiving full rehabilitation in 1956, Kaminsky was emboldened to pursue the problem of radiation sickness. He was among local experts who sought to have the region's radioactive contamination investigated. In 1956 the USSR Ministry of Health sent a commission from Moscow to examine the Vodny factory. The visiting experts deemed Vodny's facility unsafe, and radium production was immediately shut down.[59] A further commission from the Institute of Resort Studies visited and reported on the region's resort potential, minus the radioactive waters, in 1959.[60]

By the late 1950s, Soviet hygienists and industrial experts were taking a comparatively rigorous view of the health dangers of radiation. In part, this was a technocratic and humanitarian response to an obvious problem that had long been treated with criminal negligence by the security police. Transfer to civilian and military control, it was hoped, would lead to decreased danger and better systems design.[61] From the technical side, the shift at this time towards greater attention to radiation hygiene came as nuclear weaponry called for far larger and more dangerous stocks of powerfully radioactive material, uranium and plutonium. Radium-crystal distillation at Vodny was now regarded as an embarrassing irrelevance.[62] In Ukhta, medical professionals began to investigate the local impact of radiation. With Sangorodok physician Evgeny Kharechko, Kaminsky had already conducted unsanctioned dosimetry readings that revealed radiation hotspots around the district. They won funding for an official examination of long-term exposure to 'natural radiation' (clearly a euphemism) from the Komi Republic health ministry and the USSR Academy of Sciences. The project lasted three years and uncovered hundreds of cases of sickness caused by contamination.[63] Kaminsky recalls one tragic example from his practice:

> The memory of one patient refuses to give me peace even to this day. She came to me long after the factory had been closed. Maria Zykova was a surprisingly sympathetic and vibrant woman, a free employee. After an X-ray examination I immediately suspected something was not right, and sent her to Moscow, to the Radiological Institute. (She had regularly handled radium powder in her bare hands, without gloves . . .)[64]

Zykova would suffer from a complex of cancers and lost both hands to amputation, before dying of lung cancer soon after. Kaminsky comments, 'That woman was a victim of workplace negligence and medical inexperience with illnesses of this origin – I will never in my entire life forget this. I have kept her patient records to this day.'[65] Zykova's story is just one of hundreds of such tragedies from the Ukhta region's experience of mishandled radioactive substances. The scandal of the Gulag and nuclear industry's decades-long neglect of hygiene in Vodny would not be discussed publicly until the 1990s, and even then, only by local historians and the few surviving witnesses.

A final mystery

In January 1953 Yakov Kaminsky was issued a new identity card by the Ukhta Gulag camp authorities, a pass giving him access to the offices of the central camp administration. A perfectly ordinary

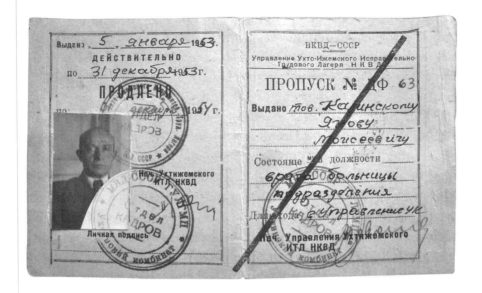

35. Moiseevich not Iosifovich: secretary's error or something more sinister? Kaminsky's Gulag identity card, 5 January 1953.

official document, it bore a strange 'error': his patronymic 'Iosifovich' (son of Joseph) was absent, unaccountably replaced by 'Moiseevich' (son of Moisey). The change might have been a busy secretary's slip, or it might have held a more sinister meaning.

In late 1952 Stalin's last terror campaign was under way, and the secret police were vigilantly fabricating a new conspiracy narrative based on the dictator's fantasies of disloyalty. The 'Doctors' Plot' targeted physicians with connections to the Kremlin's exclusive medical service, mostly Jewish ones. They were accused, falsely, of attempting to murder top Soviet leaders including Stalin himself. Soviet anti-Semitic campaigning in the last years of Stalin's dictatorship combined popular Russian xenophobia and anti-Semitism with Stalin's mistrust of any Soviet citizen with a potential second loyalty – in this case, to the new state of Israel.[66] Soviets who, during the war, had represented international Jewish relief organisations like the 'Joint' or who had worked with their foreign representatives, were now held to have taken orders from US spy agencies to commit acts of treason and medical sabotage.[67]

Ex-political prisoner Kaminsky would have been an unlikely target of this campaign: he was far from the Kremlin and its hospitals and clinics, still an 'exile' tied to Ukhta. Kaminsky was a small fish compared to the accused in the Doctors' Plot. They were publicly denounced eight days after this ID card was issued, in a sensational article in the pages of *Pravda*. And yet Kaminsky's association in the 1920s in Odesa with the 'Joint' and with the Maccabi Jewish fitness society might have been noted with a view to building a fresh case against him. The chekists in the Gulag knew how to be vigilant. Moreover, in civilian medicine the purging of Jewish doctors had begun as early as 1950, with medical researchers and lecturers subjected to reviews of identity documents and formal qualifications, leading to dismissal of half of these Jewish academics by the end of 1952.[68] When asked about how the Doctors' Plot affected her in Magadan, Anna Kliashko remarked, 'We heard about it of course – you only needed to have ears!' An atheist and not a Party member, she believed she was safe in distant Kolyma, but her gentile husband feared for her nonetheless.[69]

Was this 'mistaken' patronymic a deliberate one, intended perhaps to insist on his Jewish origins and to remind guards in an insinuating fashion to be vigilant should he try to enter the commandant's office? We cannot know from the sources at our disposal. Kaminsky avoids all discussion of the Doctors' Plot in his memoirs, which were composed at a time when interest in 'Stalin's last crime' (as it has been called) was at its peak. The Odesa Memorial researchers working with Kaminsky on his memoir would surely have included reminiscences about the anti-Semitic campaign had the old doctor mentioned it. Meanwhile, the inventory and documents in his folder at the Ukhta Museum of the History of Public Health – all assembled by local researchers in the far northern city, in the years after Kaminsky's memoir and death – say nothing about this anomalous identity document. The puzzle of this erroneous patronymic on a Jewish doctor's pass to the portals of supreme power in the Gulag camp is unsolvable. Kaminsky's identification with his Jewish heritage is proudly proclaimed in the early passages of his memoir, remembering how he overcame the tsarist quota on entrants to higher education and worked for the 'Joint' and the Maccabi society. He speaks openly about the Civil-War-era pogroms that devastated his family's fortunes, and yet he is silent about the high Stalinist anti-Semitic episode that left this trace in the archive.

Whatever his experience of the 'Doctors' Plot', Kaminsky clearly felt confident enough to pursue his investigation into the misuses of radiation, and the prospects for therapeutic bathing in the district where he was forced to serve the Gulag. Eventually, his attempts to rekindle interest in the region's resort potential, such as it was, turned to focus not on Ukhta's radioactive waters, but its sulphurous muds. Progress towards the foundation of a mud-therapy resort moved with a majestic restraint typical of the years of Soviet leader Leonid Brezhnev's rule after 1964. In 1972 Kaminsky was 75 years old, and had moved back to his native Ukraine, by the time Ministry of Health officials gave the green light for a 'mud-therapy hospital' (*griazlechebnitsa*) in Ukhta. Construction began in 1985, and the facility, capable of handling 500 visitors per shift in courses of treatment lasting 30 days, finally opened in April 1989, still serving local patients to this day.[70] No one in Moscow, however, boards a train for the 45-hour journey to Ukhta to seek out this clinic, the unlikely legacy of Gulag commandants, a Ukrainian-Jewish radiologist, and a Ukrainian prisoner-writer who once dreamed of a 'Northern Resort' and the songs that would be sung to its heroes.

CONCLUSION

'No archival materials will be gathered, and people will scatter . . .'

On 31 August 1946 young Viktor Samsonov was finally preparing to leave Ukhta, where he had been a prisoner for nine years from the age of 18, to start medical school in Ivanovo, central Russia. From a bench overlooking Vetlosian Hospital he gazed on his first, and harshest, university:

> I looked at the panorama of the camp settlement with its single-storey hospital buildings and barracks, and recalled episodes from my life here, the work I did in general labour, in the hospital departments, and even in the morgue, situated somewhere behind me [. . .] When my gaze fell upon the high camp fence with barbed wire, on the watchtower, my memory called up the vision of columns of prisoners setting off to work in the forest. Oh, how hard you had to slog there!
>
> Here they are, my little wards, where I worked and studied. Here are the medics confined to the camp zone, struggling their utmost to wrench weakened and sick sloggers from the dreaded claws of death. To me, these doctors, feldshers, and lekpoms were my selfless teachers. I silently thanked all of them, and especially Professor Vilhelm Vittenburg, and docent Yakov Kaminsky! And not only to the zeks, but to the many freely hired colleagues, who showed sympathy by sharing medical books with me. Thank you, decent people of all positions and ranks! They all helped me to

survive not just physically but morally; they helped me to start my life over from the beginning.[1]

Samsonov's memoir offers a valedictory passage, cinematic in its calm gaze passing over the hospital grounds, leading towards a darker flashback of prisoners remembered on the march to hard labour in the forests. The soon-to-be medical student puts his Gulag past behind him, with the camp's terrors recalled alongside its opportunities for learning. Somehow, he had escaped the 'dreaded claws of death'. Yet even in this farewell to a hospital that helped him to 'start my life over from the beginning' death is ubiquitous, and the morgue was a gateway to an unanticipated profession.

This literary vignette by a fortunate Gulag survivor, someone who climbed aboard the lifeboat of Gulag medicine, needs to be set against the reflection that so many prisoners did not survive and could not record their experiences. However much good the Gulag medical system could do, it could not save these millions of victims. In June 2009 in Moscow, I interviewed the daughter of the Vetlosian psychiatrist Lev Sokolovsky. Tatyana Oleinik talked to me about her childhood in the city of Ukhta and her visits back there with her own children. In 1949 her father had remarried, this time to ex-prisoner Zenoviya Mikhailovna Kazanivskaya, whom he had met as a patient in 1947; she had been a Polish laboratory student from Lviv, and he found her a post in a Vetlosian lab. Tatyana was born, grew up, and went to school in a town where Gulag memory was transforming as 'normal' life took hold. Her father's hospital, Vetlosian, was closed and demolished. Oleinik described the landscape at the Sangorodok, the town's other major labour-camp hospital that became the chief medical facility in normalising Ukhta.

I remember how I went to the Sangorodok cemetery. Now it's gone, it was all demolished. There was a cemetery for free persons; and just beyond it was a huge field. There were stakes standing up in it, like pencils – about this height [gestures: about a foot]. With a number on them. And they stretched so far that you couldn't see the horizon. I remember that. I remember how my mother said,

'What scum, what swine!' She was alone with me, and she thought I was too little to understand, but it shocked her, even as a grown-up, it was so endless this field where they buried them, and not a single one with a name. Nothing but numbers. And later they demolished it all. I went back there later, when I had two sons, and we waited until they were old enough, at least 12, to take them to Ukhta so that they would understand where we had come from, and there was nothing to see, it had all been cleared away. That was in about 1989, long after the moment I had been there as a little girl with my mother.[2]

The memory of the Gulag was fading, with the help of municipal authorities who obliterated the prisoners' cemetery with its grave markers made of wooden stakes and metal numbers. Such erasures of prisoner cemeteries were widespread around the Gulag territories, and researchers in the 'democratic' 1980s and 1990s found it difficult and sometimes impossible to identify sites of burial.[3]

The Gulag hospital could be a place of healing, compassion, and learning, while often simultaneously a portal to death after penal malnutrition, exhaustion, and systemic neglect. How can we comprehend the meaning of medical care in the forced-labour camps? It was a troubling, and extremely differentiated, feature of the Gulag's organisation and of prisoners' experience, encompassing darkness and light. It was both Alexander Solzhenitsyn's gateway to oblivion 'born of the devil and filled with the devil's blood', and Viktor Samsonov's fondly remembered 'little wards' where honourable medics struggled 'to wrench weakened and sick sloggers from the dreaded claws of death'. We can hardly be surprised that Solzhenitsyn greeted the gift of one of Samsonov's Gulag memoirs with stony silence.[4]

This book has argued that Solzhenitsyn's wholesale dismissal of Gulag medicine deprives us of deeper understanding. Looking for, and analysing, examples of the thousands of doctors, nurses, feldshers, and officials who established medical facilities and made them run in the heart of a penal empire raises questions about the nature of the camp system and the motives of the ordinary people who staffed it. This book has offered some answers, even if they are only situational and tentative, to the puzzles of their actions. The Gulag medical world was a 'grey zone' where the 'sovereign' power of commandants and guards confronted the 'disciplinary' power of medical expertise. Doctors were human – they made choices with ethical consequences when they tilted towards one form of power as they potentially undermined the other. A 'good doctor's' clinical decision to 'save' a prisoner-poet through medical 'tufta' undercut the authority of the camp commandant, work-assignment managers, and internal security police. A 'bad doctor's' physical assessment of an emaciated 'slogger' that forced him back to general labour in forests or mines contradicted conventional medical values and apparently even Soviet norms. Sorting doctors into 'good' and 'bad' professionals is simple in theory. Yet when we begin to probe concrete cases, such as those of Yan Pullerits, Nikolai Glazov, Nina Savoeva, Vadim Aleksandrovsky, Maria Kolinenko, or Lev Sokolovsky, we immediately see how the balance of good and evil in the course of a person's life is devilishly hard to weigh. Even Solzhenitsyn, in a more temperate mood, recognised that 'the line separating good and evil passes not through states, nor between classes, nor between political parties either – but right through every human heart – and through all human hearts. This line shifts. Inside us, it oscillates with the years.'[5] That shifting line, marking human decency and indifference in the face of suffering, ran through the hearts of the Gulag's doctors, nurses, feldshers, and medical workers. The line, and its shifts, were seriously affected by the penal setting and Moscow's Stalinist ideology. Our evaluation of medical workers' accomplishments, and crimes, needs to be conscious of that truth.

Features of Gulag medicine previously obscured in our histories of Stalin's forced-labour camps have been illuminated by the lives this book explores. Many of these features are entwined with the 'police colonisation' mission of the NKVD. The labour-camp system emerges as an unexpected locus of apprenticeship, of professional development, and institution-building, for both prisoner and freely hired medical workers. Prisoner-doctors were diverted by arrest and imprisonment from their familiar civilian, military, and embedded medical networks and forcibly relocated to far-flung corners of the Soviet Union where medical expertise was needed, but the state refused to pay the full costs of 'free' employment. The forced reloca-tion, extraction of labour on exploitative terms, and the distinctions in status in Gulag staff were all features of the classic definitions of internal colonisation.[6] In a period of rapid and forced-labour construction these prisoner-medics contributed to the establishment of medical infrastructure as the Gulag's enterprises and settlements grew. Prisoner medical staff who carried an unequal burden in Gulag clinics and infirmaries also ensured the collective survival of a propor-tion, probably impossible to determine, of otherwise undersupplied, malnourished, and overworked zeks, protecting them when they could against some of the hazards of labour-camp life. The survival of significant populations of ex-prisoners in former Gulag regions, initially tied by bureaucratic exile to these territories, attests to the efforts of prisoner and ex-prisoner medical staff in the camps.

Free medical workers from nurses and feldshers to qualified physicians and medical bureaucrats found opportunities for social mobility, enhanced responsibility, and career advancement in the penal setting. The case of free medical workers deserves further study to investigate how they navigated the 'original sin' of Gulag employ-ment in the post-Stalin years. In the 1950s, when other labour-camp officials in the early phase of de-Stalinisation were rattled by reformers in stormy Party meetings, how were Gulag medical leaders treated? The cases of Magadan medical managers Aleksei Khoroshev and Tatyana Repyeva suggest that their rare professional expertise in remote regions of the country earned them an escape from intense scrutiny.[7] In hospitals and clinics among ordinary physicians there was perhaps more forgiveness. Anna Kliashko recalled only respectful professional relations between freely hired doctors and those who had previously been prisoners, and she expressed passionate grati-tude for some ex-prisoner-physicians like Viktor Mikhailovich Shapiro, a doctor-zek with a fifteen-year sentence who had mentored her.[8] Lower down the medical hierarchy, the day-to-day resentments between prisoner and free nurses and feldshers (evident in Eugenia Ginzburg's account, and notably absent from the Pechora interviews with free nurses) seem unlikely to have dissipated until staff turnover and institutional reorganisation ruptured the camp system's habits.[9] Ex-prisoners like Ginzburg and Varlam Shalamov could find that their Gulag in-house nursing or feldsher training was not recognised by civilian healthcare officials. They were excluded from medical work unless, like Viktor Samsonov or Vadim Aleksandrovsky, they obtained 'legitimate' degrees from recognised institutions. The transition from Soviet labour-camp medicine to civilian practice merits further inquiry.

The reflections of Samsonov and Oleinik respectively on the landscapes of Vetlosian Central Camp Hospital and the Sangorodok's cemetery remind us of the dramatic differences in what is remembered about the Gulag and its medical system. A significant focus of this book has been on how labour-camp medicine has been commemorated as the Soviet regime came under deeper historical scrutiny. The medical history of the Gulag illustrates how regional commemoration has diverged in significant ways from conventional recollection of the camps in the Russian metropolises of Moscow and St Petersburg, as builders of 'roads to nowhere' and destroyers of human life. Medicine plays a marked and sometimes troubling role in regionally produced memory of the labour camps, advancing a narrative that often speaks about constructive contributions to the building of the region's towns, cities, and industry. In local monuments and museums, curators, activists, and historians have grappled with the legacy of the Gulag, and medical themes form an important element of this local commemoration.[10] These local medical stories often tell consoling narratives of heroism and humanity in the midst of illness and cruelty, finding 'bright' as well as 'dark' elements in individual lives. They cater to local patriotism – a primary function of certain types of regional museum – and command a significant post-Soviet residual authority as supposed purveyors of indisputable historical fact. As Sofia Gavrilova has noted in her work on Russia's regional-historical museums that present the labour camps' histories, curators and memory activists working in Gulag-built cities frequently struggled to find the right language to tell such stories.[11] Similarly, my account of Gulag medicine based on the memoirs, reminiscences, and testimony of doctors, nurses, and feldshers, finds no easy ways to weigh these stories. Instead, I suggest that they should be read as both a window into a 'grey zone' of labour-camp experience, and as a mirror, undoubtedly flawed, but no less important, that reflects how many Russians remember the Gulag.

'People will scatter . . .': Lives and fates

In the summer of 1934 Ostap Vyshnia began keeping a brief diary of his Gulag life, another sign of his remarkable privilege at this early stage in his career as a prisoner, since the zeks were normally not allowed access to writing materials, and prisoner diaries are virtually unknown. The 'forced-labour' historian was already worried that the corporate history of Ukhtpechlag was floundering. In early August the manuscript was ready, but it languished without agreement to publish on the desk of camp commandant Yakov Moroz. Despite the prisoner-editors' proposals, their 'special bureau' where the Ukrainian Vyshnia worked with the Uzbek Manon Ramzi to collect memoirs and documents was near to being shut down, making sustained historical study impossible. Of future projects to trace the history of this prison-camp region, Vyshnia wrote,

> Everything will have to be done 'campaign-style' [. . .] There won't be any systematic work, at least not on the orderly collection of materials about the history of Ukhtpechlag. Another ten years will pass [. . .] Everything will have perished, and none of the interesting facts about how people lived and worked here at the beginnings of Ukhta's industry will remain. No archival materials will be gathered, and people will scatter, get lost. If only we could collect and systematise these materials and then write interesting books about the period of Ukhta's foundation.[12]

By autumn 1934 Vyshnia's diary records that the fate of these projects is tied to Moscow's shifting priorities for Ukhtpechlag. No celebrations to mark 'five years of struggle' to build Ukhta and its industrial complex were going to be held; the corporate history he had edited would never be published. In his diary Vyshnia expresses pride in the work, even if Moroz in Ukhta, and Gulag chiefs in Moscow, block publication:

> In general it was not in vain that we worked so doggedly on the book, was it? And if the book doesn't come out, at least then the material is all assembled, put in order, and edited. Whenever the time is right – if not for our work, then for that of others, it will still be there! And be useful![13]

* * *

Yakov Kaminsky, the Jewish-Ukrainian radiologist who dreamed of a 'Northern Resort', returned to live and work in his native Odesa in 1961. He served in major hospitals in the city as director of radiology, conducting mass tuberculosis screening, popular sanitary education, and promoting the training of radiographic workers. In the 1970s he was awarded medals for his 'shockwork of Communist labour' and was designated an 'Honoured Physician of the Komi Republic'. He died in 1996. In 2000 the city of Ukhta posthumously named him a 'Citizen of the Century of Ukhta'.[14]

Lev Sokolovsky, the zek-psychiatrist who wrote so boldly about prisoners suffering from mental illness, was also designated an 'Honoured Physician of the Komi Republic' in 1961. His daughter Tatyana went to school with the children of other prisoners and labour-camp guards – 'we all studied in this school without any trouble or discrimination', she recalled, remembering that she was taught to take pride in her family's history and their service in the Gulag. In 1966 with his family Sokolovsky moved to the city of Yaroslavl in central Russia, where he worked in the provincial psychoneurological outpatient clinic. He died in 1987.[15]

Eufrosinia Kersnovskaya, the anatomist in the morgue of Norilsk Central Camp Hospital, abandoned medical jobs and served out her sentence underground as a miner in a women's brigade in Norilsk. She earned early release in August 1953. As a result of Moscow's annexation of Bessarabia (today's Moldova) into the Soviet Union during the Second World War, she was forced to accept Soviet citizenship. In retirement she relocated to Essentuki, a spa town in southern Russia in the shadow of the Caucasus mountains. A self-taught artist, she wrote and illustrated her memoirs several times over and left a vivid and unique body of documentary artwork about her Gulag years. She died in 1994.[16]

The nurse Serafima Davydenko, a 'free' employee of the Gulag, married a Soviet soldier who was sent to the camps for being taken prisoner of war. She was transferred out of Gulag medical services as the labour camps were reformed in the 1950s. She began working in the railway's sanitary service as a surgical nurse in the operating theatres of various northern hospitals. She had three children, and a happy marriage; but her husband was never rehabilitated for his 'crime'. He died in 1978, and Davydenko retired in 1988. Maria Kolinenko, another 'freely employed' Gulag nurse, married a deported Lithuanian doctor imprisoned in her camp; it was a choice that put her political reliability in the shade. They had a son, Albert, in 1946. Her husband was amnestied, and he abandoned his Russian wife and son to return to Lithuania. Albert never knew his father, and Kolinenko supported him without alimony from her ex-husband, who reportedly had a private medical practice in Lithuania.[17] Olga Klimenko wrote her memoirs about her youth and Gulag service as a prisoner-nurse, after release when she returned to her native Leningrad in the 1950s and 1960s. She is thought to have died in 1982.[18]

Viktor Samsonov completed medical school in Ivanovo and qualified as a physician in 1951. From 1952 to 1989 he worked in his native Petrozavodsk in medical facilities, defending both stages of his doctorate, specialising in pathology. He taught in the Leningrad Institute for the Professional Development of Doctors, headed the forensic-medical faculty of Petrozavodsk State University, and achieved the rank of full professor. He was named an Honoured Scientist of the Karelian Republic and later of the Russian Federation too. He wrote, and rewrote, his memoirs several times, and maintained a vigorous correspondence with friends and colleagues who shared his Gulag experience. He died in 2004.[19]

Vadim Aleksandrovsky, who was arrested in Leningrad before he could finish all his medical examinations, finally qualified as a doctor in 1956 with the timely intervention of a military-medical doctor and historian of Gulag medicine, Boris Nakhapetov. Aleksandrovsky served nine years in the Soviet Navy's medical service before discharge on health grounds; he settled in Leningrad and worked for a further twenty-eight years in the polyclinic of the Academy of Sciences. He retired in 1993. In the 1990s he conducted medical consultations for the St Petersburg department of the Association for Victims of Political Repressions, helping individuals to access welfare payments to victims of state violence. He died in 2002.[20]

Anna Kliashko, the Belarusian-Jewish girl who studied medicine while in evacuation in Siberia during the Second World War, and who chose the civilian medical system of Dalstroi as her first posting, worked in a succession of outposts in Kolyma region. She married a freely hired geologist working for Dalstroi. Eventually, they settled in Magadan where she directed the therapeutic department of the Central Provincial Hospital. She became a specialist in electrocardiogram services in the 1970s. By that time, she had been awarded medals for 'Excellence in Medical Work' and for 'Valorous Labour on the Occasion of the Centenary of the Birth of V. I. Lenin'. She was a neighbour of Nina Savoeva, and treated her for high blood pressure. After forty-four years working for the Magadan civilian medical system, Kliashko retired and emigrated with her husband and family to Canada. When her granddaughter began interviewing her for this book in June 2009, Anna had 'stopped feeling like a doctor', and her pleasure at replying to the questions we asked her resonates in the recordings. Anna died in 2018.[21]

Nina Savoeva, who 'chose Kolyma', was ejected from the Party in 1949 for marrying an ex-prisoner, Boris Lesniak. Leaving the Gulag's medical service circa 1953, she joined the civilian network in Magadan and worked as a surgeon for brain and skull trauma in the city's Central Provincial Hospital. She did not lose her edge. 'The years "beyond the zone" were neither smooth, nor peaceful. As ever I made both friends and enemies. The latter were most often among the managers, with whom I fought my entire life, and among people who were indifferent [about their work]. But that is another chapter.'[22] As far as I can determine, she did not win any labour-service awards. The couple raised a daughter in Magadan. Savoeva retired in 1972 and moved with Lesniak to Moscow. Her brief 1996 memoir won the respect of Memorial and local-history activists, despite her status as a 'freely hired' doctor and the harsh portrait of her in Eugenia Ginzburg's memoirs. Savoeva died in 2003.[23] Except for Sofia Guzikova's valorous front-line service in the Soviet army's medical branch, and hints that she practised medicine in post-war Moscow, I was unable to find any further information about her life and her decision to write her memoir of a Gulag doctor.

Nikolai Glazov was rehabilitated in May 1957, but he was not released from his last labour-camp job in Inta, Komi Republic, until 1959. In the same year he returned to his native Leningrad after winning a protracted battle to have his right to housing there restored. He also received the standard two months' back pay granted to all rehabilitated former 'political' prisoners. He very likely continued to practise medicine into the 1960s. In 1989, with the assistance of his daughter Margarita Glazova, he completed his memoirs. Glazov died not long after. Margarita participated in anti-Stalinist memory projects as a 'child of parents who were repressed', appearing with a group of activists releasing floral wreaths into the Neva River in Leningrad, in the film *The Russia We Have Lost* in 1992.[24]

Yan Pullerits, the founder of medical services in Magadan, was executed in the Great Terror in 1938. His daughter Margarita Pullerits was one of the hundreds of thousands of children who lost parents to the Stalinist repressions of 1937–38. Her mother Elena, arrested in 1938 as the 'wife of a traitor to the Motherland', would spend eight years in the camps. Margarita lived with her aunt Anna, her mother's sister, in Moscow; when the city was threatened by Nazi invaders they evacuated to live with relatives in Saratov, and never returned. They lost everything they left behind in Moscow. 'How we managed to stay alive and to survive the cold and hungry years is difficult to imagine.' Her mother returned from the Gulag only in 1946. In 1950 Margarita graduated from Saratov Pedagogic Institute and taught mathematics in Siberia and later in Saratov. A pensioner by 1989 when she wrote a memoir of her childhood and parents, she noted, 'Magadan always stayed with me with its severe but miraculous nature, the place where I spent my happy childhood.'[25]

Nikolai Viktorov, pioneering prisoner-doctor who built the medical service of Ukhta and its camp complex, was named an 'Honoured Physician of the Komi Republic' in 1961. The first modern academic historian of the industry of Ukhta region, Anna Kaneva, interviewed him in the late 1960s, in preparation for her first-stage doctoral dissertation, defended in 1970. Kaneva would later publish short biographical articles about Viktorov which cemented his reputation as the pioneer of medicine in Ukhta and the region. If he died alone in 1980 in a Syktyvkar nursing home, his memory was not forgotten in the city he helped to build. A photo and biography of Nikolai Viktorov is at the heart of a section of the exhibition entitled 'They Were the First' in the Ukhta Museum of the History of Public Health, and his is the very first chapter-length profile in a book chronicling the story of Ukhta medicine published by historians connected to the museum.[26]

Ostap Vyshnia, the 'forced-labour historian' of the Ukhta Gulag camps, was unexpectedly released from captivity in 1943. In that year, while Soviet Ukraine was still under Nazi occupation, a Ukrainian government-in-exile operated in Moscow. Two 'official artists' working for that government, Mykola Bazhan and Oleksandr Dovzhenko, were asked to nominate writers imprisoned in the Gulag who could be relied upon to assist with the war effort. They put Vyshnia on their list. He was transferred to a Moscow prison and then freed on 3 December 1943. Vyshnia first stayed with Yuri Smolych, 'who was keeping Soviet Ukrainian culture alive in the Soviet capital' and who later, in the 1960s, campaigned there for the commemoration of the generation of Ukrainian writers destroyed in the Stalinist purges.[27] During the war, Vyshnia wrote material supportive of Soviet rule over Ukraine, and attacking patriotic nationalists who opposed Moscow's rule. After 1945 he returned to writing humorous sketches about the human condition, even if some thought his work now 'lacked the depth and nuance of his earlier writing'.[28] His reputation as a powerful exponent of observational humour conveyed in Ukrainian nevertheless remained. The essence of his work, writes Mayhill Fowler, was 'larger than Ukrainian nationalism [... Vyshnia] rejected Moscow, but [...] also the capitalist West.

[He] believed in Ukraine, but a Ukraine that was not a part of the village, that was not anti-modern, but that was of the streets, and revelled in technology, jokes, and jazz melodies.'[29] Vyshnia was rehabilitated in October 1955, and died in September 1956, aged just 66. He was one of the few survivors of the Soviet Union's lethal terror that destroyed the Ukrainian cultural 'renaissance' of the 1920s, and his name is indelibly linked to the peculiar history of Gulag medicine in the Komi Republic.

NOTES

Abbreviations

GAMO   Gosudarstvennyi arkhiv Magadanskoi oblasti, State Archive of Magadan Province, Magadan

GARF   Gosudarstvennyi arkhiv Rossiiskoi Federatsii, State Archive of the Russian Federation, Moscow

GASO   Gosudarstvennyi arkhiv Sverdlovskoi oblasti, State Archive of Sverdlovsk Province, Ekaterinburg

GPU   See OGPU

MIA   Ministry of Internal Affairs Archive, Tbilisi, Georgia

MIZU   Muzei istorii zdravookhraneniia Ukhty, Ukhta Museum of the History of Public Health, Ukhta

MMA   Memorial Society Archives, Moscow

MMSPb   Memorial Society Archives, St Petersburg (now held by Nauchno-informatsionnyi tsentr 'Fond Iofe')

MOKM   Magadanskii oblastnoi kraevedcheskii muzei, Magadan Province Regional Museum, Magadan

MVD   Ministerstvo Vnutrennykh Del SSSR, Ministry of Internal Affairs of the USSR, successor to NKVD from March 1946

NAG   National Archives of Georgia, Tbilisi, Georgia

NKVD   Narodnyi Komissariat Vnutrennykh Del SSSR, People's Commissariat of Internal Affairs of the USSR; absorbed the security police (OGPU) in 1934

OGPU   Ob"edinennoe gosudarstvennoe politicheskoe upravlenie pri SNK SSSR, Unified State Political Administration attached to the Council of People's Commissars of the USSR; the security police 1923–34. During 1921–23, before the formation of the USSR, GPU (State Political Administration)

PIKM   Pechorskii istoriko-kraevedcheskii muzei, Pechora Historical-Regional Museum, Pechora

RGASPI Rossiiskii gosudarstvennyi arkhiv sotsial'no-politicheskoi istorii, Russian State Archive of Socio-Political History, Moscow
UIKM   Ukhtinskii istoriko-kraevedcheskii muzei, Ukhta Historical-Regional Museum, Ukhta

Preface and acknowledgements

1. Official deaths counted by central Gulag authorities total 1.7 million for 1930–55, or a 90 per cent survival rate; recent attempts to calculate excess deaths under 'release-to-die' (early release on medical grounds) practices add no fewer than 850,000 to this toll, bringing total deaths caused by Gulag incarceration to at least 2.5 million, equivalent to a survival rate nearer to 85 per cent. For these calculations, see Mikhail Nakonechnyi, '"They Won't Survive for Long": Soviet Officials on Medical Release Procedure', in *Rethinking the Gulag: Identities, Sources, Legacies*, ed. Alan Barenberg and Emily D. Johnson (Bloomington: Indiana University Press, 2022), 103, 121; and for an introduction to the state of the question, see idem, 'The Gulag's "Dead Souls": Mortality of Individuals Released from the Camps, 1930–55', *Kritika: Explorations in Russian and Eurasian History* 23, no. 4 (2022): 803–50; and responses by Stephen Wheatcroft and Golfo Alexopoulos in the same issue.

Introduction: A 'Ukrainian Mark Twain' and the essence of Gulag medicine

1. Rory Finnin, *Blood of Others: Stalin's Crimean Atrocity and the Poetics of Solidarity* (Toronto: University of Toronto Press, 2022), 82.
2. The most notorious of these 'corporate histories' of Gulag camps was Maksim Gor'kii, L. Averbakh, S. Firin, et al., *Belomorsko-baltiiskii kanal imeni Stalina. Istoriia stroitel'stva, 1931–1934 gg.* (Moscow: OGIZ 'Istoriia fabrik i zavodov', 1934); translated as L. Auerbach, B. Agapov, S. Alimov, et al., *The White Sea Canal: Being an Account of the Construction of the New Canal between the White Sea and the Baltic Sea* (London: John Lane, The Bodley Head, 1935). On the composition of this book see Cynthia A. Ruder, *Making History for Stalin: The Story of the Belomor Canal* (Gainesville: University Press of Florida, 1998); Julie Draskoczy, *Belomor: Criminality and Creativity in Stalin's Gulag* (Boston: Academic Studies Press, 2014).
3. I. D. Vorontsova and M. B. Rogachev, 'Neizdannaia kniga ob Ukhtpechlage: iz materialov knigi "5 let bor'by za nedra taigi i tundry"', in *Pokaianie: Martirolog. T. 8, Ch. 1*, ed. E. A. Zelenskaia and M. B. Rogachev (Syktyvkar: Komi respublikanskii blagotvoritel'nyi obshchestvennyi fond zhertv politicheskikh repressii 'Pokaianie', 2005), 163–70.
4. Ostap Vishnia, 'Doktor Ia. P. Sokolov'; 'Mens Sana in Corpore Sano'; 'Ukhtinskaia tselebnaia voda. Promysel No. II imeni OGPU', in *Pokaianie: Martirolog. T. 8, Ch. 1*, ed. E. A. Zelenskaia and M. B. Rogachev (Syktyvkar: Komi respublikanskii blagotvoritel'nyi obshchestvennyi fond zhertv politicheskikh repressii 'Pokaianie', 2005).
5. Vishnia, 'Mens Sana in Corpore Sano', 337.
6. Ibid., 338.

7. Alexander Solzhenitsyn, *The Gulag Archipelago 1918–1956: An Experiment in Literary Investigation*, trans. Thomas P. Whitney (London: Collins & Harvill Press, 1975), 2: 218.
8. Ibid., 2: 215–17.
9. Ibid., 2: 214–15.
10. On Solzhenitsyn's confinement in a *sharashka*, see Michael Scammell, *Solzhenitsyn: A Biography* (London: Hutchinson, 1985), 221–69. He portrayed *sharashka* life in his 1963–4 novel *The First Circle*; see Leona Toker, *Return from the Archipelago: Narratives of Gulag Survivors* (Bloomington & Indianapolis: Indiana University Press, 2000), 196–201.
11. On Shalamov's documentary fiction see Toker, *Return from the Archipelago*, 141–87. For his complex attitudes towards Gulag medicine, see his reminiscences in Varlam Shalamov, *Neskol'ko moikh zhiznei. Vospominaniia, zapisnye knizhki, perepiska, sledstvennye dela* (Moscow: Eksmo, 2009), 173–83, 207–11, 220–33. For examples of Shalamov's fictional approach to Gulag medicine consider 'Veismanist' (The Geneticist), which sketches a fictionalised portrait of a prisoner-doctor who retreats from the worst of medical compromises with authority by working in the camp hospital's morgue; and 'Shokovaia terapiia' (Shock Therapy), in which a zealous ex-prisoner-doctor exults in exposing malingering patients for the professional skill it displays. See Varlam Shalamov, *Preodolenie zla* (Moscow: Eksmo, 2011), 248–57, 506–13. A fuller study of Shalamov's medical tales deserves to be written.
12. A prize-winning synthesis treats the question briefly and dismisses medical care as a 'paradox': Anne Applebaum, *Gulag: A History of the Soviet Camps* (London: Allen Lane, 2003), 337–46. Recent academic studies draw upon Sanotdel records for empirical data but do not examine medical care systematically; see e.g. Alan Barenberg, *Gulag Town, Company Town: Forced Labor and its Legacy in Vorkuta* (New Haven & London: Yale University Press, 2014); Steven Anthony Barnes, *Death and Redemption: The Gulag and the Shaping of Soviet Society* (Princeton: Princeton University Press, 2011); Viktor Berdinskikh, *Istoriia odnogo lageria (Viatlag)* (Moscow: Agraf, 2001); Cynthia A. Ruder, *Building Stalinism: The Moscow Canal and the Creation of Soviet Space* (London: I. B. Tauris, 2018). I introduce the valuable work of Boris Nakhapetov and Golfo Alexopoulos, historians of the Gulag Sanotdel, later in this chapter.
13. The twentieth century's two 'totalitarian systems' resembled each other in many important ways, traced by philosophers starting notably with Hannah Arendt. Yet a range of factors made the Nazi and Soviet cases different in ways that matter for historical understanding. The main distinctions between the two totalitarian penal systems were: the short life of the Nazi case versus the longer duration and evolution of Soviet penal institutions; the ideological programmes distinguishing Nazi forms of annihilation of racial enemies versus the Soviets' ostensible intention to 'reforge' inmates into New Soviet People; the deep connection in the Soviet penal system with the Stalinist planned economy enduring for decades, as contrasted with the short-lived wartime experience of mass penal labour under the Nazis; and the relative wealth of Germany compared to Russia, which determined much about the infrastructure, organisation, and provisioning of these penal worlds. The forbidding geography of the Soviet Gulag imposed logistical challenges that invite comparison with the British transportation of prisoners to Australia a century-and-a-half earlier: by

contrast the Nazi camps had access to Europe's dense railway and transport network linking modern cities. The two systems disposed of prisoner lives by differing means. The lethal complex at Auschwitz (and the other Nazi death camps) had no Soviet analogues, although there were moments when deliberate murder of Soviet prisoners spiked (1937–38 during the nationwide Great Terror; and during the Second World War). Survival rates were higher for Soviet inmates (at approximately 85 per cent) compared to under 50 per cent for Nazi prisoners, according to recent scholarship. For discussions of the distinctions between Nazi and Soviet penal systems, see Applebaum, *Gulag*, 18–24; Jeffrey S. Hardy, *The Gulag after Stalin: Redefining Punishment in Khrushchev's Soviet Union, 1953–1964* (Ithaca & London: Cornell University Press, 2016), 6–8; Nikolaus Wachsmann, *Kl: A History of the Nazi Concentration Camps* (London: Little, Brown, 2015), 8–9. Gulag death and survival rates are discussed later in this chapter.

14. I borrow 'police colonisation' from Lynne Viola, 'The Gulag and Police Colonization in the Soviet Union', in *Stalin and Europe: Imitation and Domination, 1928–1953*, ed. Timothy Snyder and Ray Brandon (New York & Oxford: Oxford University Press, 2014).

15. On embedded medical services in Soviet institutions, see Christopher M. Davis, 'The Economics of the Soviet Health System: An Analytical and Historical Study, 1921–1978', (PhD thesis, Cambridge University, 1979), 57; idem, 'Economics of Soviet Public Health, 1928–1932: Development Strategy, Resource Constraints, and Health Plans', in *Health and Society in Revolutionary Russia*, ed. Susan Gross Solomon and John F. Hutchinson (Bloomington & Indianapolis: Indiana University Press, 1990), 150; Christopher Burton, 'Medical Welfare during Late Stalinism: A Study of Doctors and the Soviet Health System, 1945–1953' (PhD thesis, University of Chicago, 2000), 67, 113–19, 445. On the Kremlin's medical service, see S. P. Mironov, Iu. L. Perov, V. M. Tsvetkov, and V. M. Iastrebov, *Kremlevskaia meditsina (ot istokov do nashikh dnei)* (Moscow: Izvestiia; Meditsinskii tsentr Upravleniia delami Prezidenta Rossiskoi Federatsii, 2000).

16. Michael Jakobson, *Origins of the Gulag: The Soviet Prison-Camp System, 1917–1934* (Lexington: University Press of Kentucky, 1993), 119–38.

17. On tsarist exile and forced labour, see Andrew A. Gentes, *Exile to Siberia, 1590–1822* (Basingstoke & New York: Palgrave Macmillan, 2008); idem, *Exile, Murder and Madness in Siberia, 1823–61* (Basingstoke: Palgrave Macmillan, 2010); Daniel Beer, *The House of the Dead: Siberian Exile under the Tsars* (London: Allen Lane, 2016); on the tension between Russian colonisation and indigenous populations see Yuri Slezkine, *Arctic Mirrors: Russia and the Small Peoples of the North* (Ithaca & London: Cornell University Press, 1994); James Forsyth, *A History of the Peoples of Siberia: Russia's North Asian Colony, 1581–1990* (Cambridge: Cambridge University Press, 1992).

18. See Sarah Badcock, *A Prison without Walls? Eastern Siberian Exile in the Last Years of Tsarism* (Oxford: Oxford University Press, 2016).

19. On Siberia as a colony see Nikolai Mikhailovich Iadrintsev, *Sibir' kak koloniia. K iubileiu trekhsotletiia. Sovremennoe polozhenie Sibiri. Eia nuzhdy i potrebnosti. Eia proshloe i budushchee* (St Petersburg: M. M. Stasiulevich, 1882); for Kliuchevskii, see Alexander Etkind, 'Internalising Colonialism: Intellectual Endeavours and Internal Affairs in Mid-Nineteenth Century Russia,' in

Convergence and Divergence: Russia and Eastern Europe into the Twenty-First Century, ed. Peter J. S. Duncan (London: School of Slavonic and East European Studies, UCL, 2007), 104.

20. Jakobson, *Origins of the Gulag*, 16.
21. For fresh interpretations that pluralise the revolutions, and decolonise the Civil War, see e.g. Jon Smele, *The 'Russian' Civil Wars, 1916–1926: Ten Years that Shook the World* (London: Hurst & Company, 2016); Serhii Plokhy, *Lost Kingdom: The Quest for Empire and the Making of the Russian Nation, from 1470 to the Present* (London: Penguin, 2017), 213–25. Anglophone scholarship of the late twentieth century typically defined Bolshevik Russia as 'the world's first socialist state' but other socialist regimes emerged in the region in this era: see e.g. Stephen F. Jones, *Socialism in Georgian Colors: The European Road to Social Democracy 1883–1917* (Cambridge, MA, and London: Harvard University Press, 2005).
22. On Solovki and its early expansion see Nick Baron, *Soviet Karelia: Politics, Planning and Terror in Stalin's Russia, 1920–1939* (London: Routledge, 2007); Jakobson, *Origins of the Gulag*, 111–28; Iu. A. Brodskii, *Solovki. Dvadtsat' let osobogo naznacheniia* (Moscow: ROSSPEN, 2002). On canal proposals and construction, see Ruder, *Making History for Stalin*.
23. Otto J. Pohl, *The Stalinist Penal System: A Statistical History of Soviet Repression and Terror, 1930–1953* (Jefferson, NC: McFarland, 1997), 11. The figures are for camps and colonies, and exclude deportees to 'special settlements'.
24. In addition to 1.7 million officially counted deaths, a recent calculation of excess deaths caused principally by exhaustion through forced labour adds 850,000, for a total of 2.5 million prisoner lives lost through incarceration; see Mikhail Nakonechnyi, '"They Won't Survive for Long": Soviet Officials on Medical Release Procedure', in *Rethinking the Gulag: Identities, Sources, Legacies*, ed. Alan Barenberg and Emily D. Johnson (Bloomington: Indiana University Press, 2022), 103, 121. The total number of deaths attributable to Gulag imprisonment remains disputed by Western scholars, as well as a politicised and deliberately distorted discussion within Russia. On these issues see Mikhail Nakonechnyi, 'The Gulag's "Dead Souls": Mortality of Individuals Released from the Camps, 1930–55', *Kritika: Explorations in Russian and Eurasian History* 23, no. 4 (2022): 803–50, and responses by Stephen Wheatcroft and Golfo Alexopoulos in the same issue.
25. On the economics of the Gulag see Paul R. Gregory and Valery Lazarev, eds, *The Economics of Forced Labor: The Soviet Gulag* (Stanford: Hoover Institution Press, 2003).
26. Cited, in edited form, in Paul Gregory, 'An Introduction to the Economics of the Gulag', in *The Economics of Forced Labor: The Soviet Gulag*, ed. Paul R. Gregory and Valery Lazarev, (Stanford: Hoover Institution Press, 2003), 4. The full quotation cited here comes from GARF, f. R9414, op. 1, d. 368, l. 115.
27. I discuss the idea of the Gulag as 'internal colony' in Den Khili [Dan Healey], 'Nasledie Gulaga: Prinuditel'nyi trud sovetskoi epokhi kak vnutrenniaia kolonizatsiia', in *Tam, vnutri. Praktiki vnutrennei kolonizatsii v kul'turnoi istorii Rossii*, ed. Aleksandr Etkind, Dirk Uffelmann, and Il'ia Kukulin (Moscow: Novoe literaturnoe obozrenie, 2012).
28. N. V. Upadyshev, *Gulag na evropeiskom severe Rossii: Genezis, evoliutsiia, raspad* (Arkhangel'sk: Pomorskii universitet, 2007), 48.

29. N. A. Morozov, *Gulag v Komi krae 1929–1956* (Syktyvkar: Syktyvkarskii universitet, 1997), 24–5.

30. Ibid., 103–34.

31. Pavel Grebeniuk, *Kolymskii led: Sistema upravleniia na severo-vostoke Rossii 1953–1964* (Moscow: ROSSPEN, 2007), 21.

32. Upadyshev, *Gulag na evropeiskom severe Rossii*, 56–7; Morozov, *Gulag v Komi krae 1929–1956*, 25–6.

33. The volume of decrees issued by local bosses was huge; see e.g. I. D. Batsaev and A. G. Kozlov, eds, *Dal'stroi i Sevvostlag OGPU-NKVD SSSR v tsifrakh i dokumentakh. Ch. I (1931–1941)* (Magadan: SVKNII DVO RAN, 2002); Upadyshev, *Gulag na evropeiskom severe Rossii*; for the Moscow–Volga Canal Construction Camp, see GARF, f. R9489 s. ch., op. 2 holding dozens of files of decrees issued between 1933 and 1939.

34. In May 1941 the Gulag Sanotdel apparatus had 45 out of 526 central Gulag posts; see GARF, f. R9414, op. 1, d. 847, ll. 19–21. ('Utverzhdenie shtaty tsentral'nogo apparata GULAGa 1941 g.').

35. For 1939, Oleg Khlevniuk, *The History of the Gulag: From Collectivization to the Great Terror* (New Haven & London: Yale University Press, 2004), 210; wartime (1943), GARF, f. R9414, op. 1, d. 68, l. 23; for 1 January 1953, GARF f. R9414, op. 1a, d. 627, l. 62.

36. Comparison with civilian hospital bed provision: in 1939 the Gulag had over six times more beds than civilian services, with 249 beds per 10,000 prisoner population, while in 1940 the civilian network had only 40.2 beds per 10,000. There were similar disparities during and after the Second World War, although precise comparison is impossible given the available statistics. For civilian statistics see Davis, 'The Economics of the Soviet Health System', 57, 64; and for approximate comparisons with the Gulag, see B. A. Nakhapetov, *Ocherki istorii sanitarnoi sluzhby Gulaga* (Moscow: ROSSPEN, 2009), 69. Davis points out that the overall civilian bed-count masked great disparities across the country, with higher per capita numbers in urban industrial and more Westernised parts of the Soviet Union, and lower ones in rural and Central Asian regions.

37. For an example of such institutional entitlement, see the 1946 'short analysis' of Gulag medical activity and infrastructure by Major Pomerantsev of the MVD medical service, in which he boasts of the more expansive bed numbers compared to the civilian medical network, while conceding the rates are lower than other branches of the Interior Ministry's embedded medical systems: GARF, f. R9414, op. 1, d. 2796, l. 239. I am grateful to Mikhail Nakonechnyi for this source, and for his insights into Gulag statistical thinking.

38. For a commentary on article 58, see Solzhenitsyn, *The Gulag Archipelago*, 1: 60–8.

39. A 1939 statute on the camp regime explicitly permitted the employment of doctors with article 58 convictions in their professional capacity: 'Vremennaia instriuktsiia o rezhime soderzhaniia zakliuchennykh v ITL NKVD SSSR', in A. I. Kokurin and N. V. Petrov, eds, *GULAG: Glavnoe upravlenie lagerei, 1918–1960* (Moscow: Mezhdunarodnyi fond Demokratiia, 2000), 467. Three-quarters of all skilled professionals were being used in their professional specialisations in 1947, while 88.2 per cent of medical specialists were so employed; see Viktor N. Zemskov, 'GULAG (Istoriko-sotsiologicheskii aspekt)', *Sotsiologicheskie issledovaniia*, nos 6, 7 (1991): 7: 11.

40. On graduate assignments, see Burton, 'Medical Welfare during Late Stalinism', 102–8, 119. Graduate assignments to various departmental medical services and to the civilian network are detailed in GARF, f. R8009, op. 14, 'Otdel kadrov. Sektor raspredeleniia okanchivaiushchikh vuzy NKZ SSSR'.

41. GARF, f. R9414, op. 1, d. 2750, ll. 1–4, published in Iu. N. Afanas'ev et al., eds, *Istoriia stalinskogo Gulaga. Konets 1920-kh – pervaia polovina 1950-kh godov. Sobranie dokumentov v semi tomakh* (Moscow, ROSSPEN, 2004–5), 4: 485–9.

42. From these 1939 statistics there were 15.3 doctors per 10,000 Gulag prisoners; the analogous figure for 1940 in civilian medical service was 7 per 10,000 civilians. For civilian figures, see Burton, 'Medical Welfare during Late Stalinism', 64.

43. Apparently, the first courses were devised locally by individual camps (e.g. in Karaganda camp as early as 1931, GARF, f. R9414, op. 2, d. 108, ll. 220–35; in Dmitlag as early as 1933: GARF, f. R9489, op. 2, d. 25, l. 254). In 1936 a central directive from Moscow ordered camps to set up 6-month training courses for nurses and paramedics; see Nakhapetov, *Ocherki istorii*, 88. Shalamov was trained as a feldsher in Magadan in 1946; see Shalamov, *Neskol'ko moikh zhiznei*, 230. He described the courses in two short stories, 'Kursy' and 'Veismanist'.

44. See e.g. Janusz Bardach and Kate Gleeson, *Man Is Wolf to Man: Surviving Stalin's Gulag* (London: Simon & Schuster, 1998); Eugenia Ginzburg, *Within the Whirlwind*, trans. Ian Boland (London: Collins Harvill, 1989); Efrosiniia Antonovna Kersnovskaia, *Skol'ko stoit chelovek* (Moscow: ROSSPEN, 2006).

45. Golfo Alexopoulos, 'Medical Research in Stalin's Gulag', *Bulletin of the History of Medicine* 90, no. 3 (2016): 363–93. On Norilsk see chapter 6 of the present book.

46. Steven Maddox, 'Gulag Football: Competitive and Recreational Sport in Stalin's System of Forced Labor', *Kritika: Explorations in Russian and Eurasian History* 19, no. 3 (2018): 509–36; Natalia Kuziakina, *Theatre in the Solovki Prison Camp* (Luxembourg & Newark: Harwood Academic, 1995); A. N. Kaneva, *Gulagovskii teatr Ukhty* (Syktyvkar: Komi knizhnoe izdatel'stvo, 2001); A. G. Kozlov, *Ogni lagernoi rampy. Iz istorii magadanskogo teatra 30–50-kh godov* (Moscow: Raritet, 1992); idem, *Teatr na severnoi zemle: Ocherki po istorii Magadanskogo muz.-dram. teatra im. M. Gor'kogo (1933–1953 gg.)* (Magadan: Magadanskaia oblastnaia universal'naia nauchnaia biblioteka im. A. S. Pushkina, 1992).

47. A. G. Tepliakov, *Mashina terrora: OGPU-NKVD Sibiri v 1929–1941 gg.* (Moscow: Novyi khronograf, 2008) 170–6.

48. See e.g. John F. Hutchinson, *Politics and Public Health in Revolutionary Russia, 1890–1918* (Baltimore & London: Johns Hopkins University Press, 1990); Irina Sirotkina, *Diagnosing Literary Genius: A Cultural History of Psychiatry in Russia, 1880–1930* (Baltimore: Johns Hopkins University Press, 2002); Daniel Beer, *Renovating Russia: The Human Sciences and the Fate of Liberal Modernity, 1880–1930* (Ithaca & London: Cornell University Press, 2008); Daniel Philip Todes, *Pavlov's Physiology Factory: Experiment, Interpretation, Laboratory Enterprise* (Baltimore & London: Johns Hopkins University Press, 2002).

49. Nancy Mandelker Frieden, *Russian Physicians in an Era of Reform and Revolution, 1856–1905* (Princeton: Princeton University Press, 1981); Hutchinson, *Politics and Public Health in Revolutionary Russia*. For a Bolshevik doctor's memoir of *zemstvo* medical practice and revolutionary activity, see Sergei I. Mitskevich, *Zapiski vracha-obshchestvennika* (Moscow: Meditsina, 1969).

50. See Frieden, *Russian Physicians*; for an influential urban doctor's memoir, see Vikentii Veresaev, *Zapiski vracha* (Moscow: AST Zebra E, 2010).

51. Hutchinson, *Politics and Public Health in Revolutionary Russia*.

52. Neil B. Weissman, 'Origins of Soviet Health Administration', in *Health and Society in Revolutionary Russia*, ed. Susan Gross Solomon and John F. Hutchinson (Bloomington & Indianapolis: Indiana University Press, 1990); Frances L. Bernstein, Christopher Burton, and Dan Healey, 'Introduction: Experts, Expertise, and New Histories of Soviet Medicine', in *Soviet Medicine: Culture, Practice, and Science*, ed. Frances L. Bernstein, Christopher Burton, and Dan Healey (DeKalb: Northern Illinois University Press, 2010).

53. Christopher M. Davis, 'Economic Problems of the Soviet Health Service: 1917–1930', *Soviet Studies* 35, no. 3 (1983): 350; see also Sally Ewing, 'The Science and Politics of Soviet Insurance Medicine', in *Health and Society in Revolutionary Russia*, ed. Susan Gross Solomon and John F. Hutchinson (Bloomington & Indianapolis: Indiana University Press, 1990).

54. Calculated from statistics in 'Doklad nachal'nika USLONa o deiatel'nosti Upravleniia Solovetskikh lagerei osobogo naznacheniia OGPU za 1926–1927 operatsionnyi god 1927 g.', GARF, f. R9414, op. 1, d. 2918, l. 157. On the search for reductions in expenditure, see Nick Baron, 'Conflict and Complicity: The Expansion of the Karelian Gulag, 1923–1933', *Cahiers du monde russe* 22 (2001/02): 615–48.

55. Susan Gross Solomon, 'Social Hygiene and Soviet Public Health, 1921–1930', in *Health and Society in Revolutionary Russia*, ed. Susan Gross Solomon and John F. Hutchinson (Bloomington & Indianapolis: Indiana University Press, 1990).

56. Weissman, 'Origins of Soviet Health Administration', 108; Burton, 'Medical Welfare during Late Stalinism', 213–14.

57. Frances Bernstein, 'Behind the Closed Door – VD and Medical Secrecy in Early Soviet Medicine', in *Soviet Medicine: Culture, Practice, and Science*, ed. Frances L. Bernstein, Christopher Burton, and Dan Healey (DeKalb: Northern Illinois University Press, 2010).

58. Ibid.; Burton, 'Medical Welfare during Late Stalinism', 241–95. Physician Anna Kliashko recalled lessons on deontology (medical duty) and learning about the Hippocratic Oath in her Irkutsk Medical Institute lectures in the 1940s: interview, 15 September 2012, Montréal, Canada.

59. Weissman, 'Origins of Soviet Health Administration'; Susan Gross Solomon, 'The Expert and the State in Russian Public Health: Continuities and Changes across the Revolutionary Divide', in *The History of Public Health and the Modern State*, ed. Dorothy Porter (Amsterdam: Editions Rodopi B. V., 1994).

60. Davis, 'Economic Problems of the Soviet Health Service', 354–6; idem, 'Economics of Soviet Public Health, 1928–1932', 152–5.

61. Burton, 'Medical Welfare during Late Stalinism', 69–123.

62. Davis, 'Economics of Soviet Public Health, 1928–1932', 156–7, 160–1.

63. Davis, 'Economic Problems of the Soviet Health Service', 57.

64. Davis, 'Economics of Soviet Public Health, 1928–1932', 161–2; Burton, 'Medical Welfare during Late Stalinism', 153–4.

65. Christopher Burton, 'Soviet Medical Attestation and the Problem of Professionalisation under Late Stalinism, 1945–1953', *Europe-Asia Studies* 57, no. 8 (2005): 1211–30.

66. Burton demonstrates that post-1945 Soviet medical education underwent 'truncated Flexnerization', in other words adopting the style of science-led education recommended by Alexander Flexner for doctors in the USA, and widespread by the 1930s; see Burton, 'Medical Welfare during Late Stalinism', 153–64.

67. In 1950, for example, 19.3 per cent of the medical profession gave Jewish as their nationality in their identity documents, while the proportion of Jews in the Soviet population hovered around 1 per cent: Burton, 'Soviet Medical Attestation', 1221.

68. For this characterisation, see Mark G. Field, *Doctor and Patient in Soviet Russia* (Cambridge, MA: Harvard University Press, 1957), 45–61.

69. Ibid., 69–73.

70. On Chekhov's stories, see e.g. Carl Fisher, 'Doctor-Writers: Anton Chekhov's Medical Stories', in *New Directions in Literature and Medicine Studies*, ed. Stephanie M. Hilger (Basingstoke: Palgrave Macmillan, 2017). On Veresaev and Bulgakov as medical writers, see e.g. Laure Troubetzkoy, 'Récits de deux médecins: Veresaev et Bulgakov', *Revue des études slaves* 65, no. 2 (1993): 253–62.

71. For examples of the co-opting of Veresaev's medical writing for Soviet purposes, see e.g. G. Brovman, *V. V. Veresaev: zhizn' i tvorchestvo* (Moscow: Sovetskii pisatel', 1959); and I. M. Geizer, *V. V. Veresaev: Pisatel'-vrach* (Moscow: Medgiz, 1957). On the use of examples from Chekhov, see Burton, 'Medical Welfare during Late Stalinism', 248–9; for a report about Komsomol activism in Sverdlovsk Medical Institute 'to implant love for one's specialisation' including lecture-discussions on 'the figure of the doctor in Soviet literature', see GASO, f. 2195, op. 1, d. 37, ll. 16–18.

72. The account of Gulag survivor memoir here draws upon Toker, *Return from the Archipelago*. On the Soviet public engagement with de-Stalinisation, see Polly Jones, *Myth, Memory, Trauma: Rethinking the Stalinist Past in the Soviet Union, 1953–70* (New Haven & London: Yale University Press, 2013).

73. Josephine von Zitzewitz, *The Culture of Samizdat: Literature and Underground Networks in the Late Soviet Union* (London: Bloomsbury Academic, 2021).

74. Nina Tumarkin, *The Living and the Dead: The Rise and Fall of the Cult of World War II in Russia* (New York: Basic Books, 1994); Stephen F. Cohen, 'The Stalin Question since Stalin', in *An End to Silence: Uncensored Opinion in the Soviet Union from Roy Medvedev's Underground Magazine*, Political Diary, ed. Stephen F. Cohen (New York & London: W. W. Norton, 1982), 22–50.

75. 'Veiled monuments' is Tyler Kirk's term for Brezhnev-era monuments that commemorated the founding of labour-camp cities without acknowledging the prisoner status of the 'pioneers'; see Tyler C. Kirk, 'From Enemy to Hero: Andrei Krems and the Legacy of Stalinist Repression in Russia's Far North, 1964–82', *Russian Review* 82, no. 2 (2023): 292–306.

76. A. F. Khoroshev, *Ocherki istorii zdravookhraneniia Magadanskoi Oblasti* (Magadan: Magadanskoe knizhnoe izdatel'stvo, 1959).

77. Barenberg, *Gulag Town, Company Town*, 245; Grebeniuk, *Kolymskii led*, 237–40.

78. Nanci Adler, *Victims of Soviet Terror: The Story of the Memorial Movement* (Westport & London: Praeger, 1993).

79. Anne White, 'The Memorial Society in the Russian Provinces', *Europe-Asia Studies* 47, no. 8 (1995): 1343–66.

80. Vladislav Staf, 'Local Initiatives: A Historical Analysis of the Creation of Memorial Museums of the Gulag in (Post-)Soviet Russia', *Problems of Post-Communism* (2023): 1–8, https://doi.org/10.1080/10758216.2023.2166846; Sofia Gavrilova, 'Regional Memories of the Great Terror: Representation of the Gulag in Russian Kraevedcheskii Museums', *Problems of Post-Communism* (2021): 1–15, https://doi.org/10.1080/10758216.2021.1885981.

81. On the 'roadmap' for commemoration, and the Moscow museum's activity, see Staf, 'Local Initiatives'; and Andrei Zavadski and Vera Dubina, 'Eclipsing Stalin: The Gulag History Museum in Moscow as a Manifestation of Russia's Official Memory of Soviet Repression', *Problems of Post-Communism* (2021): 1–13, https://doi.org/10.1080/10758216.2021.1983444.

82. During the Soviet era and in Cold War scholarship, survivor memoirs constituted the principal sources for landmark works of historical synthesis, e.g. Solzhenitsyn, *The Gulag Archipelago 1918–1956*; Robert Conquest, *Kolyma: The Arctic Death Camps* (London: Macmillan, 1978).

83. Lynne Viola, 'The Aesthetic of Stalinist Planning and the World of the Special Villages', *Kritika: Explorations in Russian and Eurasian History* 4, no. 1 (2003): 101–28.

84. Nakhapetov, *Ocherki istorii*; Golfo Alexopoulos, *Illness and Inhumanity in Stalin's Gulag* (New Haven & London: Yale University Press, 2017).

85. Only three published memoirs by freely hired doctors of the Gulag were identified, contrasting with the several dozen published and unpublished prisoner-doctors' memoirs found in libraries or in archival collections. Two free doctors' accounts, Sofiia Guzikova's and Nina Savoeva's, are examined in chapter 3. A third, by a young graduate assigned to work in a prisoner-of-war camp, told a similar story. However, because the German soldiers she treated apparently received careful handling and quick repatriation, unlike the ordinary Gulag prisoner, I have decided to exclude it: Ina Kuznetsova, *Zona miloserdiia* (Moscow: Iz-vo im. Sabashnikovykh, 2005). I acquired testimony in interview form from two further freely hired doctors, who worked in or near the Kolyma camps, and refer to these for context and comparison. Elena Mamuchashvili related her story in Elena Mamuchashvili, 'V bol'nitse dlia zakliuchennykh', *Shalamovskii sbornik* 2 (1997): 78–88; and freely hired physician Anna Kliashko was interviewed from 2009 to 2012 as described below.

86. Such retrospective shielding bears a resemblance to forms of 'doubling' adopted by Nazi doctors while in the camps in order to function in extreme circumstances. Robert Jay Lifton describes psychological 'doubling' as a means by which Nazi doctors managed to retain their sense of professionalism as doctors but commit horrific crimes. See Robert Jay Lifton, *The Nazi Doctors: Medical Killing and the Psychology of Genocide* (New York: Basic Books, 1986), 418–29. The concentration camp 'grey zone' is a term originally devised by Primo Levi, and adapted to the Gulag case in Lynne Viola, 'The Question of the Perpetrator in Soviet History', *Slavic Review* 72, no. 1 (2013): 18. Note also Adam Brown, '"No One Will Ever Know": The Holocaust, "Privileged" Jews and the "Grey Zone"', *History Australia* 8, no. 3 (2011): 95–116.

87. I draw upon eight published prisoner-doctors' memoirs in Russian and English; and twenty-one unpublished memoirs or archival records of prisoner-doctors from historical-regional museums and the collections of Memorial in Moscow and St Petersburg.

88. Evgeniia Ginzburg, *Krutoi marshrut* (Frankfurt am Main & Milan: Possev, 1967); English edition in two volumes: Eugenia Ginzburg, *Into the Whirlwind*, trans. Paul Stevenson and Manya Harari (London: Collins Harvill, 1967); idem, *Within the Whirlwind*.

89. Miklós Nyiszli, *Auschwitz: A Doctor's Eyewitness Account* (London: Penguin, 2012); Gisela Perl, *I Was a Doctor in Auschwitz* (Lanham: Lexington Books, 2019); and note Michael J. Hargrave, *Bergen-Belsen 1945: A Medical Student's Journal* (London: Imperial College Press, 2014).

90. Ginzburg, *Within the Whirlwind*, 150. Elsewhere (ibid., 98) Ginzburg compared the Nazi and Russian character with a consoling tilt towards Russian good-heartedness: 'I strode out far more boldly now, thinking as I went along what a godsend for us all the Russian character was. By then we already knew of the Nazi bestialities. I shuddered to think how fearful the combination of cruel decrees and total, unquestioning efficiency must be. It was not quite like that with us! With us there nearly always remained some loophole for ordinary human feelings. Nearly always the decree – however devilish it may have been – was mitigated by the innate good nature of its executors, by their slackness, or simply by trust in the famous Russian "maybe".'

91. On Soviet intellectuals' autobiographies as inscriptions of the self into history, see e.g. Irina Paperno, *Stories of the Soviet Experience: Memoirs, Diaries, Dreams* (Ithaca: Cornell University Press, 2009), 1–56.

92. Alexopoulos, *Illness and Inhumanity in Stalin's Gulag*, 181. The flavour of the corporate culture is also conveyed in Nakhapetov, *Ocherki istorii*.

93. Barnes, *Death and Redemption*; Barenberg, *Gulag Town, Company Town*; Baron, *Soviet Karelia*; Wilson T. Bell, *Stalin's Gulag at War: Forced Labour, Mass Death, and Soviet Victory in the Second World War* (Toronto: University of Toronto Press, 2019); Berdinskikh, *Istoriia odnogo lageria (Viatlag)*; David J. Nordlander, 'Capital of the Gulag: Magadan in the Early Stalin Era, 1929–1941' (PhD thesis, University of North Carolina – Chapel Hill, 1997); Ruder, *Building Stalinism* relies on documents held in Moscow's central state archive – but demonstrates the value of focusing on a single camp complex.

94. On the diverging death rates given by local and central records, and the dynamics that created them, see Nakonechnyi, 'The Gulag's "Dead Souls"'.

95. Each museum had its own document classification system and I have adopted standardised citations to make identification as straightforward as possible.

96. During my research fieldwork, Memorial Moscow (MMA) used a conventional archival classification system and on first citation I give the *fond, opis'*, and *dela* numbers for these files. As the files I viewed at the International Institute for Social History all originate in MMA's collection, I have cited these using the MMA archival identifiers. At Memorial St Petersburg (MMSPb) I found that classification was by surname although since then archival file numbers have been assigned; as a result my citations refer to surnames and document titles.

97. I draw upon records of thirty-five mid-level Gulag medical staff: nineteen nurses of whom ten were freely hired; seven prisoner feldshers; five orderlies; and four other workers (pharmacists and laboratory assistants). I also observed, but did not collect, records of dentists and veterinary staff working in the Gulag in these collections.

98. Iurii Fidel'gol'ts, 'Tot Vaninskii port', in *Za chto? Proza, poeziia, dokumenty*, ed. V. A. Shentalinskii and V. N. Leonovich (Moscow: Kliuch, 1999).

99. Among Western scholars, only Golfo Alexopoulos in her ambitious study of the Sanotdel, *Illness and Inhumanity*, and Mikhail Nakonechnyi in his study of the Gulag's 'release-to-die' practices, have had the courage to address this quandary squarely, and this book is deeply indebted to both scholars' work.

100. On 'sovereign' and 'disciplinary' power within the wider framework of his evolving conception of 'biopower' and 'governmentality', see e.g. Michel Foucault, *Discipline and Punish: The Birth of the Prison*, trans. Alan Sheridan (New York: Vintage, 1979); idem, *Society Must Be Defended: Lectures at the Collège de France, 1975–76* (London: Penguin, 2004), 239–63; and see my discussion in Dan Healey, 'Lives in the Balance: Weak and Disabled Prisoners and the Biopolitics of the Gulag', *Kritika: Explorations in Russian and Eurasian History* 16, no. 3 (2015): 527–56.

Chapter 1 'They were the first': Pioneers of the Gulag medical service

1. Ostap Vishnia, 'Mens Sana in Corpore Sano', in *Pokaianie: Martirolog. T. 8, Ch. 1*, ed. E. A. Zelenskaia and M. B. Rogachev (Syktyvkar: Komi respublikanskii blagotvoritel'nyi obshchestvennyi fond zhertv politicheskikh repressii 'Pokaianie', 2005), 338.

2. My account of Viktorov's life owes much to A. N. Kaneva, 'Doktor Viktorov', in *Problemy istorii repressivnoi politiki na evropeiskom severe Rossii (1917–1956): Tezisy dokladov vserossiiskoi nauchnoi konferentsii*, ed. N. A. Morozov (Syktyvkar: Syktyvkar gosudarstvennyi universitet, 1993); idem, 'Doktor Viktorov', *Ukhta* [newspaper], 23 October 1992, 3; supplemented by materials assembled by museum researchers in MIZU. On peasant migrants in St Petersburg, see Robert Johnson, *Peasant and Proletarian: The Working Class of Moscow in the Late Nineteenth Century* (New Brunswick, NJ: Rutgers University Press, 1979); Barbara A. Engel, *Between the Fields and the City: Women, Work and Family in Russia, 1861–1914* (Cambridge: Cambridge University Press, 1994).

3. Ronald Grigor Suny, *The Making of the Georgian Nation*, 2nd edn (Bloomington: Indiana University Press, 1994), 209–36; Donald Rayfield, *Edge of Empires: A History of Georgia* (London: Reaktion, 2012), 339–46.

4. Rayfield, *Edge of Empires*, 344–5.

5. MIZU, Viktorov, Nikolai Aleksandrovich folder, 'Avtobiografiia' (31 December 1934), l. 1.

6. Ibid., l. 1 ob.

7. My account of the expedition relies upon A. N. Kaneva, 'Ukhtpechlag: Stranitsy istorii', in *Pokaianie: Martirolog. T. 8, Ch. 1*, ed. E. A. Zelenskaia and M. B. Rogachev (Syktyvkar: Komi respublikanskii blagotvoritel'nyi obshchestvennyi fond zhertv politicheskikh repressii 'Pokaianie', 2005).

8. Kaneva, 'Ukhtpechlag: Stranitsy istorii', 77. The alternative was a slow hike across country bogs and forest; by the 1940s Ukhta and its camp system would be linked to the 'mainland' by railway.

9. Applebaum suggests the *Gleb Bokii* sailed all the way to Chibyu, which would have been impossible. The expedition swapped vessels and faced hauling barges over river rapids before reaching its destination. Compare Anne Applebaum, *Gulag: A History of the Soviet Camps* (London: Allen Lane, 2003), 91–2, and Kaneva, 'Ukhtpechlag: Stranitsy istorii', 78–80.

10. See e.g. Document no. 1.12 in E. A. Zelenskaia and M. B. Rogachev, 'Ukhtinskaia ekspeditsiia OGPU v dokumentakh', in *Pokaianie: Martirolog. T. 8, Ch. 1*, ed. E. A. Zelenskaia and M. B. Rogachev (Syktyvkar: Komi respublikanskii blagotvoritel'nyi obshchestvennyi fond zhertv politicheskikh repressii 'Pokaianie', 2005), 49–50.
11. Kaneva, 'Ukhtpechlag: Stranitsy istorii', 79.
12. Vyshnia discusses the rigours of the expedition and the qualities expected of its members: 'Mens Sana in Corpore Sano', 338.
13. Ibid., 337.
14. Document no. 1.12 in Zelenskaia and Rogachev, 'Ukhtinskaia ekspeditsiia OGPU v dokumentakh', 50.
15. Vishnia, 'Mens Sana in Corpore Sano', 339.
16. Document no. 1.12 in Zelenskaia and Rogachev, 'Ukhtinskaia ekspeditsiia OGPU v dokumentakh', 49; 55–73.
17. N. G. Okhotin and A. B. Roginskii, eds, *Sistema ispravitel'no-trudovykh lagerei v SSSR, 1923–1960: Spravochnik* (Moscow: Zven'ia, 1998), 497–8.
18. Applebaum, *Gulag*, 159–72.
19. MIZU, Sokolov, Iakov Petrovich and Sokolova, Sof'ia Viktorovna folder, l. 1. Both Sokolov and his wife, also a doctor from the same graduating class, were orphans.
20. S. F. Sapolnova, T. A. Vekshina, and F. G. Kanev, eds, *Liudi v belykh khalatakh* (Ukhta & Syktyvkar: Komi respublikanskaia tipografiia, 2009), 8. It is striking how these historians who founded MIZU did not elaborate on Sokolov's career in this volume, or in their museum exhibits. For a fulsome but vacuous profile, see Ostap Vishnia, 'Doktor Ia. P. Sokolov', in *Pokaianie: Martirolog. T. 8, Ch. 1*, ed. E. A. Zelenskaia and M. B. Rogachev (Syktyvkar: Komi respublikanskii blagotvoritel'nyi obshchestvennyi fond zhertv politicheskikh repressii 'Pokaianie', 2005).
21. Kaneva, 'Doktor Viktorov' (1993), 37.
22. Vishnia, 'Doktor Ia. P. Sokolov', 360.
23. Kaneva, 'Doktor Viktorov' (1993), 37.
24. Kaneva, 'Ukhtpechlag: Stranitsy istorii', 137.
25. Ibid., 138–9 (statistics on shootings); Kaneva, 'Doktor Viktorov' (1993), 37. Charged with anti-Soviet treason, Moroz was shot in January 1940 after a long judicial process in Moscow; see Kaneva, 'Ukhtpechlag: Stranitsy istorii', 143–4.
26. Ia. I. Kaminskii, *'Minuvshee prokhodit predo mnoiu . . .': Izbrannoe iz lichnogo arkhiva* (Odesa: Aspekt, 1995), 87.
27. Ibid.; MIZU, Kaminskii, Iakov Iosifovich folder, 'Vklad zasluzhennogo vracha Komi Respubliki Ia. I. Kaminskogo v meditsinskuiu nauku i praktiku zdravookhraneniia,' ll. 1–2, 8–9; Sapolnova et al., *Liudi v belykh khalatakh*, 159–60.
28. Viktor A. Samsonov, *K tebe, Onego, vse puti. Zapiski lagernogo lekpoma, studenta, vracha, prepodavatelia* (Petrozavodsk: Iz-vo Petrozavodskogo universiteta, 2000), 45–54.
29. Kaneva, 'Doktor Viktorov' (1993), 37; MIZU, Viktorov, Nikolai Aleksandrovich folder, 'VIKTOROV, Nikolai Aleksandrovich – vrach', l. 2. For Kaneva's pioneering historical account, see A. N. Kaneva, 'Deiatel'nost' partiinoi organizatsii Komi ASSR po sozdaniiu i razvitiiu neftegazovoi promyshlennosti v 1929–1945 gg.' (Candidate's thesis, Leningrad State University, 1970).

30. M. Ia. Pullerits, 'Nemnogo o svoem detstve', *Kraevedcheskie zapiski [Magadanskii oblastnoi kraevedcheskii muzei. Magadanskoe knizhnoe izdatel'stvo]* 16 (1989): 88–9.
31. Pavel Grebeniuk, *Kolymskii led: Sistema upravleniia na severo-vostoke Rossii 1953–1964* (Moscow: ROSSPEN, 2007), 25–6.
32. See e.g. Andrea Gullotta, *Intellectual Life and Literature at Solovki 1923–1930: The Paris of the Northern Concentration Camps* (London: Legenda, 2018), 143–52; Michael David-Fox, *Showcasing the Great Experiment: Cultural Diplomacy and Western Visitors to the Soviet Union, 1921–1941* (Oxford: Oxford University Press, 2012), 142–74.
33. Grebeniuk, *Kolymskii led*, 26; for the archival research, see L. A. Obukhov, K. A. Ostal'tsev, and O. N. Safroshenko, *Khrupkaia letopis': Fotoal'bom. Iz fondov arkhivnogo otdela administratsii Krasnovisherskogo munitsipal'nogo raiona* (Perm': Liter-A, 2012), 4–11.
34. Grebeniuk, *Kolymskii led*, 26; S. V. Budnikova, 'Nekotorye dannye o repressirovannykh medikakh na Kolyme (po materialam Magadanskogo oblastnogo kraevedcheskogo muzeia)', in *Kolyma. Dal'stroi. Gulag. Skorb' i sud'by. Materialy nauchno-prakticheskoi konferentsii 13–14 iiunia 1996 goda*, ed. A. M. Biriukov (Magadan: Severnyi mezhdunarodnyi universitet, 1998), 46.
35. On Berzin's team, see David J. Nordlander, 'Capital of the Gulag: Magadan in the Early Stalin Era, 1929–1941' (PhD thesis, University of North Carolina – Chapel Hill, 1997), 147–9. For a farewell dinner organised for Berzin with Baltic comrades in Moscow in November 1931, see Semen Vilenskii and K. B. Nikolaev, eds, *Souchastniki: Arkhiv Kozlova. Tom pervyi* (Moscow: Vozvrashchenie, 2012), 201.
36. A. G. Kozlov, *Magadan: Istoriia vozniknoveniia i razvitiia. Chast' 1 (1929–1939)* (Magadan: SVKNII DVO RAN, 2002), 78, 80.
37. Ibid., 295.
38. Grebeniuk, *Kolymskii led*, 28; Oleg Khlevnyuk, 'The Economy of the OGPU, NKVD, and MVD of the USSR, 1930–1953: The Scale, Structure, and Trends of Development', in *The Economics of Forced Labor: The Soviet Gulag*, ed. Paul Gregory and Valery Lazarev (Stanford: Hoover Institution Press, 2003), 47.
39. Vilenskii and Nikolaev, eds, *Souchastniki*, 202–3; on ambulances, see A. G. Kozlov, *Iz istorii zdravookhraneniia Kolymy i Chukotki (1864–1941 gg.)* (Magadan: Magadanskoe knizhnoe iz-vo, 1989), 33.
40. Kozlov, *Iz istorii zdravookhraneniia Kolymy*, 28.
41. Grebeniuk, *Kolymskii led*, 23. During the period over 200,000 of the remaining prisoners were transferred to other camps; almost 8,000 escaped. Early release on medical grounds was typically applied to severely ill prisoners, often incurables, as a way of reducing camp death rates. Nakonechnyi argues convincingly that the degree to which early releases were tantamount to a 'release-to-die' policy varied over time according to pressures on the Gulag's supplies in famine and wartime. See Mikhail Iur'evich Nakonechnyi, 'Factory of Invalids: Mortality, Disability and Early Release on Medical Grounds from the Gulag, 1930–1955', (DPhil thesis, University of Oxford, 2020).
42. See Table 1 for prisoner stock and flow, 1932–42, in I. D. Batsaev, 'Kolymskaia griada arkhipelaga Gulag (zakliuchennye)', in *Istoricheskie aspekty severo-vostoka Rossii: Ekonomika, obrazovanie, Kolymskii Gulag*, ed. V. F. Lesniakov and V. S. Pan'shin (Magadan: SVKNII DVO RAN, 1996), 50.

43. Kozlov, *Iz istorii zdravookhraneniia Kolymy*, 15.

44. Ibid., 28.

45. Indigenous knowledge of the anti-scurvy properties of pine needles was common across the global north; French explorers in the sixteenth century learned of it from indigenous peoples in the St Lawrence River valley (modern Québec); see Don J. Durzan, 'Arginine, Scurvy and Cartier's "Tree of Life"', *Journal of Ethnobiology and Ethnomedicine* 5, no. 1 (2009): 1–16.

46. A. A. Shmidt, ed., *Tsynga i bor'ba s neiu na severe: Sbornik statei* (Moscow & Leningrad: Sanitarnoe upravlenie Gostresta Dal'stroi, Moskva; Biomedgiz, Leningrad, 1935); this title is found in the bibliography of a Noril'sk Gulag doctor S. N. Mankin's study of vitamin deficiencies, 'Vitaminizirovannyi (khvoinyi) kvas'; see GARF, f. R9414, op. 2, d. 175, l. 199. Shmidt was director of the All-Union Vitamin Research Institute; the two prisoner-doctors were F. D. Mikheev and S. A. Mazovetsky, who co-authored a chapter with E. P. Sheinker on scurvy therapies.

47. The process invented by Pullerits and team was later 'practically forgotten' and a revised version, that probably reduced the vitamin content because of boiling, was institutionalised, see Budnikova, 'Nekotorye dannye', 46–7.

48. Varlam Shalamov, *Neskol'ko moikh zhiznei. Vospominaniia, zapisnye knizhki, perepiska, sledstvennye dela* (Moscow: Eksmo, 2009), 178.

49. I. D. Batsaev and A. G. Kozlov, eds, *Dal'stroi i Sevvostlag OGPU-NKVD SSSR v tsifrakh i dokumentakh. Ch. I (1931–1941)* (Magadan: SVKNII DVO RAN, 2002), 1: 159–60 (1938 decree 'On the struggle with scurvy').

50. Vilenskii and Nikolaev, eds, *Souchastniki*, 239–65.

51. Pullerits, 'Nemnogo o svoem detstve', 90–1.

52. Kozlov, *Iz istorii zdravookhraneniia Kolymy*, 31.

53. See Vilenskii and Nikolaev, eds, *Souchastniki*, 46–7.

54. One prolific historian of Kolyma praises Pullerits for striving 'to improve the lives of repressed medical workers. Thanks to him many strong specialists were able to engage in professional duties'; see Kozlov, *Iz istorii zdravookhraneniia Kolymy*, 28–30.

55. Pullerits, 'Nemnogo o svoem detstve', 92; Vilenskii and Nikolaev, eds, *Souchastniki*, 49.

56. Budnikova, 'Nekotorye dannye', 46.

57. Pullerits, 'Nemnogo o svoem detstve', 94.

58. Vilenskii and Nikolaev, eds, *Souchastniki*, 49.

59. V. N. Khaustov, V. P. Naumov, and N. S. Plotnikova, eds, *Lubianka: Stalin i glavnoe upravlenie gosbezopasnosti NKVD, 1937–1938* (Moscow: Mezhdunarodnyi fond 'Demokratiia' [Fond A. N. Iakovleva], 2004), 541.

60. Grebeniuk, *Kolymskii led*, 29–31.

Chapter 2 'A nightmare parallel world': A chekist in the clinic?

1. N. A. Glazov, *Koshmar parallel'nogo mira: Zapiski vracha* (Novosibirsk: Iz-vo Novosibirskoi gos. obl. nauchnoi biblioteki, 1999), 14.

2. Glazov, *Koshmar parallel'nogo mira*, was published in Siberia in a run of 200 copies. My account of Glazov's life is based primarily on this published source, but I have compared it with a manuscript version held in the archives of Memorial Society, Moscow: GLAZOV, Nikolai Aleksandrovich, 'Etapy

bol'shogo puti', MMA f. 2, op. 2, d. 17. The author's daughter deposited this manuscript before publication under a different title, and with minor editorial variations.

3. The 'perpetual motion' of prisoners within the Gulag 'archipelago' was a phenomenon first discussed by Aleksandr Solzhenitsyn; see Aleksandr Solzhenitsyn, *Arkhipelag Gulag 1918–1956: Opyt khudozhestvennogo issledovaniia*, 3 vols (Ekaterinburg: U-Faktoriia, 2006), 1: 443–542 (Chast' II, 'Vechnoe dvizhenie').

4. Hooper notes that 'Gulag boss' F. M. Mochulsky evades discussion in his memoir of prisoner suffering, speculating on the causes of this evasion: continued adherence to 'political conditioning'; a refusal to care; a lack of literary skill; masculine gender norms eschewing emotionality in autobiography; or mirroring a pragmatic survival strategy of forgetting what could not be changed. Scholar Anna Krylova argues that Western scholars bring a set of misplaced expectations amounting to looking for a 'liberal subject' in Soviet ego-documents. See Cynthia V. Hooper, 'Bosses in Captivity? On the Limitations of Gulag Memoir', *Kritika: Explorations in Russian and Eurasian History* 14, no. 1 (2013): 139, quotation at 140; Anna Krylova, 'The Tenacious Liberal Subject in Soviet Studies,' *Kritika: Explorations in Russian and Eurasian History* 1, no. 1 (2000): 119–46.

5. Glazov, *Koshmar parallel'nogo mira*, 5–9. The stigma of the 'spoilt biography' was acute for those seeking to make a career, especially Party members, in the Stalin era; see e.g. Jochen Hellbeck, *Revolution on my Mind: Writing a Diary under Stalin* (Cambridge, MA & London: Harvard University Press, 2006); Igal Halfin, *Red Autobiographies: Initiating the Bolshevik Self* (Seattle: Herbert J. Ellison Center for Russian, East European, and Central Asian Studies, 2011); idem, *Terror in my Soul: Communist Autobiographies on Trial* (Cambridge, MA & London: Harvard University Press, 2003).

6. Glazov, *Koshmar parallel'nogo mira*, 9.

7. Ibid., 11.

8. Charles Shaw, 'Friendship under Lock and Key: The Soviet Central Asian Border, 1918–34', *Central Asian Survey* 30, no. 3–4 (2011): 331–48.

9. Glazov, *Koshmar parallel'nogo mira*, 19–23; 24–5. The date of transfer to Moscow OGPU work is unclear in his account, but as he patrolled Clara Zetkin's June 1933 funeral as an OGPU plain-clothes operative, I infer he was well integrated by then.

10. On border control by the OGPU, its increased presence in the early 1930s, and the increase in Party members sent to work for it, see Shaw, 'Friendship under Lock and Key', 335, 342.

11. Glazov, *Koshmar parallel'nogo mira*, 22–3. On the famine in Ukraine and Central Asia, which also affected southern Russia, see Anne Applebaum, *Red Famine: Stalin's War on Ukraine* (London: Penguin, 2017); Sarah I. Cameron, *The Hungry Steppe: Famine, Violence, and the Making of Soviet Kazakhstan* (Ithaca: Cornell University Press, 2018). On privileged distribution of food and goods to state elites under Stalin, see E. A. Osokina, *Our Daily Bread: Socialist Distribution and the Art of Survival in Stalin's Russia, 1927–1941* (Armonk & London: M. E. Sharpe, 2001).

12. Glazov, *Koshmar parallel'nogo mira*, 24–5.

13. Glazov, *Koshmar parallel'nogo mira*, 27–34.

14. Glazov, *Koshmar parallel'nogo mira*, 172. Reform after 1953 detached economic from penal operations and reduced the prisoner population drastically; see Jeffrey S. Hardy, *The Gulag after Stalin: Redefining Punishment in Khrushchev's Soviet Union, 1953–1964* (Ithaca & London: Cornell University Press, 2016).

15. Glazov, *Koshmar parallel'nogo mira*, 36. It was typical that guards appointed such doctors where they appeared among the prisoners in a transport; see e.g. A. I. Kaufman, *Lagernyi vrach. 16 let v Sovetskom Soiuze – vospominaniia sionista* (Tel Aviv: AM OVED, 1973), 31–3.

16. Glazov, *Koshmar parallel'nogo mira*, 41–4.

17. Ibid., 47. Ukhta's Sangorodok was founded in 1933; by 1938 it had 150 beds served by 194 medical workers, including 12 doctors; it was the principal medical centre for Ukhtpechlag; see S. F. Sapolnova, T. A. Vekshina, and F. G. Kanev, eds, *Liudi v belykh khalatakh* (Ukhta & Syktyvkar: Komi respublikanskaia tipografiia, 2009), 114. I have also drawn on the history of the Sangorodok found in MIZU, Eizenbraun, Emil' Vil'gel'movich folder, 'Doklad E. V. Eizenbrauna v chest' Dnia meditsinskogo rabotnika v 1966 g.'.

18. Glazov, *Koshmar parallel'nogo mira*, 48. On Gulag attempts to separate male and female prisoners, see Wilson T. Bell, 'Sex, Pregnancy, and Power in the Late Stalinist Gulag', *Journal of the History of Sexuality* 24, no. 2 (2015): 198–224.

19. Glazov, *Koshmar parallel'nogo mira*, 49. For a contrasting view of the Sangorodok's alleged order and hygiene, see Sapolnova et al., *Liudi v belykh khalatakh*, 114.

20. See e.g. the description of a first hospital assignment in N. V. Savoeva, *Ia vybrala Kolymu*, Arkhivy Pamiati. Vyp. 1 (Magadan: AO 'MAOBTI', Obshchestvo 'Poisk nezakonno repressirovannykh', 1996), 12–15.

21. For an example of a freely hired doctor who was given the opportunity to think over assuming the role of head of a Gulag hospital, see Savoeva, *Ia vybrala Kolymu*, 23. For a prisoner-physician who in protest refused to serve as a doctor in Kolyma hospital where doctors had been shot, preferring general labour, see MMSPb, GOTLIBOIM, Iosif Samoilovich, 'Vospominaniia', 31 pp., n.d. Ultimately, Gotliboim relented and joined the hospital staff in 1939.

22. Glazov, *Koshmar parallel'nogo mira*, 49–50; MMA, f. 2, op. 2, d. 17, l. 51.

23. Glazov, *Koshmar parallel'nogo mira*, 52–3.

24. MMA, f. 2, op. 2, d. 17, l. 55.

25. Glazov, *Koshmar parallel'nogo mira*, 56. The 'chekist illness' was a variant of the much wider 'Soviet exhaustion' said to affect Party, military, and managerial elites after 1917; it was an indulgent social construct rather than a genuine disorder as such, and Stalinist medical experts discredited it by the late 1930s. See e.g. Benjamin Zajicek, 'Soviet Madness: Nervousness, Mild Schizophrenia, and the Professional Jurisdiction of Psychiatry in the USSR, 1918–1936', *Ab Imperio* 2014, no. 4 (2014): 167–94; Kenneth M. Pinnow, *Lost to the Collective: Suicide and the Promise of Soviet Socialism, 1921–1929* (Ithaca & London: Cornell University Press, 2010), 44–5; Frances Lee Bernstein, *The Dictatorship of Sex: Lifestyle Advice for the Soviet Masses* (DeKalb: Northern Illinois University Press, 2007), 85–91.

26. Glazov, *Koshmar parallel'nogo mira*, 62. The releases took place under article 458 of the RSFSR Criminal Code, which set out procedures for early release on medical grounds; writing fifty years after these events, Glazov misremembers it as article 438. On these release procedures, see Golfo Alexopoulos,

Illness and Inhumanity in Stalin's Gulag (New Haven & London: Yale University Press, 2017), 134–6; Mikhail Nakonechnyi, '"They Won't Survive for Long": Soviet Officials on Medical Release Procedure', in *Rethinking the Gulag: Identities, Sources, Legacies*, ed. Alan Barenberg and Emily D. Johnson (Bloomington: Indiana University Press, 2022), 103–28.

27. Glazov, *Koshmar parallel'nogo mira*, 63.
28. Ibid., 63.
29. Nakonechnyi, '"They Won't Survive for Long"'.
30. Moscow set a quota of Gulag prisoners to be shot at 10,000 in July 1937, and these deliberate killings were conducted at specific camps by NKVD plenipotentiaries; see Oleg Khlevniuk, *The History of the Gulag: From Collectivization to the Great Terror* (New Haven & London: Yale University Press, 2004), 170–1; for NKVD order 00447 which set out the mechanisms of the mass operations in July 1937, see J. Arch Getty and Oleg V. Naumov, *The Road to Terror: Stalin and the Self-Destruction of the Bolsheviks, 1932–1939* (New Haven & London: Yale University Press, 1999), 471–81.
31. Glazov, *Koshmar parallel'nogo mira*, 63–4, 86, 92. In an August 1938 NKVD report on executions in the region, 1,112 out of 1,931 prisoners shot are said to be 'Trotskyites, Bukharinists, Kamenevites, and Zinovievites': see Iu. N. Afanas'ev et al., eds, *Istoriia stalinskogo Gulaga. Konets 1920-kh – pervaia polovina 1950-kh godov. Sobranie dokumentov v semi tomakh* (Moscow: ROSSPEN, 2004–5),1: 301. On the hunger strikes, see Alan Barenberg, *Gulag Town, Company Town: Forced Labor and its Legacy in Vorkuta* (New Haven & London: Yale University Press, 2014), 25–8; M. B. Rogachev, '"My vynuzhdeny pribegnut' k bor'be": Golodovka politzakliuchennykh v Vorkute v 1936 godu', in *Pokaianie: Komi respublikanskii martirolog zhertv massovykh politicheskikh repressii*, ed. G. V. Nevskii and V. G. Nevskii (Syktyvkar: Fond 'Pokaianie', 2004), 7: 95–106.
32. Glazov, *Koshmar parallel'nogo mira*, 70. On Eizenbraun, see MIZU, Eizenbraun, Emil' Vil'gel'movich folder.
33. Vorkuta-Vom housed weakened prisoners sent 'to recuperate' after exhaustion through labour in Vorkuta's coal mines; see Barenberg, *Gulag Town, Company Town*, 21, 24.
34. Glazov, *Koshmar parallel'nogo mira*, 86–9.
35. Barenberg, *Gulag Town, Company Town*, 31–2; A. N. Kaneva, 'Ukhtpechlag: Stranitsy istorii', in *Pokaianie: Martirolog. T. 8, Ch. 1*, ed. E. A. Zelenskaia and M. B. Rogachev (Syktyvkar: Komi respublikanskii blagotvoritel'nyi obshchestvennyi fond zhertv politicheskikh repressii 'Pokaianie', 2005), 138–9.
36. Glazov, *Koshmar parallel'nogo mira*, 92–3. Glazov says he heard from an old prisoner that when Kashketin's plane arrived, two men got out and shot the plenipotentiary; however, this is consoling legend not fact: Kashketin was decorated for his services in 1938, arrested in 1939, and shot in 1940: Barenberg, *Gulag Town, Company Town*, 286 n. 72.
37. Glazov, *Koshmar parallel'nogo mira*, 94.
38. For instances of this response, see ibid., 95, 100–2.
39. Historians have generally confined examinations of tufta to Gulag economic production, which was notoriously inflated; see e.g. Zhak Rossi, *Spravochnik po GULagu*, 2 vols (Moscow: Prosvet, 1991), 2: 414–16; Solzhenitsyn, *Arkhipelag Gulag 1918–1956*, 2: 122–32. On Gulag medical statistics and problems of

interpretation, see Mikhail Nakonechnyi, 'The Gulag's "Dead Souls": Mortality of Individuals Released from the Camps, 1930–55', *Kritika: Explorations in Russian and Eurasian History* 23, no. 4 (2022): 803–50, and the replies by Stephen Wheatcroft, Nakonechnyi, and Golfo Alexopoulos in the same issue.

40. Tatiana Afanas'eva, 'Pisateli Ukrainy na Pechore', in *Vygliadyvaias' v proshloe*, ed. T. Afanas'eva (Pechora: Pechorskoe vremia, 2010), 172–3.

41. MMA, f. 2, op. 2, d. 17, l. 115. This episode does not appear in *Koshmar parallel'nogo mira*.

42. Glazov, *Koshmar parallel'nogo mira*, 141–2.

43. Ibid., 142–3.

44. MMA, f. 2, op. 2, d. 17, ll. 119–20; cf. Glazov, *Koshmar parallel'nogo mira*, 107–8.

45. Glazov, *Koshmar parallel'nogo mira*, 143–4.

46. On these commissions, see Dan Healey, 'Lives in the Balance: Weak and Disabled Prisoners and the Biopolitics of the Gulag', *Kritika: Explorations in Russian and Eurasian History* 16, no. 3 (2015): 527–56.

47. MMSPb, KNIAZEV, Grigorii Vlasovich, 'Vospominaniia', 3 vols; 'Vorkuta (67° severnoi shiroty)', 3: 389.

48. Kniazev, 'Vospominaniia', 3: 389–90; Glazov, *Koshmar parallel'nogo mira*, 83.

49. See GARF, f. R9414, op. 1, d. 2741, l. 17. For 1932 advice to the Gulag on treatment of pellagra, and the wider context, see GARF, f. R9414, op. 1, d. 2739, ll. 8–9, 'Kratkaia instruktsiia po diagnostike i terapii pellagry'; Golfo Alexopoulos, 'Medical Research in Stalin's Gulag', *Bulletin of the History of Medicine* 90, no. 3 (2016): 363–93.

50. Glazov, *Koshmar parallel'nogo mira*, 96.

51. Ibid., 96–7.

52. Ibid., 140.

53. N. G. Okhotin and A. B. Roginskii, eds, *Sistema ispravitel'no-trudovykh lagerei v SSSR, 1923–1960: Spravochnik* (Moscow: Zven'ia, 1998), 229–30; Glazov was apparently deputy director of the Sangorodok; see N. A. Morozov, 'Istrebitel'no-trudovye gody', in *Pokaianie: Martirolog. T. 1*, ed. G. V. Nevskii (Syktyvkar: Komi knizhnoe izdatel'stvo, 1998), 1: 131.

54. Glazov, *Koshmar parallel'nogo mira*, 148; MMA, f. 2, op. 2, d. 17, ll. 168–9.

55. Soviet troops liberated Auschwitz on 27 January 1945; on the limits of awareness about Auschwitz before and after that date in the USSR, see Harvey Asher, 'The Soviet Union, the Holocaust, and Auschwitz', *Kritika: Explorations in Russian and Eurasian History* 4, no. 4 (2003): 886–912; and Alan Barenberg, '"I Would Very Much Like to Read your Story about Kolyma": Georgii Demidov, Varlam Shalamov, and the Development of Gulag Prose, 1965–67', in *Rethinking the Gulag: Identities, Sources, Legacies*, ed. Alan Barenberg and Emily D. Johnson (Bloomington: Indiana University Press, 2022), 230.

56. Glazov, *Koshmar parallel'nogo mira*, 149–50.

57. Ibid., 3.

58. Ibid., 3.

59. Hooper, 'Bosses in Captivity?'.

60. On Stalinist experience as a sharpener of survival skills, see Sheila Fitzpatrick, *Everyday Stalinism: Ordinary Life in Extraordinary Times: Soviet Russia in the 1930s* (Oxford: Oxford University Press, 1999), 218–27.

Chapter 3 'I Chose Kolyma': From the medical school benches to the hospitals of the Gulag

1. MMA, GUZIKOVA, Sof'ia Lazarevna, 'Stranitsy vospominanii', n.d., f. 2, op. 2, d. 21, l. 1.
2. Guzikova, 'Stranitsy vospominanii'.
3. On Chudnovskaya, see GARF, f. R9414, op. 9, d. 50, ll. 85–92. The statistic on freely hired doctors recruited by the Gulag is calculated from: GARF, f. R8009, op. 14, dd. 56, 246, 390, 524, 566, 753, 774, 794.
4. N. V. Savoeva, *Ia vybrala Kolymu*. Arkhivy Pamiati. Vyp. 1 (Magadan: AO 'MAOBTI', Obshchestvo 'Poisk nezakonno repressirovannykh', 1996), 9. For Savoeva's list of Moscow Medical Institute graduates sent to Magadan, see MOKM, ed. khr. 25992/17, 'Spisok vrachei vypusknikov I-go med. instituta g. Moskvy, priekhavshikh na Kolymu (arkhiv Savoevoi N. V.)' [dated 23 December 1989].
5. On graduate attitudes towards job commissions, see Christopher Burton, 'Medical Welfare during Late Stalinism: A Study of Doctors and the Soviet Health System, 1945–1953' (PhD thesis, University of Chicago, 2000), 174–240.
6. Elena Shulman, *Stalinism on the Frontier of Empire: Women and State Formation in the Soviet Far East* (Cambridge: Cambridge University Press, 2008), 130–9.
7. 'No, we didn't know anything about Kolyma, Magadan was a blank slate, I had no ideas about the place. There was one acquaintance of my mother and father who visited us from there on his way to vacation, and he told us a little bit about it, but it was so little, that you cannot say that we had any pre-existing awareness of it. It was a blank slate for me until I got there.' Interview with Anna Kliashko, 31 March 2010, Montréal, Canada.
8. Cynthia V. Hooper, 'Bosses in Captivity? On the Limitations of Gulag Memoir', *Kritika: Explorations in Russian and Eurasian History* 14, no. 1 (2013): 140.
9. GARF, f. R9414, op. 1, d. 2750, ll. 1–4, published in Iu. N. Afanas'ev et al., eds, *Istoriia stalinskogo Gulaga. Konets 1920-kh – pervaia polovina 1950-kh godov. Sobranie dokumentov v semi tomakh* (Moscow, ROSSPEN, 2004–5), 4: 485–9. From these 1939 statistics there were 15.3 doctors per 10,000 Gulag prisoners; the analogous figure for 1940 in civilian medical service was 7 per 10,000 civilians. For civilian figures, see Burton, 'Medical Welfare during Late Stalinism', 64. The 1944 Gulag doctor statistics are advisory (staff positions rather than actually filled posts); see B. A. Nakhapetov, *Ocherki istorii sanitarnoi sluzhby Gulaga* (Moscow: ROSSPEN, 2009), 92.
10. A 1939 statute on the camp regime explicitly permitted the employment of doctors with article 58 ('anti-Soviet actions') convictions in their professional capacity: 'Vremennaia instriuktsiia o rezhime soderzhaniia zakliuchennykh v ITL NKVD SSSR', in A. I. Kokurin and N. V. Petrov, eds, *GULAG: Glavnoe upravlenie lagerei, 1918–1960* (Moscow: Mezhdunarodnyi fond Demokratiia, 2000), 467. Three-quarters of all skilled prisoner-professionals were being used in their occupational fields in 1947; while 88.2 per cent of medical specialists were so employed; see Viktor N. Zemskov, 'GULAG (Istoriko-sotsiologicheskii aspekt)', *Sotsiologicheskie issledovaniia*, nos 6, 7 (1991): 6: 10–27; 7: 3–16, data at 7: 11.
11. For an example, see Elena Mamuchashvili, 'V bol'nitse dlia zakliuchennykh', *Shalamovskii sbornik* 2 (1997): 78–88. A 21 April 1938 memorandum from the

top leadership of the Gulag ordered the placement of advertisements in the medical press. The draft text read: 'Wanted. For work in construction sites and lumber works in the Far East, Baikal, and Northern regions of the USSR, doctors in all specialisations, sanitary doctors, malaria specialists, dentists, feld-shers, qualified nurses, pharmacists; pay by agreement; apply to . . .'. See GARF, f. R9414, op. 1, d. 2753, ll. 142–4.

12. Standard civilian payrates, see Mark G. Field, *Doctor and Patient in Soviet Russia* (Cambridge, MA: Harvard University Press, 1957), 104. Gulag recruiters offered Taisiia Kirillova, a graduate of Kharkiv Medical Institute in 1938, a salary of 580 roubles a month for a posting in Oneglag, with an expenses bonus of just over 1,000 roubles and a 300-rouble book allowance. Her male colleague assigned to the same camp as director of its sanitary department, Aleksei Kirienko, received 815 roubles monthly, and later a bonus of over 1,400 roubles. In the same round of assignments, doctors sent to the notoriously harsh Kotlas and Norilsk camps were offered 675 roubles 'plus a 15% bonus' monthly: see GARF, f. R8009, op. 14, d. 56, ll. 81, 86, 119.

13. MOKM, ed. khr. 21702, SAVEL'EVA, Liudmila Aleksandrovna, 'Individual'nyi trudovoi dogovor No. 2120. g. Moskva, 15 iiulia 1940 goda'.

14. See MOKM, ed. khr. 25973/15, USHAKOVA, Aleksandra Petrovna, 'Avtobiografiia Ushakovoi A. P. 22.vi.1985 g.' (who arrived as a Komsomol recruit in Pevek, Chukotka, in 1939, and took her first holiday and attended courses in Moscow in 1948); Savoeva, *Ia vybrala Kolymu*, 37. Anna Kliashko laughed when asked what her starting salary was: 'I can say that I survived several currency reforms and I simply forget now what the money meant back then, and now it's hard to say what we got. I can simply say that working in the Far North, our salaries were not bad in comparison to the average wages in the Soviet Union. We were able to live reasonably comfortably, to travel, to raise a family, so our salaries were pretty good – that was the policy in the North.' Interview, 23 June 2009.

15. On the higher status and pay of 'embedded' medical services over the civilian one in the Soviet economy, see Christopher M. Davis, 'The Economics of the Soviet Health System: An Analytical and Historical Study, 1921–1978' (PhD thesis, Cambridge University, 1979), 57; Burton, 'Medical Welfare during Late Stalinism', 119.

16. Yakov Petrovich Sokolov was an orphan who studied medicine at the First Moscow Medical Institute in 1925–31, during which time he also worked voluntarily for the OGPU. On graduation his first job was as director of the sanitary department (Sanotdel) of Ukhtizhemlag. His wife, Sofia Viktorovna, also a student at the same institute, was assigned a job as clinic manager under him. See MIZU, Sokolov, Iakov Petrovich and Sokolova, Sof'ia Viktorovna folder, autobiographical extracts from Arkhiv MVD g. Ukhta, A-41393, d. 336/304; A-46560, d. 454/263.

17. Such examples are numerous. Isai Yakovlevich Usminsky, on graduation from Vitebsk Medical Institute, was assigned to Ukhta camp hospitals in 1951, and transferred to civilian hospitals in 1956, eventually becoming 'the chief otolaryngology specialist in Ukhta' and an 'Honoured Physician of the Komi Republic' in 1968; see MIZU, Usminskii, Isai Iakovlevich folder, ed. khr. GIKM 3029/5. Note the careers of camp clinic manager Tatiana Repyeva, and medical administrator-physician Aleksei Khoroshev, in A. G. Kozlov, *Iz istorii*

zdravookhraneniia Kolymy i Chukotki (1941–1954 gg.) (Magadan: Magadanskii oblastnoi dom sanitarnogo prosveshcheniia, Magadanskii oblastnoi kraevedcheskii muzei, 1991), 24, 114.

18. The best-known example of the labour-camp employee memoir is Fyodor Vasilevich Mochulsky and Deborah A. Kaple, *Gulag Boss: A Soviet Memoir* (Oxford and New York: Oxford University Press, 2011); on the genre, see Hooper, 'Bosses in Captivity?'. Guzikova mentions signing her non-disclosure pledge: Guzikova, 'Stranitsy vospominanii', l. 1. MIKM displays a typical non-disclosure agreement (*Ob"iazatel'stvo*) in its Dal'stroi Trust public-facing history room described in the Introduction.

19. On 'veiled' commemoration in the 1960s–1980s, see Tyler C. Kirk, 'From Enemy to Hero: Andrei Krems and the Legacy of Stalinist Repression in Russia's Far North, 1964–82', *Russian Review* 82, no. 2 (2023): 292–306.

20. In her introduction to Mochulsky's memoir, Kaple notes that he wrote his text after 1988, and apparently felt confusion and remorse about his role as a Gulag commandant; see Mochulsky, *Gulag Boss*, xx–xxi. On medical fiction writing in the Russian tradition, see Elena Fratto, *Medical Storyworlds: Health, Illness, and Bodies in Russian and European Literature at the Turn of the Twentieth Century* (New York: Columbia University Press, 2021).

21. Guzikova, 'Stranitsy vospominanii'. An extract was published as 'Iz vospominanii S. L. Guzikovoi', in Oleg Khlevniuk, V. A. Kozlov, and S. V. Mironenko, eds, *Zakliuchennye na stroikakh kommunizma. Gulag i ob"ekty energetiki v SSSR. Sobranie dokumentov i fotografii* (Moscow: ROSSPEN, 2008), 427–32.

22. Date and place of birth found on a war decoration citation for Guzikova at https://www.polkmoskva.ru/people/985287/ (accessed 6 March 2020).

23. Guzikova, 'Stranitsy vospominanii', l. 6.

24. Guzikova, 'Stranitsy vospominanii', l. 25. Discrepancies exist between the date of mobilisation Guzikova gives in this memoir, and those found on a citation document for war service. The citation says she joined the army in February 1942 in Cherdyn, Molotov Oblast, i.e. within 15 kilometres of Bulatovo camp. In the same document, the accompanying narrative describing her service says she 'was a participant in the Great Patriotic War from 1941'. These confusions and possible fabrications suggest that Guzikova, or the military, sought to conceal her Gulag service even in April 1945 when the citation was produced. I found her war record at https://www.polkmoskva.ru/people/985287/ (accessed 6 March 2020); the site has since been removed, apparently in connection with the Kremlin's anxieties about war commemoration during the current phase of its war against Ukraine.

25. The memoir's content suggests Guzikova must have survived to the late 1980s to have written this account. Guzikova figures in 1947 in Moscow as the friend and doctor of Lidiia Ivanovna Smirnova, a government official whose biography is found at http://zavjalov.okis.ru/smirnovaL2.html (accessed 6 March 2020).

26. On the memory politics of Russia's online veteran commemoration see Julie Fedor, 'Memory, Kinship, and the Mobilization of the Dead: The Russian State and the "Immortal Regiment" Movement', in *War and Memory in Russia, Ukraine and Belarus*, ed. J. Fedor, M. Kangaspuro, J. Lassila, T. Zhurzhenko, and A. Etkind (Cham: Springer, 2017).

27. Guzikova, 'Stranitsy vospominanii', 9. On Petkevich, a nurse in the Gulag (as well as her headline profession in Gulag theatres), see Tamara Petkevich, *Memoir of a Gulag Actress* (DeKalb: Northern Illinois University Press, 2011).

28. The Memorial's archival indexes and annotations often refer to a younger family member's assistance in getting a senior relative to tell their story. Nikolai Glazov's prisoner-doctor memoir was the product of his daughter's encouragement, as discussed in chapter 2.

29. Savoeva's name and Komsomol membership in 1940 is found in health commissariat lists of medical school graduates, see GARF, f. R8009, op. 14, d. 128, l. 4.

30. Savoeva evades revealing her own Party membership, only mentioning it when she admits she was excluded from the Party in the late 1940s after a dispute with a corrupt official (*Ia vybrala Kolymu*, 44). Shalamov says she was a full Party member while running Belichya, and that she was expelled for marrying an ex-zek, Lesniak; see Varlam Shalamov, *Neskol'ko moikh zhiznei. Vospominaniia, zapisnye knizhki, perepiska, sledstvennye dela* (Moscow: Eksmo, 2009), 210.

31. See Panikarov's foreword to Savoeva, *Ia vybrala Kolymu*, 3; Boris N. Lesniak, *Ia k vam prishel!* (Magadan: MAOBTI, 1998), 3–5. On Panikarov see Vladislav Staf, 'Local Initiatives: A Historical Analysis of the Creation of Memorial Museums of the Gulag in (Post-)Soviet Russia', *Problems of Post-Communism* (2023): 6, https://doi.org/10.1080/10758216.2023.2166846.

32. Semen Vilenskii, ed., *Dodnes' tiagoteet: v 2-kh tomakh* (Moscow: Vozvrashchenie, 2004), 2: 295–309.

33. Another free doctor spoke about her work as a freely hired doctor when literary historians solicited her reminiscences. See the interview from Dr Elena Mamuchashvili, who worked alongside the prisoner-feldsher Varlam Shalamov; Mamuchashvili, 'V bol'nitse dlia zakliuchennykh'.

34. On promotion and its discontents, see Sheila Fitzpatrick, *Education and Social Mobility in the Soviet Union 1921–1934* (Cambridge: Cambridge University Press, 1979); idem, *Everyday Stalinism: Ordinary Life in Extraordinary Times: Soviet Russia in the 1930s* (Oxford: Oxford University Press, 1999).

35. GARF, f. R9414, op. 1, d. 2753, l. 318, dated 9 November 1938.

36. Ibid., ll. 318–19.

37. Savoeva, *Ia vybrala Kolymu*, 12. Despite working in civilian medical services, Kliashko likewise met Nikishov upon arrival in 1948; he told her to avoid fraternisation with ex-prisoners, but she claims it was impossible to follow this order because of the large number of such people among her colleagues and patients: interview, 15 September 2012. Guzikova recalled a similar reception at her first camp: Guzikova, 'Stranitsy vospominanii', l. 2.

38. Apparently, women were selected firstly because they overwhelmingly dominated the ranks of newly trained physicians in the Stalin era; it was probably assumed they would be more compliant employees too. Another rationale was to encourage the colonisation of these remote regions; Gulag planners were aware of the huge gender imbalance in these 'construction sites' and female workers would expand opportunities for marriage and influence more workers to stay in these regions. On the problems of gender imbalance in the Gulag settlements and 'family-lessness', see Dan Healey, *Russian Homophobia from Stalin to Sochi* (London: Bloomsbury Academic, 2017), 31–2.

39. Guzikova, 'Stranitsy vospominanii', ll. 3, 5, 12.
40. Such decrees on winter preparations became routine. Senior judicial officials monitored Gulag camps for fulfilment of these decrees. For procuracy commentary on the 1940 winter preparations decree noting the failure of camp commandants 'to treat it seriously', see GARF, f. R8131, op. 37, d. 357, ll. 1–1 ob.
41. Guzikova, 'Stranitsy vospominanii', l. 12. This episode followed one in which bosses humiliated Dr Guzikova for trying to stop distribution of food she deemed unsafe for prisoner consumption.
42. Ibid.
43. See e.g. A. G. Tepliakov, *Mashina terrora: OGPU-NKVD Sibiri v 1929–1941 gg.* (Moscow: Novyi khronograf, 2008), 170–6.
44. This episode resembles the plot of a perestroika-era drama film, *Defence Counsel Sedov* (Evgenii Tsymbal, director, 1988), in which a champion of falsely accused agronomists in the 1937 Terror unwittingly brings a widening circle of innocents to their doom. Savoeva describes the atmosphere in the Moscow Medical Institute during the Terror: Savoeva, *Ia vybrala Kolymu*, 8–9.
45. Leona Toker, *Return from the Archipelago: Narratives of Gulag Survivors* (Bloomington & Indianapolis: Indiana University Press, 2000), 94–8; Solzhenitsyn asserts the absolute right of the hunger-striker in the face of authority: Aleksandr Solzhenitsyn, *Arkhipelag Gulag 1918–1956: Opyt khudozhestvennogo issledovaniia*, 3 vols (Ekaterinburg: U-Faktoriia, 2006), 3: 473.
46. Guzikova, 'Stranitsy vospominanii', l. 5.
47. Ibid., ll. 2, 3.
48. Ibid., l. 10.
49. Mark Field cites Virchow in relation to Soviet civilian doctors: see *Doctor and Patient*, 159.
50. Savoeva, *Ia vybrala Kolymu*, 14.
51. Ibid., 14–19.
52. Ibid., 21.
53. Ibid.
54. Ibid. A graduate of Gorky Medical Institute, Repyeva arrived in Kolyma to work in indigenous medical services in 1936; she soon ran mining-camp clinics for Dal'stroi: see A. G. Kozlov, *Iz istorii zdravookhraneniia Kolymy i Chukotki (1864–1941 gg.)* (Magadan: Magadanskoe knizhnoe iz-vo, 1989), 24.
55. On the corporate language of the Sanotdel, see Golfo Alexopoulos, *Illness and Inhumanity in Stalin's Gulag* (New Haven & London: Yale University Press, 2017), 160–82.
56. Sevlag means 'Northern Camp'; on the institutional complexity of Dalstroi, see N. G. Okhotin and A. B. Roginskii, eds, *Sistema ispravitel'no-trudovykh lagerei v SSSR, 1923–1960: Spravochnik* (Moscow: Zven'ia, 1998), 117–20. For bed numbers, see Savoeva, *Ia vybrala Kolymu*, 29.
57. 'Unguarded' (*beskonvoinye*) prisoners increased in number during the war because guards were diverted to the army; see Wilson Bell, 'Was the Gulag an Archipelago? De-Convoyed Prisoners and Porous Borders in the Camps of Western Siberia', *Russian Review* 72, no. 1 (2013): 116–41.
58. Shalamov, *Neskol'ko moikh zhiznei*, 207.
59. She also regretted having to leave Belichya in 1946; see Eugenia Ginzburg, *Within the Whirlwind*, trans. Ian Boland (London: Collins Harvill, 1989), 133, 155–6.

60. On the episode, see 'Nastoiashchie liudi (o magadanskom vrache Nine Vladimirovne Savoevoi)', http://temnyjles.ru/LK/ocherki.shtml (accessed 25 March 2020).

61. Shalamov, *Neskol'ko moikh zhiznei*, 210; Savoeva, *Ia vybrala Kolymu*, 44.

62. Savoeva, *Ia vybrala Kolymu*, 40–6.

63. Ibid., 17.

64. Guzikova, 'Stranitsy vospominanii', ll. 8, 9.

65. Ibid., l. 8.

66. Ibid.

67. Ibid., l. 10.

68. Ibid., l. 25.

69. On this point see, e.g., Zuzanna Bogumił, *Gulag Memories: The Rediscovery and Commemoration of Russia's Repressive Past*, trans. Philip Palmer (New York: Berghahn Books, 2018), 86–7.

70. On the victim's perspective in Gulag studies see, e.g., Nanci Adler, *Victims of Soviet Terror: The Story of the Memorial Movement* (Westport & London: Praeger, 1993); Stephen F. Cohen, *The Victims Return: Survivors of the Gulag after Stalin* (Exeter, NH: Publishing Works, 2010). For reflections on the complexity of representing these victim perspectives, see Alexander Etkind, *Warped Mourning: Stories of the Undead in the Land of the Unburied* (Stanford: Stanford University Press, 2013), 7–12, 23–4, 35–9.

71. Savoeva, *Ia vybrala Kolymu*, 30. Savoeva's attitude towards Shalamov was more indulgent and gender dynamics, including the possibility of a sexual liaison, may account for the difference. Shalamov wrote a short story implying Savoeva initiated an encounter, 'Chernaia mama' in Shalamov, *Neskol'ko moikh zhiznei*, 217–20.

72. Ginzburg, *Within the Whirlwind*, 134–6. Queen Tamara was Georgia's extraordinarily successful monarch, 1184 to 1213, renowned for a golden age of political and literary achievement. Ginzburg's taunt rides roughshod over the ethnic differences of the Caucasus.

73. Ibid., 137, 142–3.

74. Ginzburg describes the string-pulling she worked to get the transfer to Belichya: ibid., 130–2.

75. Savoeva, *Ia vybrala Kolymu*, 31, 33; 'hysterical fit', Ginzburg, *Within the Whirlwind*, 142–3.

76. 'These texts are far from indisputable. Ginzburg's memoirs and Shalamov's short stories are often subjective. Perhaps one should not expect anything other than prejudgement from those who passed through the Kolyma camps about those who stood on the other side of the barbed wire. However, having experienced many horrors of the camps, both V. T. Shalamov and E. S. Ginzburg survived them thanks to the humane attitude towards them shown by people such as N. V. Savoeva. Savoeva's own memoirs, like those of several other freely hired Dal'stroi employees and formerly repressed people, are completely contradictory to the evaluations of medical workers given in "Kolyma Tales" and "Krutoi marshrut".' See Kozlov, *Iz istorii zdravookhraneniia Kolymy i Chukotki (1941–1954 gg.)*, 66–7.

77. Savoeva kept annual reports of Belichya hospital's activity but her husband Lesniak destroyed them under threat of rearrest in the late 1940s; Lesniak, *Ia k vam prishel!*, 123.

78. Mortality in the entire Gulag peaked in 1942; see Applebaum, *Gulag*, 519. On war's impact on the camps, see Wilson T. Bell, *Stalin's Gulag at War: Forced Labour, Mass Death, and Soviet Victory in the Second World War* (Toronto: University of Toronto Press, 2019), 94–5; the broader context is exposed in Wendy Z. Goldman and Donald A. Filtzer, *Fortress Dark and Stern: The Soviet Home Front during World War II* (New York: Oxford University Press, 2021), and Wendy Z. Goldman and Donald A. Filtzer, eds, *Hunger and War: Food Provisioning in the Soviet Union during World War II* (Bloomington: Indiana University Press, 2015). Numerous wartime decrees of Sevvostlag (Dal'stroi's camp complex) attest to starvation and high mortality in Kolyma. See I. D. Batsaev and A. G. Kozlov, eds, *Dal'stroi i Sevvostlag OGPU-NKVD SSSR v tsifrakh i dokumentakh. Ch. 2 (1941–1945)* (Magadan: SVKNII DVO RAN, 2002).

79. For a study grounded in regional Gulag records, which traces the evolution and scale of early release on health grounds with empirical rigour, see Mikhail Iur'evich Nakonechnyi, 'Factory of Invalids: Mortality, Disability and Early Release on Medical Grounds from the Gulag, 1930–1955' (DPhil thesis, University of Oxford, 2020); and idem, '"They Won't Survive for Long": Soviet Officials on Medical Release Procedure', in *Rethinking the Gulag: Identities, Sources, Legacies*, ed. Alan Barenberg and Emily D. Johnson (Bloomington: Indiana University Press, 2022), 103–28. For a reading of the central Gulag records, Alexopoulos, *Illness and Inhumanity in Stalin's Gulag*.

80. Solzhenitsyn mocked the notion that Gulag morgues performed medically useful work, emphasising the desecration of corpses by ghoulish thugs; see Solzhenitsyn, *Arkhipelag Gulag*, 2: 176–7. A December 1941 Gulag order permitted burial without coffins but still foresaw individual graves: GARF, f. R9414, op. 1, d. 2762, ll. 190–1. Gulag chief V. G. Nasedkin issued a detailed decree on burial procedures on 2 February 1943; it permitted common graves for naked corpses: GARF, f. R9414, op. 1, d. 2785, ll. 18–18 ob. Also note V. N. Triakhov, *Gulag i voina: Zhestokaia pravda dokumentov* (Perm': Pushka, 2004), 188–9.

81. Alexopoulos, *Illness and Inhumanity in Stalin's Gulag*, 160–82.

82. Shalamov, *Neskol'ko moikh zhiznei*, 215–16.

83. Savoeva, *Ia vybrala Kolymu*, 28–9; for Magadan's first transfusion in December 1939, see A. F. Khoroshev, *Ocherki istorii zdravookhraneniia Magadanskoi Oblasti* (Magadan: Magadanskoe knizhnoe izdatel'stvo, 1959), 23; Kozlov, *Iz istorii zdravookhraneniia Kolymy i Chukotki (1941–1954 gg.)*, 53–4. Blood transfusions and a Soviet donor system were well established by the late 1930s; see N. L. Krementsov, *A Martian Stranded on Earth: Alexander Bogdanov, Blood Transfusions, and Proletarian Science* (Chicago & London: University of Chicago Press, 2011).

84. Kalembet had worked under founder of Soviet epidemiology Daniil Kirillovich Zabolotny and served as a Soviet embassy physician in the West before arrest in 1937; he was a resourceful organiser and adviser to Savoeva on all questions of hospital management. See Savoeva, *Ia vybrala Kolymu*, 24–7. Evidently, decisions he made enabled Shalamov to remain in Belichya as an orderly, the first step towards his feldsher course; Shalamov, *Neskol'ko moikh zhiznei*, 209–11. Kalembet figures in Shalamov's 1972 story 'Perchatka' (The Glove) in which Shalamov also acknowledges that he owes his survival to Savoeva and Lesniak; see Varlam Shalamov, *Preodolenie zla* (Moscow: Eksmo, 2011), 727–56.

85. Kozlov, *Iz istorii zdravookhraneniia Kolymy i Chukotki (1941–1954 gg.)*, 55, 114; Khoroshev, *Ocherki istorii zdravookhraneniia Magadanskoi Oblasti.*
86. See Kozlov, *Iz istorii zdravookhraneniia Kolymy i Chukotki (1864–1941 gg.)*, 24.
87. See MOKM, ed. khr. 21698, SAVEL'EVA, Liudmila Aleksandrovna, 'Avtobiografiia 23.vi.1948 g.'; ed. khr. 25973/15, USHAKOVA, Aleksandra Petrovna, 'Avtobiografiia Ushakovoi A. P. 22.vi.1985 g.'.

Chapter 4 'Feeling my way': Apprenticeships behind barbed wire

1. Vadim Aleksandrovskii, *Zapiski lagernogo vracha* (Moscow: Vozvrashchenie, 1996), 4–5; B. A. Nakhapetov, *Ocherki istorii sanitarnoi sluzhby Gulaga* (Moscow: ROSSPEN, 2009), 95. Afanasyev is not mentioned in Aleksandrovsky's memoir despite their simultaneous arrest; Nakhapetov was a first-year student in the same course, knew both victims, and finds the memoirist's silence about Afanasyev 'a great surprise'. He remembers Afanasyev as 'foppish' for wearing a bow tie in Imperial naval style, and describes him as 'a fair-haired good-looking man with a charming smile on a welcoming Russian face'. He was released but never rehabilitated and thus unable to return to military service; he completed his medical degree at I Leningrad Medical Institute; Nakhapetov, *Ocherki*, 97. On the Leningrad Affair, see David Brandenberger, 'Stalin, the Leningrad Affair, and the Limits of Postwar Russocentrism', *Russian Review* 63, no. 2 (2004): 241–55.
2. Aleksandrovskii, *Zapiski*, 7, 55.
3. On Shalamov's medical education, see e.g. Elena Mamuchashvili, 'V bol'nitse dlia zakliuchennykh', *Shalamovskii sbornik* 2 (1997): 78–88; Leona Toker, *Return from the Archipelago: Narratives of Gulag Survivors* (Bloomington & Indianapolis: Indiana University Press, 2000), 141–8. For Ginzburg's, see Toker, *Return from the Archipelago*, 52–5; Eugenia Ginzburg, *Within the Whirlwind*, trans. Ian Boland (London: Collins Harvill, 1989), 7–8. Bardach's education began in transit camp on the way to Kolyma; see Janusz Bardach and Kate Gleeson, *Man Is Wolf to Man: Surviving Stalin's Gulag* (London: Simon & Schuster, 1998), 171–80. In 1950, 20-year-old Yuri Fidelgolts was in Vanino transit camp where a doctor vouched to authorities that he was a 'feldsher' despite a lack of training (because he was a political prisoner and a safer choice than any criminal preferred by the bosses); he learned on the fly to assist his prisoner-doctor patron in the clinic: interview, 23 March 2009, Moscow.
4. Shalamov started a law degree in the 1920s but was arrested before qualifying; he worked as a journalist in the mid-1930s before arrest again in 1937 and detention in Kolyma. Varlam Shalamov, *Neskol'ko moikh zhiznei. Vospominaniia, zapisnye knizhki, perepiska, sledstvennye dela* (Moscow: Eksmo, 2009), 13; Toker, *Return from the Archipelago*, 141–8.
5. Samsonov was an enthusiastic memoirist in retirement. He consolidated three memoirs released in 1990, 1993, and 1997 in a single volume, and most references to his life will cite it: Viktor A. Samsonov, *K tebe, Onego, vse puti. Zapiski lagernogo lekpoma, studenta, vracha, prepodavatelia* (Petrozavodsk: Iz-vo Petrozavodskogo universiteta, 2000). A further book summarised his medical career: *Preodoleniia: V nelegkom puti v nauku ot medbrata-zakliuchennogo do professora universiteta* (Petrozavodsk: Petrozavodskii gosudarstvennyi univer-sitet, 2004). Samsonov published his correspondence with readers and other

Gulag survivors in Viktor A. Samsonov, *V perezhitom nenast'e: O lagernykh vrachakh i drugikh znakomykh medikakh, a takzhe o zemliakakh-kondopozhanakh, postradavshikh ot repressii 30–40-kh godov (dokumenty i pis'ma iz arkhiva avtora)* (Petrozavodsk: Petrozavodskii gosudarstvennyi universitet, 2001).

6. Samsonov, *K tebe*, 27–34.
7. Ibid., 45.
8. Ibid., 45–8.
9. Ibid., 52.
10. Ibid., 54.
11. Samsonov, *V perezhitom nenast'e*, 55.
12. Ilkka Mäkinen, 'Libraries in Hell: Cultural Activities in Soviet Prisons and Labor Camps from the 1930s to the 1950s', *Libraries and Culture* 28, no. 2 (1993): 117–42. On reforging, see Steven Anthony Barnes, *Death and Redemption: The Gulag and the Shaping of Soviet Society* (Princeton: Princeton University Press, 2011), 57–68.
13. Anna Kliashko lent books to a book-loving orderly, a former 'criminal' prisoner; she was able to buy or order Soviet medical literature without restrictions: interview, 24 June 2009, Montréal, Canada.
14. Samsonov, *K tebe*, 53. The book was M. S. Ikhteiman, *Rukovodstvo dlia srednego meditsinskogo personala* (Leningrad: Biomedgiz, 1935).
15. Samsonov, *K tebe*, 55, 57.
16. M. V. Chernorutskii, *Diagnostika vnutrennykh boleznei*, 1st edn (Leningrad: Medgiz, 1938).
17. The latest edition in 1940 was A. F. Berdiaev, *Khirurgiia ambulatornogo vracha*, 5th edn (Moscow & Leningrad: Medgiz, 1939). Earlier editions were published in 1928, 1930, 1931, 1935, and there would be 1944 and 1949 editions after Gaav made this present.
18. S. F. Sapolnova, T. A. Vekshina, and F. G. Kanev, eds, *Liudi v belykh khalatakh* (Ukhta & Syktyvkar: Komi respublikanskaia tipografiia, 2009), 66–7.
19. Samsonov, *K tebe*, 55–6. For Shalamov's story, see 'Perchatka' in Varlam Shalamov, *Preodolenie zla* (Moscow: Eksmo, 2011), 727–56.
20. On Vittenburg, see Sapolnova et al., *Liudi v belykh khalatakh*, 165–7.
21. Samsonov, *K tebe*, 59–65. Collective discussions of autopsies were part of medical routine in Dalstroi according to Anna Kliashko, interview, 15 September 2012, Montréal, Canada.
22. Samsonov, *K tebe*, 72. These were likely G. G. Genter, *Uchebnik akusherstva: Dlia studentov medvuzov* (Leningrad: Biomedgiz, 1937); and the hugely popular Ernst Bumm, *Rukovodstvo k izucheniiu akusherstva*, 3rd edn (Moscow & Leningrad: Gos. izd-vo, 1930).
23. Samsonov, *K tebe*, 73–7. His certificate is reproduced in Samsonov, *V perezhitom nenast'e*, 10.
24. Samsonov, *K tebe*, 79.
25. Vyshnia was investigated in 1940 for his friendships in camp; see N. A. Morozov, *Gulag v Komi krae 1929–1956* (Syktyvkar: Syktyvkarskii universitet, 1997), 39. The boundary between prisoners with salvageable and hopeless degeneration of their physical condition pervaded Gulag medical instructions; see Dan Healey, 'Lives in the Balance: Weak and Disabled Prisoners and the Biopolitics of the Gulag', *Kritika: Explorations in Russian and Eurasian History* 16, no. 3 (2015): 540–1.

26. Samsonov, *K tebe*, 83–5, 87.
27. Ibid., 100.
28. Ibid., 58–9, 87, 116, 214.
29. Ibid., 89–91, 114, 134. His rations were upgraded from category IV (feldshers') to III (low-tier staff in charge of wards/clinics) in October 1944, in line with a 1943 decree; see Nakhapetov, *Ocherki istorii sanitarnoi sluzhby Gulaga*, 140–1.
30. Samsonov, *K tebe*, 103–4.
31. Ibid., 136–8. On Skakunovskaia, see Sapolnova et al., *Liudi v belykh khalatakh*, 110–11.
32. Samsonov, *K tebe*, 143–6, 148–51.
33. Ibid., 169.
34. Ibid., 74.
35. Ibid., 117–25.
36. Ibid., 125.
37. The brochure was I. A. Kassirskii, *Alimentarnaia distrofiia i pellagra (diagnostika, klinika, terapiia)* (Ryblaga NKVD SSSR: Sanotdel Ryblaga NKVD SSSR, 1943). See Samsonov, *K tebe*, 126.
38. Samsonov, *K tebe*, 125.
39. For a list of Gulag medical conferences from neighbouring Pechora camp system, see GARF, f. R9414, op. 2, d. 168, ll. 5–5 ob; for a list of such meetings in Norilsk, see Z. I. Rozenblium [Kand. medits. nauk], 'Otchet o nauchnykh soveshchaniiakh vrachei Noril'ska v 1940–1947 gg.', GARF, f. R9414, op. 2, d. 175, ll. 248–58. For an emotive conference reception for a prisoner-doctor's presentation in the Kolyma camps, see MMSPb, DUBININ, Dmitrii Vasil'evich, 'Vospominaniia' [n.d., *c.* 1956], 78. Anna Kliashko recalled a range of medical conferences, intramural and regional, in Kolyma in the early 1950s with no distinctions between prisoners and free employees: interviews, 31 March 2010, 15 September 2012, Montréal, Canada.
40. Samsonov, *K tebe*, 199. Samsonov does not explain the reason for this restriction. He petitioned the Supreme Court to quash his conviction and enable a wider choice of institutes, unsuccessfully. The restriction likely derived from rules about residency excluding ex-prisoners from major cities.
41. Ibid., 214.
42. Aleksandrovskii, *Zapiski*, 3.
43. On the use of prisoner labour across the Soviet economy in this era, see Paul Gregory, 'An Introduction to the Economics of the Gulag', in *The Economics of Forced Labor: The Soviet Gulag*, ed. Paul R. Gregory and Valery Lazarev (Stanford: Hoover Institution Press, 2003), 19–21.
44. N. G. Okhotin and A. B. Roginskii, eds, *Sistema ispravitel'no-trudovykh lagerei v SSSR, 1923–1960: Spravochnik* (Moscow: Zven'ia, 1998), 287–8.
45. I. M. Fil'shtinskii, *My shagaem pod konvoem. Rasskazy iz lagernoi zhizni* (Nizhnii Novgorod: Dekom, 2005), 17.
46. Nakonechnyi consistently cites forestry camps as the deadliest during war and famine emergencies; in 1941–45 he notes 11,316 prisoners died in Kargopollag, with another 6,193 invalids released, of which 90 per cent were likely to die within days of being freed: Mikhail Iur'evich Nakonechnyi, 'Factory of Invalids: Mortality, Disability and Early Release on Medical Grounds from the Gulag, 1930–1955' (DPhil thesis, University of Oxford, 2020), 53–4, 117–23.
47. Aleksandrovskii, *Zapiski*, 41; Fil'shtinskii, *My shagaem*, 17.

48. Suzanne Poirier, *Doctors in the Making: Memoirs and Medical Education* (Iowa City: University of Iowa Press, 2009).

49. See Judith Pallot, 'Forced Labour for Forestry: The Twentieth Century History of Colonisation and Settlement in the North of Perm' Oblast', *Europe-Asia Studies* 54, no. 7 (2002): 1055–83; Nakonechnyi, 'Factory of Invalids'; N. V. Upadyshev, *Gulag na evropeiskom severe Rossii: Genezis, evoliutsiia, raspad* (Arkhangel'sk: Pomorskii universitet, 2007).

50. Aleksandrovskii, *Zapiski*, 7–8.

51. Ibid., 9.

52. Ibid., 11.

53. Ibid.

54. Ibid., 12.

55. Ibid., 13.

56. Ibid., 14.

57. Ibid., 14–15. Convalescent rest stations were reserves within camps where prisoners were released from work, fed better, and gained weight; good behaviour and productive work habits were the standard criteria for entry but memoirists report plenty of abuse of the privilege: see Healey, 'Lives in the Balance', 551–3.

58. Aleksandrovskii, *Zapiski*, 17.

59. Ibid., 21.

60. Ibid., 22.

61. Ibid., 23.

62. Ibid., 24.

63. Mikhail Bulgakov, 'Kreshchenie povorotom', *Izbrannaia proza* (Moscow: Sovetskaia Rossiia, 1983), 280.

64. Aleksandrovskii, *Zapiski*, 40.

65. Ibid., 26–7.

66. Ibid., 27.

67. Aleksandrovsky enlisted the help of a laboratory technician to study cases, and he plunged into his medical textbooks to understand their causes and treatment; ibid., 29–30. In 1944 worm infestation affected one-third of the population of the USSR, according to official sources; see Donald Filtzer, *The Hazards of Urban Life in Late Stalinist Russia: Health, Hygiene, and Living Standards, 1943–1953* (Cambridge: Cambridge University Press, 2010), 203.

68. Aleksandrovskii, *Zapiski*, 27, 32.

69. Ibid., 34.

70. Ibid., 37.

71. Soviet penicillin was first developed in 1942–43, but not mass-manufactured until after 1945; factories producing the drug in Riga, Minsk, and Moscow were operating in 1948; see Mary Schaeffer Conroy, *Medicines for the Soviet Masses during World War II* (Lanham & Plymouth: University Press of America, 2008), 129–33; Robert Bud, *Penicillin: Triumph and Tragedy* (Oxford: Oxford University Press, 2007), 81–2. Soviets received limited supplies from Canada and distribution reached Magadan: see GAMO, f. 45, op. 1, d. 5, ll. 1a–1b ob. (instructions in English and French for use from a bottle of sodium penicillin manufactured by Aerst, McKenna & Harrison Ltd, Montréal, Canada); for instructions from Ministry of Healthcare, 1951, on administering penicillin, see GAMO, f. 45, op. 1, d. 23, ll. 38–41. Anna Kliashko first encountered penicillin

as a student in Irkutsk in 1948; it was of Soviet manufacture, and she recalled that in Magadan 'commissions' of doctors were convened to determine who should receive it: interview, 24 June 2009, Montréal, Canada.

72. Aleksandrovskii, *Zapiski*, 39–40, 46.

73. Ibid., 41.

74. Ibid., 27.

75. Ibid., 47.

76. Ibid., 55.

77. Ibid., 71–5.

78. Nakhapetov, *Ocherki*, 97; Aleksandrovskii, *Zapiski*, 4, 76. On the sixth-year curriculum and its introduction, see Christopher Burton, 'Medical Welfare during Late Stalinism: A Study of Doctors and the Soviet Health System, 1945–1953' (PhD thesis, University of Chicago, 2000), 154–66.

79. Aleksandrovskii, *Zapiski*, 41.

80. 'I wrote about this in a letter to A. I. Solzhenitsyn of 23 March 1995. In confirmation of the humanity and mercy of doctors I enclosed with the letter a copy of my book (of a documentary-fictional type) with my memoirs of work with camp doctors. My letter did not receive a reply. I particularly wanted to emphasise their noble actions in my memoirs': Samsonov, *V perezhitom nenast'e*, 27. See also Viktor A. Samsonov, 'Opyt osvoeniia nachal'nykh osnov meditsiny i prozektorskoi praktiki v usloviiakh Ukhtizhemlaga (vospominaniia)', *Arkhiv patologii*, no. 1 (1999): 59–63, at 63.

81. Samsonov, *K tebe*, 146. At this point, Samsonov had only known three homes: his father's house, the Petrozavodsk boarding school as a teenager, and the camps. He cannot be blamed for choosing to live in 'normal' surroundings upon release from the Gulag.

82. On the porosity of the Gulag, see e.g. Wilson Bell, 'Was the Gulag an Archipelago? De-Convoyed Prisoners and Porous Borders in the Camps of Western Siberia', *Russian Review* 72, no. 1 (2013): 116–41; and Oleg Khlevniuk and Simon Belokowsky, 'The Gulag and the Non-Gulag as One Interrelated Whole', *Kritika: Explorations in Russian and Eurasian History* 16, no. 3 (2015): 479–98.

83. Aleksandrovskii, *Zapiski*, 78.

Chapter 5 Sisters of mercy and Komsomol girls: Nursing in the Gulag

1. Eugenia Ginzburg, *Within the Whirlwind*, trans. Ian Boland (London: Collins Harvill, 1989), 3.

2. Ibid., 8.

3. Ibid. The handbook Ginzburg mentions ('Spravochnik fel'dshera') is impossible to identify. Unlike Samsonov, she says little about medical literature in her memoir.

4. Ibid., 121.

5. Ibid., 423. On Ginzburg's transformation, see Leona Toker, *Return from the Archipelago: Narratives of Gulag Survivors* (Bloomington & Indianapolis: Indiana University Press, 2000), 52–5, 260–1; Natasha Kolchevska, 'The Art of Memory: Cultural Reverence as Political Critique in Evgeniia Ginzburg's Writing of the Gulag', in *The Russian Memoir: History and Literature*, ed. Beth Holmgren (Evanston: Northwestern University Press, 2003); Dariusz Tolczyk, 'Politics of

Resurrection: Evgeniia Ginzburg, the Romantic Prison, and the Soviet Rhetoric of the Gulag', *Canadian-American Slavic Studies* 39, no. 1 (2005): 53–70.

6. Laurie Stoff, *Russia's Sisters of Mercy and the Great War: More Than Binding Men's Wounds* (Lawrence: University Press of Kansas, 2015); Susan Grant, 'From War to Peace: The Fate of Nurses and Nursing under the Bolsheviks', in *Russia's Home Front, 1917–1922: The Experience of War and Revolution*, ed. A. Lindenmeyr, C. J. Read, and P. Waldron (Bloomington: Slavica, 2016); idem, *Soviet Nightingales: Care under Communism* (Ithaca & London: Cornell University Press, 2022).

7. Susan Grant, 'Creating Cadres of Soviet Nurses, 1936–1941', in *Russian and Soviet Health Care from an International Perspective: Comparing Professions, Practice and Gender, 1880–1960*, ed. Susan Grant (Basingstoke: Palgrave Macmillan, 2017), 60.

8. On feldshers, see Samuel C. Ramer, 'Feldshers and Rural Health Care in the Early Soviet Period', in *Health and Society in Revolutionary Russia*, ed. Susan Gross Solomon and John F. Hutchinson (Bloomington & Indianapolis: Indiana University Press, 1990); idem, 'The Russian Feldsher: A PA Prototype in Transition', *Journal of the American Academy of PAs* 31, no. 11 (2018): 1–6.

9. In 1928 there were 114,000 'mid-level medical personnel' in the USSR; by 1940 this number was 472,000; see Christopher M. Davis, 'The Economics of the Soviet Health System: An Analytical and Historical Study, 1921–1978' (PhD thesis, Cambridge University, 1979), 57.

10. Grant, 'Creating Cadres of Soviet Nurses', 59, 64–5.

11. D. Gorfin, 'Sestra meditsinskaia', in *Bol'shaia meditsinskaia entsiklopediia*, ed. N. A. Semashko (Moscow: Sovetskaia entsiklopediia, 1934), 30: 345–52.

12. Susan Grant argues that the gender order in medicine was shifting in the 1930s as new physicians were predominantly female, and the nursing career when tied to national defence and patriotism gained in status and allure for those serving in military and aviation, for example. See Susan Grant, 'Nurses in the Soviet Union: Explorations of Gender in State and Society', in *Palgrave Handbook of Women and Gender in Twentieth-Century Russia and the Soviet Union*, ed. Melanie Ilic (London: Palgrave, 2018).

13. Grant, *Soviet Nightingales*, 47–8, 96–7. Grant says little about male nurses but they were evidently rare in Soviet civilian medicine. For Gulag male nurses drinking and stealing morphine, see E. A. Kersnovskaia, *Skol'ko stoit chelovek* (Moscow: ROSSPEN, 2006), 567.

14. On pre-revolutionary debates about feldsher status, see Ramer, 'The Russian Feldsher', 2–4.

15. Grant, 'Creating Cadres of Soviet Nurses', 63.

16. GARF, f. R9414, op. 2, d. 108, ll. 220–31.

17. GARF, f. R9489, op. 2, d. 25, l. 254.

18. See e.g. 'Imeiut spetsial'nost'', *Kanaloarmeika*, 21 November 1934, no. 8, 1; 'Lager' daet im kvalifikatsiiu', *Perekovka na stroitel'stve kanala Moskva-Volga*, 8 December 1934, no. 86 (179), 2.

19. B. A. Nakhapetov, *Ocherki istorii sanitarnoi sluzhby Gulaga* (Moscow: ROSSPEN, 2009), 88–9. For the orders to run these courses in 1939, see GARF, f. R9414, op. 1, d. 2756, ll. 498–9, 534.

20. Shalamov was trained as a feldsher in Magadan in 1946; see Varlam Shalamov, *Neskol'ko moikh zhiznei. Vospominaniia, zapisnye knizhki, perepiska, sledstvennye*

dela (Moscow: Eksmo, 2009), 230. Another self-trained nurse who convinced a Gulag doctor to train her was Liudmila Miklashevskaia; see Elaine MacKinnon, 'Motherhood and Survival in the Stalinist Gulag', *Aspasia* 13, no. 1 (2019): 76.

21. Nakhapetov, *Ocherki istorii sanitarnoi sluzhby Gulaga*, 92.

22. The numbers available are 325 mid-level medical personnel recruited to the MVD in 1946; 1,100 in 1948; 152 in 1949; 696 in 1950; and 311 in 1951; sources: GARF, f. R8009, op. 14, dd. 390 (l. 42), 566 (l. 21), 753 (l. 15), 774 (l. 7), 794 (l. 62 ob). No statistics for 1947 are found in these records. Ginzburg noted how frequently she worked with 'Komsomol girls on contract' or competed with them for nursing posts: Ginzburg, *Within the Whirlwind*, 213.

23. MMSPb, KLIMENKO, Ol'ga Konstantinovna, 'Desiat' let' (154 pp., typed). Leningrad, 1978. Extracts of this manuscript were published in *Grani: zhurnal literatury, iskusstva, nauki i obshchestvenno-politicheskoi mysli*, 1990–91, nos 157 to 159. Klimenko wrote a separate memoir about her youth up to 1919; see M. F. Kosinskii, *Pervaia polovina veka: Vospominaniia* (Paris: YMCA-press, 1995), 35–6.

24. Klimenko, 'Desiat' let', l. 61.

25. Vologda Province was a hive of penal canal-building, timber-felling, and railway construction operations that opened and shut rapidly, answering to differing Gulag 'glavki' or industrial management divisions: see N. G. Okhotin and A. B. Roginskii, eds, *Sistema ispravitel'no-trudovykh lagerei v SSSR, 1923–1960: Spravochnik* (Moscow: Zven'ia, 1998), 188–9, 197–9, 259, 298–300, 348–9, 508, 512–13.

26. Klimenko, 'Desiat' let', l. 55.

27. Ibid., ll. 59–60.

28. Ibid., l. 60.

29. Olga Mane, a prisoner at Solovki, worked two weeks 'in general labour, according to the rules' before being admitted to work as a nurse in Solovki's main, Kremlin, hospital in 1935: MMSPb, MANE, Ol'ga Meerovna, 'Interv'iu s Mane Ol'goi Meerovnoi'. Zapis' 15.09.1991, Moskva (Morgacheva, T. V.), kasetka 3, l. 2. At Yaia camp for wives of political prisoners, Maria Sandratskaya worked in general labour assignments before falling ill with pellagra; when she recovered, she was given a nursing post in the late 1930s: MMA, SANDRATSKAIA, Mariia Karlovna [Vospominaniia] Leningrad, 1964, f. 2, op. 1, d. 105, ll. 52–3.

30. Klimenko, 'Desiat' let', ll. 88–9.

31. Ibid., l. 101.

32. In a series of interviews with former freely hired Gulag nurses, orderlies, and other mid-level medical staff, conducted in the early 2000s, Pechora regional museum curator Tatyana Afanasyeva asked a variety of open questions about work, but some interview subjects were evidently unprepared to recall in detail the 'uninteresting' aspects of their jobs. They emphasised the well-known local doctors and professors of medicine they worked under, or the places where they worked. See PIKM, papka 31/39/8, 'Medsestry'.

33. One justifiably bitter prisoner-petitioner to Viacheslav Molotov in 1953 wrote of the Norilsk Sanotdel leadership's 'psychosis' about clean floors, which were the focus of inspection tours, while the obvious desperate illness and disability of hard-labour prisoners went ignored: MMA, f. 2, op. 1, d. 25, 'Bernshtein, Lev Borisovich. [Zapiski] Vanino, 1953', l. 53.

34. Donald Filtzer, *The Hazards of Urban Life in Late Stalinist Russia: Health, Hygiene, and Living Standards, 1943–1953* (Cambridge: Cambridge University Press, 2010), 129–30.

35. For example, *Kanaloarmeika*, 3 July 1934, no. 5, 1 (photograph of a shock-worker laundress); *Prorvinskii lovets: Organ KVO Prorvinskogo isprav.-trud. lageria NKVD*, 28 May 1936, no. 27(59), 3 (two laundresses who fulfilled 230 per cent of the planned norm).

36. Klimenko, 'Desiat' let', ll. 66–7. For Shalamov's bitter documentary short story about the bathhouses of the Kolyma camps, see 'V bane' in Varlam Shalamov, *Sobranie sochinenii v chetyrekh tomakh*. 4 vols (Moscow: Khudozhestvennaia literatura; Vagrius, 1998), 1: 519–24. On the Russian bath, see Ethan Pollock, *Without the Banya We Would Perish: A History of the Russian Bathhouse* (New York: Oxford University Press, 2019).

37. Klimenko, 'Desiat' let', ll. 68, 104.

38. Ibid., l. 84; on water supply and sewerage, see Filtzer, *The Hazards of Urban Life in Late Stalinist Russia*, 66–126.

39. Klimenko, 'Desiat' let', l. 80. Like many civilian construction projects, the L'nostroi factory complex, initiated in 1936 and interrupted by the war, used prisoner labour; see the Vologda Discovery VKontakte pages of local historian Gury Ninoruov (dated 26 February 2013): https://vk.com/topic-39003234_27689885?offset=0 (accessed 19 August 2020).

40. For examples, see GARF, f. R9489, op. 2, d. 5, ll. 443–443 ob. (1933); ibid., f. R9489, op. 2, d. 89, ll. 338–46 (1936); ibid., f. R9412, op. 1, d. 143, l. 18 (1948).

41. Klimenko, 'Desiat' let', l. 66.

42. Ibid., l. 124.

43. Ibid., l. 21.

44. Ibid., ll. 85–6.

45. Ibid., ll. 101, 104.

46. On the famine, see Veniamin F. Zima, *Golod v SSSR 1946–1947 godov: Proiskhozhdenie i posledstviia* (Moscow: Institut rossiiskoi istorii RAN, 1996).

47. Klimenko, 'Desiat' let', l. 90. Sheksna was a canal-building camp with timber-felling tracts, places of significant prisoner wastage: see Okhotin and Roginskii, eds, *Sistema ispravitel'no-trudovykh lagerei*, 513.

48. Klimenko, 'Desiat' let', l. 93.

49. Infectious wards were probably avoided by freely hired medical staff. For prisoner-nurses and -orderlies working in TB wards, see e.g. MMSPb, KONO, Mariia L'vovna, 'Vospominaniia' (n.d., n.p.), ll. 15–16; MMA, ZAITSEV, Aleksandr Georgievich, 'Pervyi i vtoroi aresty. Lageria' Vospominaniia. Gor'kii, 1989, Rukopis' 189 pp., f. 2, op. 2, d. 32 ll. 109–13.

50. Helen Bynum, *Spitting Blood: The History of Tuberculosis* (Oxford: Oxford University Press, 2012), 142–4; on Soviet labour therapy for various illnesses, see the anonymous article, 'Trudoterapiia', in *Bol'shaia sovetskaia entsiklopediia*, ed. B. A. Vvedenskii (Moscow: Bol'shaia sovetskaia entsiklopediia, 1956), 43: 333–4.

51. Klimenko, 'Desiat' let', ll. 94, 101–2. Calcium chloride was a routine remedy for TB before widespread use of antibiotics in the USSR; see Mary Schaeffer Conroy, *Medicines for the Soviet Masses during World War II* (Lanham & Plymouth: University Press of America, 2008), 118, 124. Pneumothorax was and is occasionally treated with a needle or tube to drain the air causing the collapse, from the ribcage; Bynum, *Spitting Blood*, 152–6.

52. Klimenko, 'Desiat' let', l. 98.

53. Ibid., l. 99.

54. On Ginzburg, see Kolchevska, 'The Art of Memory'.

55. Klimenko, 'Desiat' let', l. 67.

56. Ibid., l. 75.

57. Ibid., condemnation, ll. 89–93, 108, 124, 132; quotation, l. 61.

58. Ginzburg, *Within the Whirlwind*, 162.

59. Ginzburg comments on a freely hired Gulag doctor she encountered as a nurse in Kolyma: '. . . I felt sympathy for this typical beneficiary of the era of adult education and women's rights who had learned to make out prescriptions in Latin. Somehow it seemed to me that my own efforts all those years ago must have contributed to the transformation of Dusya, the medical orderly, into Eudokia Ivanovna, our head doctor. Sometimes I had a clear picture of this Dusya devotedly following my lectures from one of the front rows in a large workers education auditorium.' Ginzburg, *Within the Whirlwind*, 25.

60. Ibid., 162, 216.

61. Elena Shulman, *Stalinism on the Frontier of Empire: Women and State Formation in the Soviet Far East* (Cambridge: Cambridge University Press, 2008); Jonathan A. Bone, 'À la recherche d'un Komsomol perdu: Who Really Built Komsomol'sk-Na-Amure, and Why', *Revue des études slaves* 71, no. 1 (1999): 59–92.

62. Tatiana Afanas'eva, ed., *Vgliadyvaias' v proshloe* (Pechora: Pechorskoe vremia, 2010), 102; see also PIKM, 'Vospominaniia Deriabinoi, Liubovi Mikhailovna [Medsestra], g. Pechora. Zapis' T. Afanas'evoi, 6.07.2000 g., l. 1.'

63. Afanas'eva, *Vgliadyvaias' v proshloe*, 104; see also PIKM, f. 31, op. 39, d. 6, 'Komlev B. V. i Komleva M. I.', Fonozapis' 1989, g. Pechora, l. 5.

64. PIKM, f. 31, op. 39, d. 8 'Medsestry', 'Davydenko, Serafima Stepanovna' [interview, n.d., n.p.], l. 1.

65. Afanas'eva, *Vgliadyvaias' v proshloe*, 186; see also PIKM, f. 31, op. 39, d. 8 'Medsestry', 'Sokolova (Smirnova), Iuliia Grigor'evna, Zapis' T. Afanas'evoi, ianvar' 2001 g., g. Pechora', l. 1.

66. Feldsher Mariia P. Kolinenko arrived in Pechora in 1941; see PIKM, f. 31, op. 39, d. 8 'Medsestry', 'Kolinenko, Mariia Petrovna'.

67. Doctors assigned to the Gulag did contest their postings, as central and republican health commissariat and local medical institute archives illustrate. See discussions of ruses used by some doctors to avoid assignments in GARF, f. R8009, op. 14, d. 56, ll. 1–5 (1939); ibid., f. R8009, op. 14, d. 390, l. 67 (1946); NAG, f. 289, op. 1, d. 3155, ll. 1–39 (1940); for Sverdlovsk Medical Institute graduates objecting to work assignments, see GASO, f. 2195, op. 1, d. 33, ll. 1, 80–2, 123–6, 135, 186–7.

68. Afanas'eva, *Vgliadyvaias' v proshloe*, 104. For withholding of diplomas, see also 'Davydenko, Serafima Stepanovna' [interview, n.d., n.p.], l. 2.

69. PIKM, f. 31, op. 39, d. 8 'Medsestry', 'Davydenko, Serafima Stepanovna', 'Trudovoi dogovor'. A similar story of escape from a collective farm was recalled by Nina Naleeva, a 'sanitarka' or hospital cleaner in Pechora Gulag camps. 'Mother convinced me to run away from the starving village to my brother' who already worked in Pechora on the railway as a contracted technician. PIKM, f. 31, op. 39, d. 8 'Medsestry', 'Naleeva (Ivanova), Nina Stepanovna' interview with T. Afanas'eva, 16 June 2010, Pechora, l. 1.

70. PIKM, 'Kollektsiia dokumentov Akal'zina Alekseia Ivanovicha i Akal'zinoi Raisy Ivanovny KP4017/1-31, NV 2707/1-5; see also Afanas'eva, *Vgliadyvaias' v proshloe*, 134–5.

71. PIKM, 'Kollektsiia dokumentov Akal'zina Alekseia Ivanovicha i Akal'zinoi Raisy Ivanovny KP4017/1-31, NV 2707/1-5, 'Trudovoi dogovor'.

72. MIZU, Khar'kova (Panina), Elena Ivanovna, vol'nonaemnaia folder, l. 5.

73. PIKM, f. 31, op. 39, d. 8 'Medsestry', 'Kolinenko, Maria Petrovna' [interview], l. 2.

74. Ibid., 'Davydenko, Serafima Stepanovna' [interview], l. 2.

75. Ibid., 'Sokolova (Smirnova), Iuliia Grigor'evna, Zapis' T. Afanas'evoi, ianvar' 2001 g., g. Pechora', l. 1.

76. See the Virtual Gulag Museum, 'Nekropoli. Kladbishche lazareta No. 2 SANO Sevpechlag', http://www.gulagmuseum.org/showObject. do?object=48060&language=1 (accessed 7 September 2020). Sokolova also escorted a transport of prisoners to the far northern camp of Mul'da in 1947 ('Sokolova', l. 4).

77. PIKM, f. 31, op. 39, d. 8 'Medsestry', 'Sokolova (Smirnova), Iuliia Grigor'evna, Zapis' T. Afanas'evoi, ianvar' 2001 g., g. Pechora', l. 2; ibid., 'Davydenko, Serafima Stepanovna' [interview], l. 2.

78. Ibid., 'Belova, K. P. Iz otcheta o rabote klinicheskoi laboratorii bol'nitsy N. 8 laborant Belova Klavdiia Petrovna'.

79. Afanas'eva, *Vgliadyvaias' v proshloe*, 104–5.

80. Ibid., 102.

81. PIKM, f. 31, op. 39, d. 8 'Medsestry', 'Kolinenko, Maria Petrovna', l. 2.

82. MIZU, Khar'kova folder, 'Trudovaia kniga'.

83. On incentives, see E. A. Osokina, *Our Daily Bread: Socialist Distribution and the Art of Survival in Stalin's Russia, 1927–1941* (Armonk & London: M. E. Sharpe, 2001); Lewis H. Siegelbaum, *Stakhanovism and the Politics of Productivity in the USSR, 1935–1941* (Cambridge: Cambridge University Press, 1988).

84. PIKM, 'Deriabina, Liubov' Mikhailovna, medsestra': 'Protokol No. 6 Zasedaniia shtaba 'O' 4-go otdeleniia 30 iiulia 1943 goda', l. 4; 'Postanovlenie nachal'nika Upravleniia i nachal'nika Politotdela Pechorskogo zheleznodorozhnogo stroitel'stva i lageria NKVD SSSR, 29 fevralia 1944 g.'; *Proizvodstvennyi biulleten'*, 18 November 1942, p. 2; 'Iz postanovliia tsentral'nogo shtaba', *Proizvodstvennyi biulleten'*, 18 November 1942, p. 2; 'Itogi obshchelagernogo konkursa', *Proizvodstvennyi biulleten'*, 27 July 1943, p. 2.

85. PIKM, f. 31, op. 39, d. 8 'Medsestry', 'Sokolova (Smirnova), Iuliia Grigor'evna, Zapis' T. Afanas'evoi, ianvar' 2001 g., g. Pechora', l. 3.

86. Ibid., ll. 2–4.

87. Sokolova had well-developed literary tastes, somewhat unusually for this group of nurses. She loved reading and borrowed books from prisoner-patients and medical staff; she says she knew some inmates mentioned by Solzhenitsyn in his *Gulag Archipelago*.

88. Viktor A. Samsonov, *K tebe, Onego, vse puti. Zapiski lagernogo lekpoma, studenta, vracha, prepodavatelia* (Petrozavodsk: Iz-vo Petrozavodskogo universiteta, 2000), 119–20.

89. Afanas'eva, *Vgliadyvaias' v proshloe*, 104.

90. Ibid., 103–4; PIKM, f. 31, op. 39, d. 6, 'Komlev B. V. i Komleva M. I.'.

91. PIKM, f. 31, op. 39, d. 8, 'Medsestry', Davydenko, Serafima Stepanovna [interview, n.d., n.p.], ll. 1–3; ibid., Kolinenko, Maria Petrovna [interview, n.d., n.p.], ll. 1–4.
92. Grant, *Soviet Nightingales*, 109–15.

Chapter 6 The place where Death delights in helping Life: A prisoner in the morgue

1. E. A. Kersnovskaia, *Naskal'naia zhivopis'*. *Al'bom. Redaktor-sostavitel' V. Vigilianskii* (Moscow: S. P. 'Kvadrat', 1991), 293.
2. Vladimir Vigilianskii, 'Zhitie Evfrosinii Kersnovskoi', in Kersnovskaia, *Naskal'naia zhivopis'*, 13.
3. Vigilianskii, 'Zhitie Evfrosinii Kersnovskoi', 13.
4. Construction in Norilsk was hard labour, and many women were deployed in this work during and after the war. See e.g. MMA, f. 2, op. 2, d. 66, ODOLINSKAIA, Nina Fominichna. Sovetskie katorzhniki. Vospominaniia. Odessa, 1989, ll. 26–34.
5. Biographical information from Kersnovskaya's own writing is often loosely dated, but a helpful summary is found on a website devoted to her work: https://www.gulag.su/about/index.php?eng=&page=1&list=1&foto=1 (accessed 23 September 2020). See also Vigilianskii, 'Zhitie Evfrosinii Kersnovskoi', 8–17.
6. Simon Ertz, 'Building Norilsk', in *The Economics of Forced Labor: The Soviet Gulag*, ed. Paul Gregory and Valery Lazarev (Stanford: Hoover Institution Press, 2003); I. N. Trofimenko, 'Noril'skii ispravitel'no-trudovoi lager': Otbor kontingenta i uroven' smertnosti zakliuchennykh (1935–1950 gg.)', in *Noril'skaia Golgofa*, ed. O. L. Podborskaia (Krasnoiarsk: Obshchestvo 'Memorial'; Regional'noe ob"edinenie 'Sibir'', 2002); N. G. Okhotin and A. B. Roginskii, eds, *Sistema ispravitel'no-trudovykh lagerei v SSSR, 1923–1960: Spravochnik* (Moscow: Zven'ia, 1998), 338–9. On contemporary Norilsk, see Marlene Laruelle and Sophie Hohmann, 'Biography of a Polar City: Population Flows and Urban Identity in Norilsk', *Polar Geography* 40, no. 4 (2017): 306–23; David Humphreys, 'Challenges of Transformation: The Case of Norilsk Nickel', *Resources Policy* 36, no. 2 (2011): 142–8. An invaluable source of reminiscences and essays about Norilsk is G. I. Kasabova, *O vremeni, o Noril'ske, o sebe* . . . 11 vols (Moscow: Polimediia, 2004–2010).
7. For a 1939 order from the Sanotdel directorate in Moscow to prison governors requiring them to conduct medical examinations on prisoners 'who can be used in labour in the conditions of the Far North' before being sent to Norilsk and Kolyma, see GARF, f. R9414, op. 1, d. 2756, ll. 230–2. For a Gulag prisoner's recollection of his designation in 1942 by a medical commission as unfit for transfer to Noril'sk, see MMA, f. 2, op. 3, d. 57 SEMAKIN, Nikolai Kuz'mich. Vospominaniia ostavshegosia zhivym nevol'nika. 1996, l. 69; and for a prisoner, Zigurd Liudvig, who was selected, see Kasabova, *O vremeni*, 9: 54.
8. Leonid Borodkin and Simon Ertz, 'Coercion Versus Motivation: Forced Labor in Norilsk', in *The Economics of Forced Labor: The Soviet Gulag*, ed. Paul Gregory and Valery Lazarev (Stanford: Hoover Institution Press, 2003); on interruptions of food shipments to Norilsk in 1943, see GARF, f. R8131, op. 37, d. 2063, ll. 31 ob.–32 ob.

9. On Eremeev, in this post from July 1943 to September 1945, see his entry on Memorial's 'Kadrovyi sostav organov gosudarstvennoi bezopasnosti SSSR. 1935–1939': https://nkvd.memo.ru/index.php/ (accessed 24 September 2020); his positive reception of medics: MMA, f. 2, op. 1, d. 125, CHEBURKIN, Pavel Vladimirovich [Vospominaniia] Shchekino, b.d., ll. 15–16. On conferences, see GARF, f. R9414, op. 2, d. 175, ll. 248–58 (Z. I. Rozenblium, 'Otchet o nauchnykh soveshchaniiakh vrachei Noril'ska v 1940–1947 gg.').

10. For a bitter account of Norilsk Sanotdel manipulation of statistics, abuse of labour categorisations, and other corrupt practices between 1948 and 1953 by administrator-medics with scanty qualifications 'so illiterate they could not even correctly spell [their titles as] doctor-officers of the MVD', see MMA, f. 2, op. 1, d. 25, BERNSHTEIN, Lev Borisovich. [Zapiski] Vanino, 1953, ll. 48–54. This was a prisoner petition for release written to Viacheslav M. Molotov in 1953 after Stalin's death.

11. W. F. Bynum, Anne Hardy, Stephen Jacyna, Christopher Lawrence, and E. M. (Tilli) Tansey, *The Western Medical Tradition 1800 to 2000* (Cambridge: Cambridge University Press, 2006), 61–3, 120–3; Georges Canguilhem, *The Normal and the Pathological* (New York: Zone Books, 1991), 203–26; Michel Foucault, *The Birth of the Clinic: An Archaeology of Medical Perception* (London: Routledge Classics, 2003), 152–82. On the cultural meanings of the traffic in corpses and autopsy practices, see Mary Fissell, 'Making Meaning from the Margins: The New Cultural History of Medicine', in *Locating Medical History: The Stories and their Meanings*, ed. Frank Huisman and John Harley Warner (Baltimore: Johns Hopkins University Press, 2004), 380–5.

12. A. Abrikosov, 'Patologicheskaia anatomiia', in *Bol'shaia meditsinskaia entsiklopediia*, ed. N. A. Semashko (Moscow: Sovetskaia entsiklopediia, 1932), 24: 115–28; Grigorii A. Batkis, *Organizatsiia zdravookhraneniia* (Moscow: Medgiz, 1948), 330–4.

13. Batkis, *Organizatsiia zdravookhraneniia*, 334.

14. Christopher Burton, 'Vseokhvatnaia pomoshch' pri stalinizme? Sovetskoe zdravookhranenie i dukh gosudarstva blagodenstviia, 1945–1953', in *Sovetskaia sotsial'naia politika: Tseny i deistvuiushchie litsa, 1940–1985*, ed. Elena Iarskaia-Smirnova and P. V. Romanov (Moscow: Variant, TsSPGI, 2008), 176.

15. 'Vskrytie trupa', in *Bol'shaia sovetskaia entsiklopediia*, ed. B. A. Vvedenskii (Moscow: Bol'shaia sovetskaia entsiklopediia, 1951), 9: 351. A sense of the less regulated 1920s comes in the analogous article in the first edition of the Soviet medical encyclopedia with its focus on the medical expert's technique: A. Abrikosov, I. Davydovskii, and A. Kriukov, 'Vskrytie', in *Bol'shaia meditsinskaia entsiklopediia*, ed. N. A. Semashko (Moscow: Sovetskaia entsiklopediia, 1928) 5: 762–76.

16. Interview with Anna Kliashko, 15 September 2012, Montréal, Canada.

17. Batkis, *Organizatsiia zdravookhraneniia*, 331.

18. 'Vskrytie trupa', 351.

19. Aleksandr Solzhenitsyn, *Arkhipelag Gulag 1918–1956: Opyt khudozhestvennogo issledovaniia*. 3 vols (Ekaterinburg: U-Faktoriia, 2006), 2: 176–7. I have adapted Thomas P. Whitney's English translation to convey the contrast between medical and violent terminology.

20. For an account of dying in the Gulag that virtually ignores morgues and autopsy, see Anne Applebaum, *Gulag: A History of the Soviet Camps* (London: Allen Lane, 2003), 307–15.

21. E. A. Kersnovskaia, *Skol'ko stoit chelovek* (Moscow: ROSSPEN, 2006), 489. A procurator's investigation of causes of death in Norilsk in 1943 presented a table analysing the conclusions of 1,442 autopsies for that year: GARF, f. R8131, op. 37, d. 2063, ll. 30 ob–31. Sofia Guzikova, discussed in chapter 3, came under pressure to grapple with a backlog of autopsies in her infirmary.

22. Kersnovskaia's in-camp drafts were confiscated. After release, she feared confiscation of the completed version, and revised, recopied, and concealed varying versions of the text and almost 700 illustrations in several locations. Editors of the published versions make varying choices about which texts and illustrations to include. In this chapter I rely principally on the 2006 text-rich version. New editions in 2016 and 2018 contain some exclusions, evidently to soften Kersnovskaia's assessments of some colleagues. It has not been possible to include examples of the illustrations but they can readily be found at https://archive.gulag.su/project/index.php?eng=&page=0 (accessed 12 May 2023). On Kersnovskaia's memoirs, see Catherine Viollet, 'L'œuvre autobiographique de Evfrosinija Kersnovskaya: Chronique illustrée du Gulag', *AvtobiografiЯ: Journal on Life Writing and the Representation of the Self in Russian Culture*, no. 1 (2012): 223–36; Vigilianskii, 'Zhitie Evfrosinii Kersnovskoi'. On her illustrations, see also Katya Pereyaslavska, 'Gulag Art: Elusive Evidence from the Forbidden Territories', *Art Documentation: Journal of the Art Libraries Society of North America* 30, no. 1 (2011): 37–8.

23. Kasabova, *O vremeni*, 9: 54–62; Kersnovskaia, *Skol'ko stoit chelovek*, 559–60.

24. GARF, f. R9414, op. 2, d. 175, ll. 5–17, 'S. M. Smirnov, Zdravookhranenie v Noril'ske'.

25. Ibid., ll. 7–8. Soviet medical officials, responding to global trends after the Second World War, wanted healthcare to be more consciously science-led, and hospitals were trusted more to deliver this agenda than smaller, dispersed, facilities; on the modern scientific hospital, see Bynum et al., *The Western Medical Tradition 1800 to 2000*, 441; for the USSR: Burton, 'Vseokhvatnaia pomoshch' pri stalinizme?', 176–7.

26. GARF, f. R9414, op. 2, d. 175, ll. 7, 13–14.

27. In 1944 the proportion of freely hired to prisoner-doctors, dentists, nurses, and feldshers across the Gulag medical service was about 50:50; see B. A. Nakhapetov, *Ocherki istorii sanitarnoi sluzhby Gulaga* (Moscow: ROSSPEN, 2009), 92 (Tablitsa 19. Chislennost' vol'nonaemnykh i zakliuchennykh meditsinskikh rabotnikov GULAGa).

28. Kersnovskaia, *Skol'ko stoit chelovek*, 434.

29. Ibid., 432.

30. Kasabova, *O vremeni*, 9: 54–5, 60.

31. Kuznetsov allegedly abused his male privilege flagrantly. Kersnovskaya deemed him not just a typical ladies' man but 'a clever perverted-blackmailer' of women; see Kersnovskaia, *Skol'ko stoit chelovek*, 432–3, 436, 443.

32. Ibid., 454. Mardna's reports were varied: one on abscesses, another on lung cancer incidence – high in Norilsk; and one on hypoglycaemia.

33. Ibid., 446–7. Liudvig remembered Mardna warmly as 'a leading medic' in the hospital; Kasabova, *O vremeni*, 9: 56–7.

34. Kersnovskaia, *Skol'ko stoit chelovek*, 460–1. 'Dysentery' figures as the leading cause of death in procurators' reports about mortality in Norilsk in 1943 and 1944, with 'alimentary dystrophy' in combination or separately; the two

combined causes accounted for almost 40 per cent of all deaths that year: GARF, f. R8131, op. 37, d. 2063, ll. 30 ob–31, 122 ob–23.

35. Kersnovskaia, *Skol'ko stoit chelovek*, 466.

36. Ibid., 467–70.

37. Ibid., 474.

38. Ibid., 489.

39. Kasabova, *O vremeni*, 9: 57.

40. See the depiction of prisoner-pathological anatomist Professor Umansky in short stories 'Veismanist', Varlam Shalamov, *Preodolenie zla* (Moscow: Eksmo, 2011), 506–13; and 'Kursy', idem, *Sobranie sochinenii v chetyrekh tomakh*, 4 vols (Moscow: Khudozhestvennaia literatura; Vagrius, 1998), 1: 445–85. On the real Yakov Mikhailovich Umansky see S. V. Budnikova, 'Nekotorye dannye o repressirovannykh medikakh na Kolyme (po materialam Magadanskogo oblastnogo kraevedcheskogo muzeia)', in *Kolyma. Dal'stroi. Gulag. Skorb' i sud'by. Materialy nauchno-prakticheskoi konferentsii 13–14 iiunia 1996 goda*, ed. A. M. Biriukov (Magadan: Severnyi mezhdunarodnyi universitet, 1998), 49.

41. Kersnovskaia, *Skol'ko stoit chelovek*, 477, 480, 499. Liudvig recalled Nikishin's excellence as an educator but said nothing about his personal character. On his three-month nursing courses and his instruction in pathological anatomy, see also see Georgii Popov, 'Opiat' ozhivet potusknevshee vremia' [memoir], https://www.memorial.krsk.ru/Public/1989/19891230.htm (accessed 12 October 2020).

42. Kersnovskaia, *Skol'ko stoit chelovek*, 484. An inspection by a procurator of Kalagron ('Kollorgon') penal camp subdivision in late 1943 revealed that all prisoners were emaciated because the bread ration was only distributed once a day, and most inmates were lice-infested; mortality, he implied, was extremely high. Even though this investigation led to an improvement in ration distribution it seems doubtful that mortality improved dramatically after the war; see GARF, f. R8131, op. 37, d. 2063, l. 31 ob.

43. Kersnovskaia, *Skol'ko stoit chelovek*, 482.

44. Ibid., 476.

45. Ibid., 485–6. The changed attitude she ascribes to economic and ideological factors: by wartime the Norilsk complex had finally been built so rations could be reduced; and the war and post-war influx of non-Soviet prisoners were seen as new 'enemies' unworthy of better treatment. Norilsk was, in fact, a place of punishment for prisoners deemed especially dangerous – a location for so-called *katorgi* or hard-labour camps. On *katorgi*, see Steven Anthony Barnes, *Death and Redemption: The Gulag and the Shaping of Soviet Society* (Princeton: Princeton University Press, 2011), 140–3; Alan Barenberg, *Gulag Town, Company Town: Forced Labor and its Legacy in Vorkuta* (New Haven & London: Yale University Press, 2014), 64–5, 97–9.

46. Kersnovskaia, *Skol'ko stoit chelovek*, 494–5. Kersnovskaya says that the guards brought 'their own doctor' – a prisoner with a political sentence – but he coolly produced conclusions with unmistakable significance for the guards: bullets entered the front of bodies, in the chest, neck, and face, which contradicted the guards' account of prisoners running away. Kersnovskaya was already suspicious about their story of a mass escape, having noted the prisoners' lack of outerwear necessary for a planned trek away from Norilsk. She says nothing about the consequences for the guards, but she imagines the doctor was sent to

general labour and died of starvation disease. 'Accidents of daily life' constituted 5.2 per cent of deaths investigated by autopsy in 1943: GARF, f. R8131,
op. 37, d. 2063, ll. 30 ob–31.

47. One pre-archival source, Jacques Rossi, claims, 'Hundreds of thousands of
    prisoners of Noril'sk camp are buried on Shmidt Mountain.' Zhak Rossi,
    Spravochnik po GULagu, 2 vols (Moscow: Prosvet, 1991), 2: 457.

48. For a prisoner memoir describing common graves with five to ten bodies each
    in 1938 in a Kolyma camp, see MMSPb, GOTLIBOIM, Iosif Samoilovich.
    Vospominaniia, l. 19. A December 1941 Gulag order permitted burial without
    coffins but still foresaw individual graves: GARF, f. R9414, op. 1, d. 2762, ll.
    190–1. The order about gold prostheses was issued by the deputy head of the
    Gulag Zavgorodny on 17 November 1941: GARF, f. R9414, op. 1, d. 2771, ll.
    1–2. Gulag chief Nasedkin issued a detailed decree on burial procedures on 2
    February 1943; it permitted common graves for naked corpses: GARF, f.
    R9414, op. 1, d. 2785, ll. 18–18 ob. Also note V. N. Triakhov, *Gulag i voina:
    Zhestokaia pravda dokumentov* (Perm': Pushka, 2004), 188–9.

49. A. B. Bezborodov and V. M. Khrustalev, eds, *Istoriia stalinskogo Gulaga. Konets
    1920-kh – pervaia polovina 1950-kh godov. Tom 4: Naselenie Gulaga: Chislennost'
    i usloviia soderzhaniia* (Moscow: ROSSPEN, 2004–5), 4: 534–5, citing GARF,
    f. R9414, op. 1, d. 2809, ll. 89–89 ob.

50. Kersnovskaia, *Skol'ko stoit chelovek*, 485. If such punctiliousness with spring
    reburials was observed in a Norilsk burial ground close to the camps and town,
    less salubrious winter disposal was recalled by an inmate of a remote Komi
    camp in the late 1930s: 'brigades of shockworker-gravediggers' were sent to
    bury corpses of prisoners; they dumped them into rivers that flowed past no
    human habitations. Skeletons were found in the spring by lone hunters tracking
    in the woods, but who would investigate 'when a human life was worth less
    than a bent penny'? See MMA, f. 2, op. 3, d. 17, GURSKII, Konstantin
    Petrovich. 'Po dorogam GULAGa. Vospominaniia'. Kniga 3-aia, 'Ukhtpechlag'.
    Ialta, b.d., ll. 111–12.

51. Georgii Demidov, 'Dubar'', *Chudnaia planeta. Rasskazy* (Moscow:
    Vozvrashchenie, 2008), 41.

52. Ibid., 41.

53. Kersnovskaia, *Skol'ko stoit chelovek*, 486–7.

54. Ibid., 477.

55. Ibid., 477–8, 492.

56. Ibid., 484.

57. Shalamov's portrait of Kolyma anatomist Umansky ascribed to the doctor a
    talent for leading diagnosticians to the hard facts of Gulag conditions without
    bruising their professional pride, although it cost him his own self-regard as a
    healer. Umansky 'looked deeper, farther, with more principle. He saw his obli-
    gations not to catch doctors with trifles, in little mistakes, but to make them
    see – and show others! – the large things that stood behind these trifles, the
    "backdrop" of starvation and emaciation that affected the disease picture as
    studied by the doctor in his textbook. The textbook of prisoners' diseases had
    not yet been written. It would never be written.' Shalamov, 'Veismanist', 507–8.

58. Kersnovskaia, *Skol'ko stoit chelovek*, 489–90.

59. Ibid., 491–2.

60. Batkis, *Organizatsiia zdravookhraneniia*, 334.

61. Baev had been arrested in 1937; released in 1944, he defended his dissertation in 1947, and was briefly rearrested in 1949. Kersnovskaya remembers him as a 'freely hired' doctor; for this episode, see Kersnovskaia, *Skol'ko stoit chelovek*, 493–4. On Baev in these years, see Aleksandr Aleksandrovich Baev, *Ocherki. Perepiska. Vospominaniia* (Moscow: Nauka, 1998), 81–4; E. V. Markova, *Gulagovskie tainy osvoeniia severa* (Moscow: Stroiizdat, 2001), 130–1; Stephen F. Cohen, *The Victims Return: Survivors of the Gulag after Stalin* (Exeter, NH: Publishing Works, 2010), 12–14.

62. See, for example, E. A. Kersnovskaia, *Skol'ko stoit chelovek* (Moscow: Kolibri, 2018). It appears in the notebook (*tetrad'*) transcripts on the official Kersnovskaia website: https://archive.gulag.su/copybook/index.php?eng=0&page=8&list=26 (accessed 12 May 2023).

63. Kersnovskaia, *Skol'ko stoit chelovek*, 497.

64. Ibid. Prisoner S. N. Liandres was a 'qualified pharmacist' who ran the Central Camp Hospital pharmacy during the war; see Popov, 'Opiat' ozhivet potusknevshee vremia'.

65. Kersnovskaia, *Skol'ko stoit chelovek*, 502–5.

66. Ibid., 523.

67. Shalamov, 'Veismanist', 507.

68. Ibid., 507–8. Reportedly anticipating the Great Terror in 1935, the real Umanskii volunteered for the Gulag medical service in Kolyma, but this did not save him from arrest in Magadan in 1937 and a ten-year sentence, which he served working as a doctor. By 1951 he was the pathological anatomist in the Magadan Province Central Hospital. On his education and career, see Budnikova, 'Nekotorye dannye', 49–50; Boris N. Lesniak, *Ia k vam prishel!* (Magadan: MAOBTI, 1998), 112–20.

69. Kersnovskaia, *Skol'ko stoit chelovek*, 474.

Chapter 7 'I do not assist simulators': A prisoner-psychiatrist challenges Gulag conventions

1. The case history of L.F.S. is found in GARF, f. R9414, op. 2, d. 166, 'Nauchnaia rabota L. G. Sokolovskogo 'O simuliatsii psikhozov i nevrozov'. Vypusk 15. Rukopisnyi ekz-r dlia sluzhebnogo pol'zovaniia. 1944.' See l. 11.

2. On these studies see Golfo Alexopoulos, 'Medical Research in Stalin's Gulag', *Bulletin of the History of Medicine* 90, no. 3 (2016): 363–93.

3. This discussion of malingering in Soviet and Gulag medicine is based on Dan Healey, '"Dramatological" Trauma in the Gulag: Malingering and Self-Inflicted Injuries and the Prisoner-Patient', in *Geschichte(n) des Gulag – Realität und Fiktion*, ed. Felicitas Fischer von Weikersthal and Karoline Thaidigsmann (Heidelberg: Winter-Verlag, 2013).

4. According to some contemporary attempts to track this demand, it was not unusual in 1933–34, for example, for inmates to visit the outpatient clinic over twenty times per year; in 1936 this had dropped to eighteen times annually, but under the pressure of the Great Terror and the massive influx of prisoners in the system, visits rose to twenty-three per prisoner in 1938. For 1933–34: GARF, f. R9414, op. 1, d. 2742; 1936: GARF, f. R9414, op. 1, d. 2740, l. 38; 1938: GARF, f. R9414, op. 1, d. 2740, l. 56.

5. On medical inspection, see Dan Healey, 'Lives in the Balance: Weak and Disabled Prisoners and the Biopolitics of the Gulag', *Kritika: Explorations in Russian and Eurasian History* 16, no. 3 (2015): 538–40.

6. Golfo Alexopoulos, *Illness and Inhumanity in Stalin's Gulag* (New Haven & London: Yale University Press, 2017), 96–103.

7. A. Iu. Zhukov and V. G. Makurov, eds, *Gulag v Karelii. Sbornik dokumentov i materialov 1930–1941* (Petrozavodsk: Karel'skii nauchnyi tsentr RAN, 1992), 42–4, 122–5; on the link between prisoners' living conditions and reforging, see Christopher Joyce, 'The Gulag in Karelia: 1929 to 1941', in *The Economics of Forced Labor: The Soviet Gulag*, ed. Paul Gregory and Valery Lazarev (Stanford: Hoover Institution Press, 2003), 182. For other examples, from the Moscow–Volga Canal camp in this period, see GARF, f. R9489, op. 2, d. 25, l. 39; and f. R9489, op. 2, d. 5, l. 474.

8. *Perekovka*, 27 May 1933, no. 29, 2.

9. F. N. Baranovskii, 'Son otkazchika: P'esa v 3-kh kartinakh'. *Pod znamenem Belomorstroia: Lit.-khudozh. [ezhemes.] zh-l: Izd. BBK NKVD* no. 1, (1936): 46–9, quoted at 47.

10. See e.g. Konstantin Sobolevsky: 'Pozor', in: Kul'turno-vospitatel'nyi otdel, *Kanaloarmeitsy plakat* [from the Reforging Library, No. 27] (Dmitlag: Izdanie Dmitlaga NKVD SSSR, 1936), 34. On prisoner Sobolevsky and this 'Library' series, see Cynthia A. Ruder, *Building Stalinism: The Moscow Canal and the Creation of Soviet Space* (London: I. B. Tauris, 2018), 79–109.

11. GARF, f. R9414, op. 1, d. 2753, ll. 134–5.

12. GARF, f. R9414, op. 1, d. 2756, ll. 64–9; see also Oleg Khlevniuk, *The History of the Gulag: From Collectivization to the Great Terror* (New Haven & London: Yale University Press, 2004), 220–1.

13. See e.g. cases of wartime 'systematic work-refusal' by women prisoners, 1942, PIKM, Kedrovyi Shor archive, 'Knigi prikazanii. KP3153/1, KP2457/1', decrees no. 63, 142; GARF, f. 9407, op. 1, d. 1501, l. 108 for a 1950 report about women who self-harmed when separated from men they had adopted as 'camp husbands' (my thanks to Emily Johnson for this source); and comments in 1951 on 'unrepentant simulators' at one women's division of a construction camp: GARF, f. R9414, op. 1a, d. 147, ll. 132–5.

14. GARF, f. R9413, op. 1, d. 9, ll. 106–31.

15. See e.g. GARF, f. R9414, op. 1a, d. 628, l. 21; GARF, f. R9414, op. 1a, d. 630, ll. 75, 179; f. R9414, op. 1, d. 2894, l. 128.

16. A moving example of a political prisoner who imagined visits to his family in Moscow to preserve his mental health is found in MMA, DEIAGER, Ivan Isaakovich, Pis'ma zhene i detiam 1935–1938, f. 2, op. 3, dd. 19–20, e.g. at d. 19, ll. 7–8.

17. Dan Healey, *Bolshevik Sexual Forensics: Diagnosing Disorder in the Clinic and Courtroom, 1917–1939* (DeKalb: Northern Illinois University Press, 2009), 104–12.

18. On 'genius' studies, see Irina Sirotkina, *Diagnosing Literary Genius: A Cultural History of Psychiatry in Russia, 1880–1930* (Baltimore: Johns Hopkins University Press, 2002), 145–80; on worker mental hygiene and psychotherapies, see Lewis H. Siegelbaum, 'Okhrana Truda: Industrial Hygiene, Psychotechnics, and Industrialization in the USSR', in *Health and Society in Revolutionary Russia*, ed. Susan Gross Solomon and John F. Hutchinson

(Bloomington & Indianapolis: Indiana University Press, 1990); Frances Lee Bernstein, *The Dictatorship of Sex: Lifestyle Advice for the Soviet Masses* (DeKalb: Northern Illinois University Press, 2007).

19. Benjamin Zajicek, 'Scientific Psychiatry in Stalin's Soviet Union: The Politics of Modern Medicine and the Struggle to Define "Pavlovian" Psychiatry, 1939–1953' (PhD thesis, University of Chicago, 2009), 6; idem, 'Soviet Madness: Nervousness, Mild Schizophrenia, and the Professional Jurisdiction of Psychiatry in the USSR, 1918–1936', *Ab Imperio* 2014, no. 4 (2014): 167–94; idem, 'A Soviet System of Professions: Psychiatry, Professional Jurisdiction, and the Soviet Academy of Medical Sciences, 1932–1951', in *Russian and Soviet Health Care from an International Perspective: Comparing Professions, Practice and Gender, 1880–1960*, ed. Susan Grant (Cham: Springer International Publishing, 2017), 97–117.

20. Zajicek, 'Scientific Psychiatry in Stalin's Soviet Union', 208–10.

21. Dan Healey, 'Russian and Soviet Forensic Psychiatry: Troubled and Troubling', *International Journal of Law and Psychiatry* 37, no. 1 (2014): 71–81.

22. For 1931, see Iu. N. Afanas'ev et al., eds, *Istoriia stalinskogo Gulaga. Konets 1920-kh – pervaia polovina 1950-kh godov. Sobranie dokumentov v semi tomakh* (Moscow: ROSSPEN, 2004–5), 4: 462; for 1935, see GARF, f. R9414, op. 1, d. 2744, l. 66. In 1939 a high Gulag official in Moscow castigated camp commandants for 'forgetting about prisoners' placed in civilian psychiatric hospitals and ordered them to check all cases and bring them back to camp industries if they had been cured: see GARF, f. R9414, op. 1, d. 2756, l. 234.

23. For the statistics in this paragraph, see Afanas'ev et al., eds, *Istoriia stalinskogo Gulaga*, 4: 485–9.

24. For 1941, see GARF, f. R9414, op. 1, d. 2762, l. 110; for 1949, see ibid., op. 1, d. 2827, l. 75. For the 1952 situation, see ibid., op. 1, d. 326, l. 128.

25. Unless otherwise stated, Sokolovsky's biography is drawn from F. G. Kanev, 'Doktor Sokolovskii – osnovatel' psikhonevrologicheskoi sluzhby v g. Ukhty', in S. F. Sapolnova, T. A. Vekshina, and F. G. Kanev, eds, *Liudi v belykh khalatakh* (Ukhta & Syktyvkar: Komi respublikanskaia tipografiia, 2009), 74–9.

26. Sokolovsky's nationality is stated as Jewish on a 1947 identity document reproduced in Sapolnova et al., eds, *Liudi v belykh khalatakh*, 79.

27. On Sokolovsky's unnamed wife's decision to divorce him upon arrest, see Ia. I. Kaminskii, *'Minuvshee prokhodit predo mnoiu . . .': Izbrannoe iz lichnogo arkhiva* (Odesa: Aspekt, 1995), 124. On the 1937 decree and the fate of the 'wives' of enemies, see Emma Mason, 'Women in the Gulag of the 1930s', in *Women in the Stalin Era*, ed. Melanie Ilic (Basingstoke: Palgrave Macmillan, 2001), 131–50; and 'Operativnyi prikaz NKVD no. 00486', in A. I. Kokurin and N. V. Petrov, eds, *GULAG: Glavnoe upravlenie lagerei, 1918–1960* (Moscow: Mezhdunarodnyi fond Demokratiia, 2000), 106–10.

28. Kaminskii, *'Minuvshee prokhodit predo mnoiu . . .'*, 124.

29. The date can be established in Sokolovsky's study, with the earliest case of a prisoner with epileptic symptoms admitted 11 April 1941, by which time the psychiatric department was evidently operating; see GARF, f. R9414, op. 2, d. 166, l. 5 (case no. 9).

30. See maps of Vetlosian drawn from memory in the 2000s by ex-prisoners: Sapolnova et al., eds, *Liudi v belykh khalatakh*, 43–4.

31. See chapter 4 in this book on apprenticeships at this hospital; and note the account of Vetlosian in Sapolnova et al., *Liudi v belykh khalatakh*, 26–42.

32. Alexopoulos, 'Medical Research in Stalin's Gulag', 389.
33. GARF, f. R9414, op. 2, d. 166, l. 1. Sokolovsky attributes the second quotation here to a textbook he undoubtedly used in Kazan lectures and probably had access to in Vetlosian camp hospital: V. A. Vnukov and Ts. M. Feinberg, *Sudebnaia psikhiatriia. Uchebnik dlia iuridicheskikh vuzov* (Moscow: OGIZ, 1936), 291. Among the medical works Sokolovsky cites – with page numbers suggesting he was able to consult them in the camp – are M. O. Gurevich and M. Ia. Sereiskii, *Uchebnik psikhiatrii*, 2nd edn (Moscow: Gos. med. iz-vo, 1932); V. Nadezhdin, 'Simuliatsiia', in *Bol'shaia meditsinskaia entsiklopediia*, ed. N. A. Semashko (Moscow: Sovetskaia entsiklopediia, 1934), 30: 425–85; M. I. Astvatsaturov, *Uchebnik nervnykh boleznei*, 6th edn (Leningrad: Biomedgiz, 1935); V. A. Giliarovskii, *Psikhiatriia. Rukovodstvo dlia vrachei i studentov*, 3rd edn (Moscow & Leningrad: Medgiz, 1938).
34. GARF, f. R9414, op. 2, d. 166, l. 2.
35. Alexopoulos, 'Medical Research in Stalin's Gulag', 389.
36. Another research paper on malingering and self-harm in prisoners in the same central Gulag collection by a prisoner-physician displays a harsh determination to unmask the simulator: K. P. Bogolepov, 'Opisanie metodov organo- i chlenovreditel'stva sredi prestupnogo mira' (1948, MS 'for internal use only'), GARF, f. R9414, op. 2, d. 174. On this paper, see Healey, '"Dramatological" Trauma in the Gulag', 57–8; Alexopoulos, 'Medical Research in Stalin's Gulag', 378.
37. GARF, f. R9414, op. 2, d. 166, ll. 4–5.
38. Cases 2 to 5, GARF, f. R9414, op. 2, d. 166, ll. 3–4.
39. Cases 7 to 9, GARF, f. R9414, op. 2, d. 166, l. 5.
40. Cases 10 to 13, GARF, f. R9414, op. 2, d. 166, l. 6.
41. Cases 19, 15 in GARF, f. R9414, op. 2, d. 166, ll. 7, 11.
42. During the Second World War, 'alimentary' or 'nutritional' dystrophy was studied by Soviet doctors treating civilians in the Siege of Leningrad. Rebecca Manley traces how the term migrated from civilian to Gulag medicine, in Rebecca Manley, 'Nutritional Dystrophy: The Science and Semantics of Starvation in World War II', in *Hunger and War: Food Provisioning in the Soviet Union during World War II*, ed. Wendy Z. Goldman and Donald Filtzer (Bloomington: Indiana University Press, 2015), 251–4.
43. Case 17, GARF, f. R9414, op. 2, d. 166, l. 7.
44. 'Emaciation' (*istoshchenie*) was permitted for use in diagnostics within camps, in a May 1941 decree from the Gulag's chief director Nasedkin; but for external reporting to avoid 'undesirable impressions about the cause of death' among relatives and the courts, the same decree banned it on death certificates, ordering the use of secondary effects such as 'heart failure, weakening heart function, pulmonary tuberculosis, etc.' instead. See GARF, f. R9414, op. 1, d. 2762, l. 103.
45. Case 20, GARF, f. R9414, op. 2, d. 166, l. 12.
46. GARF, f. R9414, op. 2, d. 166, l. 22.
47. GARF, f. R9414, op. 2, d. 166, l. 9. 'Catamnesis' is the follow-up medical history of a patient, after initial diagnosis or following treatment.
48. In a culture where literature enjoyed great cultural and moral authority, 'literary diagnosis' imparted Russian psychiatry with greater esteem; for this argument, see Sirotkina, *Diagnosing Literary Genius*.

49. Frederick White, *Degeneration, Decadence and Disease in the Russian Fin de Siècle: Neurasthenia in the Life and Work of Leonid Andreev* (Manchester: Manchester University Press, 2014).
50. Aleksei Yanishevsky read and then published his lecture, 'The hero of Leonid Andreev's "The Thought" from the perspective of a doctor-psychiatrist', in Kazan; see Frederick H. White, 'Leonid Andreev's Release from Prison and the Codification of Mental Illness', *New Zealand Slavonic Journal* 41 (2007): 18–41.
51. GARF, f. R9414, op. 2, d. 166, l. 10. On Soviet critics and Andreev, see White, *Degeneration, Decadence and Disease in the Russian Fin de Siècle*, 1–6.
52. GARF, f. R9414, op. 2, d. 166, l. 10, citing Konstantin S. Stanislavskii, *Rabota aktera nad soboi v tvorcheskom protsesse perezhivaniia: Dnevnik uchenika* (Moscow: Khudozhestvennaia literatura, 1938). Giliarovsky is credited with coining the term 'timogenic', publishing it in 1946; see Zajicek, 'Scientific Psychiatry in Stalin's Soviet Union', 163.
53. Stanislavsky revised the text of this book constantly in the 1930s, taking account of his changing approach, and also ideological constraints. English translations abridged and domesticated the book, removing obscure references to Russian details, for American drama students; see Sharon Marie Carnicke, 'Stanislavsky: Uncensored and Unabridged', *TDR (1988–)* 37, no. 1 (1993): 22–37.
54. MMSPb, GURVICH Oskar Iosifovich (psevd. Pavel Irinin), 'Tropinki vospominanii', l. 143.
55. Ibid., ll. 143–4.
56. Ibid., ll. 144–5.
57. One was a Polish woman, 'Stenia', suffering from alimentary dystrophy; according to Gurvich, Sokolovsky treated her then found her work. 'Stenia' was evidently Sokolovsky's second wife, Zenoviya Kazanivskaya, who recounted to Viktor Samsonov that she had been a prisoner arrested in Lviv as a student, transported to Ukhta, and hospitalised at Vetlosian for severe emaciation; Sokolovsky met her as a patient-prisoner in 1947 and found her a laboratory job; see Viktor A. Samsonov, *V perezhitom nenast'e: O lagernykh vrachakh i drugikh znakomykh medikakh, a takzhe o zemliakakh-kondopozhanakh, postradavshikh ot repressii 30–40-kh godov (dokumenty i pis'ma iz arkhiva avtora)* (Petrozavodsk: Petrozavodskii gosudarstvennyi universitet, 2001), 56. Another patient Sokolovsky saved was Maria Mikhailovna Ioffe, the widow of Trotsky ally Adolph Abramovich Ioffe, who committed suicide in 1927. Maria Ioffe suffered from apparent paralysis when Gurvich encountered her in Vetlosian. When he met her in 1954 on the eve of her political rehabilitation her paralysis had disappeared and she told him that Sokolovsky and chief of Vetlosian Hospital Yakov Kaminsky had helped her survive, implying that their assistance included a favourable false diagnosis: Gurvich, 'Tropinki vospominanii', ll. 145–7. Kaminsky notes in his memoirs that he was investigated by a 'a big commission from the Gulag' for his part in protecting Ioffe; see Kaminskii, 'Minuvshee prokhodit predo mnoiu . . .', 100–1.
58. Gurvich, 'Tropinki vospominanii', l. 143.

Chapter 8 'You will be singing these songs': The radium-water spa of the zeks

1. Ostap Vishnia, 'Ukhtinskaia tselebnaia voda. Promysel No. II imeni OGPU', in *Pokaianie: Martirolog. T. 8, Ch. 1*, ed. E. A. Zelenskaia and M. B. Rogachev (Syktyvkar: Komi respublikanskii blagotvoritel'nyi obshchestvennyi fond zhertv politicheskikh repressii 'Pokaianie', 2005), 271.

2. I. D. Vorontsova and M. B. Rogachev, 'Neizdannaia kniga ob Ukhtpechlage: iz materialov knigi "5 let bor'by za nedra taigi i tundry"', in *Pokaianie: Martirolog. T. 8, Ch. 1*, ed. E. A. Zelenskaia and M. B. Rogachev (Syktyvkar: Komi respublikanskii blagotvoritel'nyi obshchestvennyi fond zhertv politicheskikh repressii 'Pokaianie', 2005), 163–70.

3. John McCannon, 'Tabula Rasa in the North: The Soviet Arctic and Mythic Landscapes in Stalinist Popular Culture', in *The Landscape of Stalinism: The Art and Ideology of Soviet Space*, ed. Evgeny Dobrenko and Eric Naiman (Seattle: University of Washington Press, 2003), 241–60.

4. G. M. Danishevskii, 'Kurortologiia', in *Bol'shaia meditsinskaia entsiklopediia*, ed. A. N. Bakulev (Moscow: Sovetskaia entsiklopediia, 1960), 14: 1060–87; 'The Cult of Water Cures in Germany', *British Medical Journal* (20 Aug. 1927): 320–2.

5. On Soviet workers' sanatoria and the class politics, and medical perspectives, that made them distinctive from capitalist resorts, see Tricia Starks, *The Body Soviet: Propaganda, Hygiene, and the Revolutionary State* (Madison: University of Wisconsin Press, 2008).

6. A. F. Khoroshev, *Ocherki istorii zdravookhraneniia Magadanskoi oblasti* (Magadan: Magadanskoe knizhnoe izdatel'stvo, 1959), 38–41. For a 1951 report on misallocation to undeserving workers of tickets to Talaya's resort, see GAMO, f. 45, op. 1, d. 23, l. 147. The Gulag also used forced labour to build and reconstruct civilian resorts. In 1949 the Georgian Communist Party ordered a new hotel and spa facility be constructed at Tskhaltubo by 4,000 prisoners guarded and managed by 500 Gulag staff; MIA, f. 14, op. 23, d. 291, ll. 3, 16–17.

7. Interview with Anna Kliashko, 15 September 2012, Montréal, Canada.

8. Ia. I. Kaminskii, *Dokladnaia zapiska ob organizatsii severnogo kurorta v gorode Ukhta Komi ASSR* (Ukhta, 1944), MIZU, Kaminskii, Iakov Iosifovich folder.

9. Ia. I. Kaminskii, '*Minuvshee prokhodit predo mnoiu . . .': Izbrannoe iz lichnogo arkhiva* (Odesa: Aspekt, 1995), which was produced with the help of chief district archivist G. L. Malinova, a member of the Odesa Memorial board of directors.

10. From Kropyvnytskyi, Varun-Sekret was a conservative Duma deputy in the Oktobrist and later Landowners fractions. Kaminskii, '*Minuvshee prokhodit predo mnoiu . . .*', 13.

11. On Odesa's lively Maccabi activity and its political dimensions, see Igor Yeykelis, 'Odessa Maccabi 1917–20: The Development of Sport and Physical Culture in Odessa's Jewish Community', *East European Jewish Affairs* 28, no. 2 (1998): 83–101.

12. Kaminskii, '*Minuvshee prokhodit predo mnoiu . . .*', 15–18.

13. Ibid., 16.

14. Ibid., 17. Kaminsky does not mention having read *Doctor Zhivago*.

15. Kaminskii, *'Minuvshee prokhodit predo mnoiu . . .'*, 19–28; the statistics come from an official's report on the pogrom, reproduced in this memoir. On Hryhoriv, see Christopher Gilley, 'Pogroms and Imposture: The Violent Self-Formation of Ukrainian Warlords', in *In the Shadow of the Great War: Physical Violence in East-Central Europe, 1917–1923*, ed. Jochen Böhler, Ota Konrád, and Rudolf Kučera (New York: Berghahn Books, 2021).

16. Kaminskii, *'Minuvshee prokhodit predo mnoiu . . .'*, 48.

17. Adrian Thomas and Arpan K. Banerjee, *The History of Radiology* (Oxford: Oxford University Press, 2013), 11–36; for a Stalin-era history of radiology in Odesa, which ignores mention of then-disgraced Yakov Kaminsky, see I. Ia. Balaban, E. D. Dubovyi, and E. E. Eram, 'Istoriia rentgenologii na Odesshchine', in *Materialy po istorii rentgenologii v SSSR*, ed. S. A. Reinberg (Moscow: Minzdrav RSFSR; Ts. nauchno-issledovatel'skii institut rentgenologii i radiologii im. V. M. Molotova, 1948), 250–61.

18. Thomas and Banerjee, *The History of Radiology*, 20; Balaban et al., 'Istoriia rentgenologii', 255–6; Kaminskii, *'Minuvshee prokhodit predo mnoiu . . .'*, 47–9.

19. Kaminskii, *'Minuvshee prokhodit predo mnoiu . . .'*, 40; the pamphlet appeared in the 1920s popular-science 'The sex question in accessible sketches' series: Ia. I. Kaminskii, *Polovaia zhizn' i fizicheskaia kul'tura* (Odessa: Svetoch, 1927); a second, illustrated edition was published in the same year.

20. For Kaminsky's recollections of Sakhnovsky, and Sakhnovsky's of Kaminsky, see Kaminskii, *'Minuvshee prokhodit predo mnoiu . . .'*, 49–60.

21. Ibid., 63–82.

22. Ibid., 86–7. For a similar description of the journey to Ukhta and selection for medical work, see the reminiscences of Romanian surgeon Aleksandr Tsetsulesku, in S. F. Sapolnova, T. A. Vekshina, and F. G. Kanev, *Liudi v belykh khalatakh* (Ukhta & Syktyvkar: Komi respublikanskaia tipografiia, 2009), 24–5.

23. On Loidin, see RGASPI, f. 17, op. 100, d. 101450.

24. Anne Applebaum, *Gulag: A History of the Soviet Camps* (London: Allen Lane, 2003), 519.

25. Kaminskii, *'Minuvshee prokhodit predo mnoiu . . .'*, 99.

26. For analysis of his input at the September 1945 conference, see Golfo Alexopoulos, *Illness and Inhumanity in Stalin's Gulag* (New Haven & London: Yale University Press, 2017), 160–82 (quoted at 163).

27. 'Sluzhebnaia kharakteristika [nachal'nik podrazdelneiia maior v/s Balaev, 6 March 1954]', MIZU, Iakov Iosifovich Kaminskii folder, l. 76.

28. A. I. Kichigin and A. I. Taskaev, '"Vodnyi Promysel": Proizvodstvo radiia v Respublike Komi (1931–1956 gg.)', *Voprosy istorii estestvoznaniia i tekhniki*, no. 4 (2004): 3–30, radium statistics at 29; see also A. I. Taskaev and A. I. Kichigin, *Istoriia radiatsionnoi gigieny i radiatsionnoi bezopasnosti v SSSR na primere ukhtinskogo radievogo promysla* (Syktyvkar: Komi nauchnyi tsentr Uralskogo otdeleniia RAN, 2006). Population statistics: see E. A. Zelenskaia, *Lagernoe proshloe Komi Kraia (1929–55 gg.) v sud'bakh i vospominaniiakh sovremennikov* (Ukhta & Kirov: Blagotvoritel'nyi fond 'Tochka opora'; KOGUP Kirovskaia oblastnaia tipografiia 2004), 37.

29. On Sokolov's direction of the first human trials, see V. V. Iurchenko, 'K istorii promyshlennogo razvitiia evropeiskogo severa: Proekt ispol'zovaniia ukhtin-skoi radioaktivnoi vody v lechebnykh tseliakh (1932–1938)', in *Liudi v belykh*

khalatakh, ed. S. Sapolnova, T. A. Vekshina, and F. G. Kanev (Ukhta & Syktyvkar: Komi respublikanskaia tipografiia, 2009), 152.

30. Kichigin and Taskaev, '"Vodnyi Promysel"', citing decrees from the National Archive of the Komi Republic in Syktyvkar, 10–11; G. M. Danishevskii, ed., *Ukhtinskie mineral'nye radievy vody (Radium-Mineralwässer von Uchta)* (Ukhta & Moscow: Ukhto-Pecherskii Trest; Gosudarstvennyi Tsentral'nyi Institut Kurortologii, 1933); for a French summary, see G. M. Danichevsky, ed., *Analyses des travaux de l'Institut Central de Balnéologie et des [sic] Climatologie* (Moscow & Leningrad: Édition médicale et biologique d'état, 1933).

31. The classified report is found at GARF, f. R9414, op. 2, d. 103; nevertheless, copies of the document are accessible in libraries in the Komi Republic.

32. V. A. Aleksandrov, 'Bal'neologicheskoe znachenie mineral'nykh vod Ukhtinskogo raiona', in Danishevskii, ed., *Ukhtinskie mineral'nye radievye vody*, 3–8. Reconstitution of radioactive water from radium was also attempted, but rejected because of the high cost, at the Perm' branch of the Moscow Resort Studies Institute: see V. K. Modestov, P. A. Iasnitskii, and M. A. Rozentul, eds, *Sbornik rabot permskogo otdeleniia Ural'skogo filiala Tsentral'nogo instituta kurortologii* (Perm': Permskoe otdelenie Ural'skogo filiala Tsentral'nogo instituta kurortologii, 1934).

33. Aleksandrov, 'Bal'neologicheskoe znachenie', 6.

34. Kichigin and Taskaev, '"Vodnyi Promysel"', 8; Taskaev and Kichigin, *Istoriia radiatsionnoi gigieny*, 27.

35. Taskaev and Kichigin, *Istoriia radiatsionnoi gigieny*, 6–9.

36. Ibid., 13. The effect of the waters on animals and yeast products was also studied.

37. One account, citing Komi Republic archival sources, gives the following numbers of persons treated annually: 1932 = 49; 1933 = 117; 1934 = 82; 1935 = 161; 1936 = 174; elsewhere the same account gives the total number of patients served before the war as 1,500, this time citing a prisoner-doctor, Lev L. Davydov, who was the last director of the physiotherapy laboratory; see MIZU, Kaminskii folder, ll. 5, 8.

38. Vishnia, 'Ukhtinskaia tselebnaia voda', 269; Iurchenko, 'K istorii promyshlennogo razvitiia evropeiskogo severa', 152.

39. For descriptions of various bathing routines, see Danishevskii, ed., *Ukhtinskie mineral'nye radievye vody*. The Moscow patient samples came principally from factory and office workers and their dependants.

40. Iurchenko, 'K istorii promyshlennogo razvitiia evropeiskogo severa', 154–5. Nurse Elena Kharkova, discussed in chapter 5, worked in Vodny from 1933 to 1938, perhaps in the civilian clinic, because her workbook records her entering Gulag service from 1938 in Vetlosian Hospital; see MIZU, Khar'kova (Panina), Elena Ivanovna, vol'nonaemnaia folder, l. 5.

41. The directors were doctors A. A. Titaev (1932–34), A. A. Liubushin (1934–38), and O. A. Stepun (1939–41); see Taskaev and Kichigin, *Istoriia radiatsionnoi gigieny*, 13–14. On dispensarisation, see Grigorii A. Batkis, *Organizatsiia zdravookhraneniia* (Moscow: Medgiz, 1948), 374–92.

42. Taskaev and Kichigin, *Istoriia radiatsionnoi gigieny*, 20–5; Iurchenko, 'K istorii promyshlennogo razvitiia evropeiskogo severa', 18–25; Zelenskaia, *Lagernoe proshloe Komi Kraia*, 38.

43. Iurchenko, 'K istorii promyshlennogo razvitiia evropeiskogo severa', 156.

44. Taskaev and Kichigin, *Istoriia radiatsionnoi gigieny*, 27–9.

45. For the geologist's report, see UIKM, 'Ukhtinskie radionosnye vody' folder, A. V. Kulevskii, 'Kratkaia istoriia Ukhtinskogo mestorozhdeniia radionosnykh vod i osnovnye dannye po geologii mestorozhdeniia. Materialy dlia brigady Akademii nauk SSSR. SEKRETNO. 1940 god' (quoted at l. 15).

46. Ostap Vishnia, 'Dnevnik Pavla Mikhailovicha Gubenko (Ostap Vishnia)', in *Pokaianie: Martirolog. T. 8, Ch. 1*, ed. E. A. Zelenskaia and M. B. Rogachev (Syktyvkar: Komi respublikanskii blagotvoritel'nyi obshchestvennyi fond zhertv politicheskikh repressii 'Pokaianie', 2005), 424.

47. Kaminskii, *'Minuvshee prokhodit predo mnoiu . . .'*, 114. Stepun's research after Vodny concentrated on techniques for reviving emaciated prisoners through intramuscular injections of sterilised milk, or the patient's own blood; see Viktor A. Samsonov, *K tebe, Onego, vse puti. Zapiski lagernogo lekpoma, studenta, vracha, prepodavatelia* (Petrozavodsk: Iz-vo Petrozavodskogo universiteta, 2000), 60–1.

48. Kaminskii, *Dokladnaia zapiska*. The copy signed by Kaminsky at MIZU was one of three that were created by 'our calligraphers' as the prisoner had no access to a typewriter (Kaminskii, *'Minuvshee prokhodit predo mnoiu . . .'*, 114). No copy appears in the archival inventories of the Gulag in Moscow.

49. Kaminskii, *Dokladnaia zapiska*, 4.

50. Ibid., 5–6.

51. Ibid., 6–7.

52. Ibid., 8–10; he cited 1939 Party Congress resolutions and an article by the director of the USSR Resort Administration in *Pravda* that year for his reading of government resort policy.

53. Taskaev and Kichigin, *Istoriia radiatsionnoi gigieny*, 15.

54. Ibid., 15, 30. The Soviet Union's reliance on distillation of radium from naturally radioactive waters at Ukhta meant it did not have a ready supply of uranium (a by-product of radium-mining in other countries). The expertise developed at Vodny factory would need to be redeployed to securing a useable supply of the rare metal uranium. See David Holloway, *Stalin and the Bomb: The Soviet Union and Atomic Energy, 1939–1956* (New Haven & London: Yale University Press, 1994), 63–4.

55. UIKM, TOROPOV, Fedor Aleksandrovich fond (Vodny), 'Kharakteristika na nachal'nika TsKhL'; I. I. Kolotii, 'Glavnyi tekhnolog' ll. 1–10. Kolotii was a young physical chemistry graduate assigned to Vodny in 1951; he composed this biography of Toropov in post-Soviet times as the chairman of the Museum of the History and Labour Glory of the Progress Factory – the successor to the Vodny radium factory.

56. Kaminskii, *'Minuvshee prokhodit predo mnoiu . . .'*, 113–14.

57. The Vodny factory was transferred from Gulag jurisdiction to the Ministry of Medium-Machine Building, a cover for nuclear-industry production, in 1952; see UIKM, TOROPOV, Fedor Aleksandrovich fond (Vodny), Kolotii, 'Glavnyi tekhnolog' l. 3.

58. Taskaev and Kichigin, *Istoriia radiatsionnoi gigieny*, 15–18; Kaminskii, *'Minuvshee prokhodit predo mnoiu . . .'*, 113; Sapolnova et al., eds, *Liudi v belykh khalatakh*, 161.

59. Taskaev and Kichigin, *Istoriia radiatsionnoi gigieny*, 30–3; Kaminskii, *'Minuvshee prokhodit predo mnoiu . . .'*, 113. The 'factory' evidently remained operational,

and a successor producing electronic components, 'Progress', retains an archive of the radium factory.

60. Kaminskii, 'Minuvshee prokhodit predo mnoiu . . .', 114–15; Sapolnova et al., eds, Liudi v belykh khalatakh, 161.

61. The optimism of this moment, and the failures of technocratic control, are vividly recounted in Kate Brown, Plutopia: Nuclear Families, Atomic Cities, and the Great Soviet and American Plutonium Disasters (Oxford & New York: Oxford University Press, 2013).

62. Kaminskii, 'Minuvshee prokhodit predo mnoiu . . .', 115; Taskaev and Kichigin, Istoriia radiatsionnoi gigieny, 30–3. One Soviet academic reportedly remembered how, during the Second World War era of scientific co-operation, Canadian counterparts burst into laughter at the Soviets when they described obtaining radium from mineral waters; see Kichigin and Taskaev, '"Vodnyi Promysel"', 29.

63. Kaminskii, 'Minuvshee prokhodit predo mnoiu . . .', 117–18.

64. Ibid., 113.

65. Ibid.

66. For a review of archival scholarship on the Doctors' Plot, see David Brandenberger, 'Stalin's Last Crime? Recent Scholarship on Postwar Soviet Antisemitism and the Doctor's Plot', Kritika: Explorations in Russian and Eurasian History 6, no. 1 (2005): 187–204. An institutional history of the Kremlin's medical service treats the episode with scant mention of the anti-Semitic tone of the campaign; see S. P. Mironov, Iu. L. Perov, V. M. Tsvetkov, and V. M. Iastrebov, Kremlevskaia meditsina (ot istokov do nashikh dnei) (Moscow: Izvestiia; Meditsinskii tsentr Upravleniia delami Prezidenta Rossiiskoi Federatsii, 2000), 144–7.

67. Iakov L. Rappoport, The Doctors' Plot (London: Fourth Estate, 1991), 75, 79.

68. Christopher Burton, 'Soviet Medical Attestation and the Problem of Professionalisation under Late Stalinism, 1945–1953', Europe-Asia Studies 57, no. 8 (2005): 1219–25.

69. Interview, 15 September 2012, Montréal, Canada. In this interview, when asked what her religious convictions were as a young adult, Anna explained: 'None whatsoever – we were atheists.' She ignored anti-Semitic jokes as irrelevant to her sense of identity; her husband, '100 per cent Russian from a centuries-old Urals family', worried on her behalf more than she did during the anti-Semitic campaign. Anna acquired a firmer Jewish identity in the wake of the collapse of the Soviet Union.

70. Sapolnova et al., eds, Liudi v belykh khalatakh, 161–3; MIZU, Kaminskii, Iakov Iosifovich folder, ll. 8–10.

Conclusion: 'No archival materials will be gathered, and people will scatter . . .'

1. Viktor A. Samsonov, K tebe, Onego, vse puti. Zapiski lagernogo lekpoma, studenta, vracha, prepodavatelia (Petrozavodsk: Iz-vo Petrozavodskogo universiteta, 2000), 214.

2. Interview with Tatyana Oleinik, 26 June 2009, Moscow. See also letters to Samsonov from Sokolovsky's wife, and his daughter, in Viktor A. Samsonov, V perezhitom nenast'e: O lagernykh vrachakh i drugikh znakomykh medikakh, a takzhe o zemliakakh-kondopozhanakh, postradavshikh ot repressii 30–40-kh godov

(dokumenty i pis'ma iz arkhiva avtora) (Petrozavodsk: Petrozavodskii gosudarst-vennyi universitet, 2001), 56–7.

3. Irina Flige, 'The Necropolis of the Gulag as a Historical-Cultural Object: An Overview and Explication of the Problem', in *Rethinking the Gulag: Identities, Sources, Legacies*, ed. Alan Barenberg and Emily D. Johnson (Bloomington: Indiana University Press, 2022).

4. Samsonov, *V perezhitom nenast'e*, 27.

5. Alexander Solzhenitsyn, *The Gulag Archipelago 1918–1956: An Experiment in Literary Investigation*, trans. Thomas P. Whitney (London: Collins & Harvill Press, 1975), 2: 615.

6. Michael Hechter, *Internal Colonialism: The Celtic Fringe in British National Development* (London: Routledge, 1975); John Liu, 'Towards an Understanding of the Internal Colonial Model', in *Postcolonialism: Critical Concepts in Literary and Cultural Studies*, ed. Diana Brydon (London & New York: Routledge, 2000), 1347–64.

7. Reforming Party and government leaders challenged Dalstroi's old guard in Magadan between 1954 and 1957: see Pavel Grebeniuk, *Kolymskii led: Sistema upravleniia na severo-vostoke Rossii 1953–1964* (Moscow: ROSSPEN, 2007), 45–74. Khoroshev and Repyeva are discussed in chapter 3.

8. '[Shapiro] knew so very much, and he so generously shared his knowledge, he revealed his professional secrets to us, he coached us, so well that it all yielded results: I think that the fact that I gained a first professional classification [*pervaia professional'naia kategoriia*], that I was considered, when I was working in the Magadan Province Hospital, a very good doctor, that I always had a long queue of patients coming to see me, all that I owe to Viktor Mikhailovich Shapiro, all that he gave me as a specialist.' Interview, 24 June 2009; and for more examples, interview, 15 September 2012; Montréal, Canada.

9. Eugenia Ginzburg, *Within the Whirlwind*, trans. Ian Boland (London: Collins Harvill, 1989), 162, 215–16.

10. On regional-historical museums, see Sofia Gavrilova, *Russia's Regional Museums: Representing and Misrepresenting Knowledge about Nature, History and Society* (London: Routledge, 2022). For insight into museum treatments of the Gulag, see Sofia Gavrilova, 'Regional Memories of the Great Terror: Representation of the Gulag in Russian Kraevedcheskii Museums', *Problems of Post-Communism* (2021): 1–15, https://doi.org/10.1080/10758216.2021.1885981; Andrei Zavadski and Vera Dubina, 'Eclipsing Stalin: The Gulag History Museum in Moscow as a Manifestation of Russia's Official Memory of Soviet Repression', *Problems of Post-Communism* (2021): 1–13, https://doi.org/10.1080/10758216.2021.1983444; Alena Kravtsova and Elena Omelchenko, 'Public Perceptions of Russia's Gulag Memory Museums', *Problems of Post-Communism* (2022): 1–11, https://doi.org/10.1080/10758216.2022.2152052; Vladislav Staf, 'Local Initiatives: A Historical Analysis of the Creation of Memorial Museums of the Gulag in (Post-)Soviet Russia', *Problems of Post-Communism* (2023): 1–8, https://doi.org/10.1080/10758216.2023.2166846.

11. Gavrilova, 'Regional Memories of the Great Terror', 12–14.

12. Ostap Vishnia, 'Dnevnik Pavla Mikhailovicha Gubenko (Ostap Vishnia)', in *Pokaianie: Martirolog. T. 8, Ch. 1*, ed. E. A. Zelenskaia and M. B. Rogachev (Syktyvkar: Komi respublikanskii blagotvoritel'nyi obshchestvennyi fond zhertv politicheskikh repressii 'Pokaianie', 2005), 421.

13. Ibid., 423.
14. MIZU, Kaminskii, Iakov Iosifovich folder; Ia. I. Kaminskii, *'Minuvshee prokhodit predo mnoiu . . .': Izbrannoe iz lichnogo arkhiva* (Odesa: Aspekt, 1995), 142–56.
15. S. F. Sapolnova, T. A. Vekshina, and F. G. Kanev, eds, *Liudi v belykh khalatakh* (Ukhta & Syktyvkar: Komi respublikanskaia tipografiia, 2009), 74–7; interview with Tatyana Oleinik, 26 June 2009, Moscow.
16. Catherine Viollet, 'L'œuvre autobiographique de Evfrosinija Kersnovskaya: Chronique illustrée du Gulag', *Avtobiografi*Я: *Journal on Life Writing and the Representation of the Self in Russian Culture*, no. 1 (2012): 223–36.
17. PIKM, f. 31, op. 39, d. 8, 'Medsestry', 'Kolinenko, Maria Petrovna' [interview]; 'Davydenko, Serafima Stepanovna [interview, n.d., n.p.]'.
18. Her death is apparently commemorated online; see https://www.geni.com/people/ольга-клименко/6000000107661993960 (accessed 29 April 2023).
19. In addition to his own memoirs, see https://www.sakharov-center.ru/asfcd/auth/?t=author&i=7 (accessed 29 April 2023).
20. Vadim Aleksandrovskii, *Zapiski lagernogo vracha* (Moscow: Vozvrashchenie, 1996), 3–4; B. A. Nakhapetov, *Ocherki istorii sanitarnoi sluzhby Gulaga* (Moscow: ROSSPEN, 2009), 95–9.
21. Interviews with Anna Kliashko, 23–24 June 2009; 31 March 2010; 15 September 2012; all in Montréal, Canada. See a short biography and photograph of Anna at http://www.kolymastory.ru/glavnaya/istoriya-magadana/istoriya-magadanskoj-bolnitsy/1946-1959-gody/ (accessed 18 March 2020).
22. N. V. Savoeva, *Ia vybrala Kolymu*, Arkhivy Pamiati. Vyp. 1 (Magadan: AO 'MAOBTI', Obshchestvo 'Poisk nezakonno repressirovannykh', 1996), 46.
23. For extracts from Savoeva's memoir, see Semen Vilenskii, ed., *Dodnes' tiagoteet: v 2-kh tomakh* (Moscow: Vozvrashchenie, 2004), 2: 294–309.
24. N. A. Glazov, *Koshmar parallel'nogo mira: Zapiski vracha* (Novosibirsk: Iz-vo Novosibirskoi gos. obl. nauchnoi biblioteki, 1999); see the back cover of this book for a still from *Rossiia, kotoruiu my poteriali* including Glazova.
25. M. Ia. Pullerits, 'Nemnogo o svoem detstve', *Kraevedcheskie zapiski [Magadanskii oblastnoi kraevedcheskii muzei. Magadanskoe knizhnoe izdatel'stvo]* 16 (1989): 88.
26. A. N. Kaneva, 'Deiatel'nost' Partiinoi organizatsii Komi ASSR po sozdaniiu i razvitiiu neftegazovoi promyshlennosti v 1929–1945 gg.' (Candidate's thesis, Leningrad State University, 1970); Sapolnova et al., *Liudi v belykh khalatakh*, 17–21.
27. Mayhill Courtney Fowler, *Beau Monde on Empire's Edge: State and Stage in Soviet Ukraine* (Toronto, Buffalo & London: University of Toronto Press, 2017), 207.
28. Maxim Tarnawsky, 'Introduction', in *Hard Times* by Ostap Vyshnia (London: Glagoslav Publications, 2018), 10.
29. Fowler, *Beau Monde on Empire's Edge*, 213. On Vyshnia, see also Rory Finnin, *Blood of Others: Stalin's Crimean Atrocity and the Poetics of Solidarity* (Toronto: University of Toronto Press, 2022), 82–3.

SELECT BIBLIOGRAPHY

Primary Sources

Archives and museum collections

Gosudarstvennyi arkhiv Rossiiskoi Federatsii, GARF, State Archive of the Russian Federation, Moscow

Rossiiskii gosudarstvennyi arkhiv sotsial'no-politicheskoi istorii, RGASPI, Russian State Archive of Socio-Political History, Moscow

Gosudarstvennyi arkhiv Magadanskoi oblasti, GAMO, State Archive of Magadan Province, Magadan

Gosudarstvennyi arkhiv Sverdlovskoi oblasti, GASO, State Archive of Sverdlovsk Province, Ekaterinburg

Magadanskii oblastnoi kraevedcheskii muzei, MOKM, Magadan Province Regional Museum, Magadan

Muzei istorii zdravookhraneniia Ukhty, MIZU, Ukhta Museum of the History of Public Health, Ukhta

Pechorskii istoriko-kraevedcheskii muzei, PIKM, Pechora Historical-Regional Museum, Pechora

Ukhtinskii istoriko-kraevedcheskii muzei, UIKM, Ukhta Historical-Regional Museum, Ukhta

Memorial Society Archives, MMA, Moscow

Memorial Society Archives, MMSPb, St Petersburg (now held by Nauchno-informatsionnyi tsentr 'Fond Iofe')

Ministry of Internal Affairs Archive, MIA, Tbilisi, Georgia. Central Committee of the Communist Party of the Georgian Soviet Socialist Republic, f. 14

National Archives of Georgia, NAG, Tbilisi, Georgia

Reference works, websites, periodicals

Semashko, N. A., ed. *Bol'shaia meditsinskaia entsiklopediia*. 1–e izd. 35 vols. Moscow: Sovetskaia entsiklopediia, 1928–1936.

Vavilov, S. I., ed. *Bol'shaia sovetskaia entsiklopediia*. 2-e izd. 53 vols. Moscow: Gosudarstvennoe nauchnoe izdatel'stvo, 1949–1958.

SELECT BIBLIOGRAPHY

Evfrosiniia Kersnovskaia official website: https://gulag.su/

Kadrovyi sostav organov gosudarstvennyi bezopasnosti SSSR 1935–1939: nkvd.memo.ru

Krasnoiarskoe obshchestvo 'Memorial': https://www.memorial.krsk.ru/index.htm

Moia rodina – Magadan: http://www.kolymastory.ru/

Virtual Gulag Museum: http://www.gulagmuseum.org (now offline)

Vospominaniia o GULAGe i ikh avtory (formerly Sakharov Centre): https://vgulage.name/

British Medical Journal

Kanaloarmeika

Perekovka na stroitel'stve kanala Moskva-Volga

Pod znamenem Belomorstroia: Lit.-khudozh. [ezhemes.] zh-l: Izd. BBK NKVD

Proizvodstvennyi biulleten' (Pechorskogo zheleznodorozhnogo stroitel'stva i lageria NKVD)

Prorvinskii lovets: Organ KVO Prorvinskogo isprav.-trud. lageria NKVD

Unpublished theses

Burton, Christopher. 'Medical Welfare during Late Stalinism: A Study of Doctors and the Soviet Health System, 1945–1953'. PhD thesis, University of Chicago, 2000.

Davis, Christopher M. 'The Economics of the Soviet Health System: An Analytical and Historical Study, 1921–1978'. PhD thesis, Cambridge University, 1979.

Kaneva, A. N. 'Deiatel'nost' partiinoi organizatsii Komi ASSR po sozdaniiu i razvitiiu neftegazovoi promyshlennosti v 1929–1945 gg.'. Candidate's thesis, Leningrad State University, 1970.

Nakonechnyi, Mikhail Iur'evich. 'Factory of Invalids: Mortality, Disability and Early Release on Medical Grounds from the Gulag, 1930–1955'. DPhil thesis, University of Oxford, 2020.

Nordlander, David J. 'Capital of the Gulag: Magadan in the Early Stalin Era, 1929–1941'. PhD thesis, University of North Carolina – Chapel Hill, 1997

Zajicek, Benjamin. 'Scientific Psychiatry in Stalin's Soviet Union: The Politics of Modern Medicine and the Struggle to Define "Pavlovian" Psychiatry, 1939–1953'. PhD thesis, University of Chicago, 2009.

Published works

Afanas'ev Iu. N. et al., eds. *Istoriia stalinskogo Gulaga. Konets 1920-kh – pervaia polovina 1950-kh godov. Sobranie dokumentov v semi tomakh.* 7 vols. Moscow: ROSSPEN, 2004–5.

Aleksandrovskii, Vadim. *Zapiski lagernogo vracha.* Moscow: Vozvrashchenie, 1996.

Astvatsaturov, Mikhail Ivanovich. *Uchebnik nervnykh boleznei.* 6th edn. Leningrad: Biomedgiz, 1935.

Baev, Aleksandr Aleksandrovich. *Ocherki. Perepiska. Vospominaniia.* Moscow: Nauka, 1998.

Balaban, I. Ia., E. D. Dubovyi, and E. E. Eram. 'Istoriia rentgenologii na Odesschine'. In *Materialy po istorii rentgenologii v SSSR*, ed. S. A. Reinberg,

250–61. Moscow: Minzdrav RSFSR; Ts. nauchno-issledovatel'skii institut rent-genologii i radioilogii im. V. M. Molotova, 1948.

Bardach, Janusz and Kate Gleeson. *Man Is Wolf to Man: Surviving Stalin's Gulag.* London: Simon & Schuster, 1998.

Batkis, Grigorii A. *Organizatsiia zdravookhraneniia.* Moscow: Medgiz, 1948.

Batsaev, I. D. and A. G. Kozlov, eds. *Dal'stroi i Sevvostlag OGPU-NKVD SSSR v tsifrakh i dokumentakh. Ch. I (1931–1941).* Magadan: SVKNII DVO RAN, 2002.

———. *Dal'stroi i Sevvostlag OGPU-NKVD SSSR v tsifrakh i dokumentakh. Ch. II (1941–1945).* Magadan: SVKNII DVO RAN, 2002.

Berdiaev, Arkadii Fedorovich. *Khirurgiia ambulatornogo vracha.* 5th edn. Moscow & Leningrad: Medgiz, 1939.

Brodskii, Iu. A. *Solovki. Dvadtsat' let osobogo naznacheniia.* Moscow: ROSSPEN, 2002.

Bulgakov, Mikhail. *Izbrannaia proza.* Moscow: Sovetskaia Rossiia, 1983.

Bumm, Ernst. *Rukovodstvo k izucheniiu akusherstva.* 3rd edn. Moscow & Leningrad: Gos. izd-vo, 1930.

Chernorutskii, Mikhail Vasil'evich. *Diagnostika vnutrennykh boleznei.* 1st edn. Leningrad: Medgiz, 1938.

Chirkov, Iu. I. *A bylo vse tak. . . .* Moscow: Iz-vo politicheskoi literatury, 1991.

Chistiakov, Ivan. *Sibirskoi dal'nei storonoi. Dnevnik okhrannika BAMa, 1935–1936.* Moscow: AST, CORPUS, 2014.

Danichevsky, G. M., ed. *Analyses des travaux de l'Institut Central de Balnéologie et des [sic] Climatologie.* Moscow & Leningrad: Édition médicale et biologique d'état, 1933.

Danishevskii, G. M., ed. *Ukhtinskie mineral'nye radievy vody (Radium-Mineralwässer von Uchta).* Ukhta & Moscow: Ukhto-Pecherskii Trest; Gosudarstvennyi Tsentral'nyi Institut Kurortologii, 1933.

Demidov, Georgii. *Chudnaia planeta. Rasskazy.* Moscow: Vozvrashchenie, 2008.

Dolgun, Alexander and Patrick Watson. *Alexander Dolgun's Story: An American in the Gulag.* New York: Ballantine Books, 1975.

Fidel'gol'ts, Iurii. 'Tot Vaninskii port'. In *Za chto? Proza, poeziia, dokumenty*, ed. V. A. Shentalinskii and V. N. Leonovich, 114–54. Moscow: Kliuch, 1999.

Fil'shtinskii, I. M. *My shagaem pod konvoem. Rasskazy iz lagernoi zhizni.* Nizhnii Novgorod: Dekom, 2005.

Genter, German Genrikhovich. *Uchebnik akusherstva: Dlia studentov medvuzov.* Leningrad: Biomedgiz, 1937.

Giliarovskii, V. A. *Psikhiatriia. Rukovodstvo dlia vrachei i studentov.* 3rd edn. Moscow & Leningrad: Medgiz, 1938.

Ginzburg, Eugenia. *Into the Whirlwind,* trans. Paul Stevenson and Manya Harari. London: Collins Harvill, 1967.

———. *Within the Whirlwind,* trans. Ian Boland. London: Collins Harvill, 1989.

Ginzburg, Evgeniia. *Krutoi marshrut.* Frankfurt am Main & Milan: Possev, 1967.

Glazov, N. A. *Koshmar parallel'nogo mira: Zapiski vracha.* Novosibirsk: Iz-vo Novosibirskoi gos. obl. nauchnoi biblioteki, 1999.

Gor'kii, Maksim. 'Po soiuzu sovetov'. In *Sobranie sochinenii v vosemnadtsati tomakh.* Moscow: Gos. izd. khudozhestvennoi literatury, 1962.

Gor'kii, Maksim, L. Averbakh, and S. Firin et al. *Belomorsko-baltiiskii kanal imeni Stalina. Istoriia stroitel'stva, 1931–1934 gg.* Moscow: OGIZ 'Istoriia fabrik i zavodov', 1934.

Gurevich, M. O. and M. Ia. Sereiskii. *Uchebnik psikhiatrii.* 2nd edn. Moscow: Gos. med. iz-vo, 1932.

Iadrintsev, Nikolai Mikhailovich. *Sibir' kak koloniia. K iubileiu trekhsotletiia. Sovremennoe polozhenie Sibiri. Eia nuzhdy i potrebnosti. Eia proshloe i budushchee.* St Petersburg: M. M. Stasiulevich, 1882.

Ikhteiman, M. S. *Rukovodstvo dlia srednego meditsinskogo personala.* Leningrad: Biomedgiz, 1935.

Kaminskii, Ia. I. *'Minuvshee prokhodit predo mnoiu . . .': Izbrannoe iz lichnogo arkhiva.* Odesa: Aspekt, 1995.

Kasabova, G. I. *O vremeni, o Noril'ske, o sebe . . .* 11 vols. Moscow: Polimediia, 2004–2010.

Kassirskii, I. A. *Alimentarnaia distrofiia i pellagra (diagnostika, klinika, terapiia).* Ryblaga NKVD SSSR: Sanotdel Ryblaga NKVD SSSR, 1943.

Kaufman, A. I. *Lagernyi vrach. 16 let v Sovetskom Soiuze – vospominaniia sionista.* Tel Aviv: AM OVED, 1973.

Kersnovskaia, Evfrosiniia Antonovna. *Naskal'naia zhivopis'. Al'bom. Redaktor-sostavitel' V. Vigilianskii.* Moscow: S. P. 'Kvadrat', 1991.

———. *Skol'ko stoit chelovek.* Moscow: ROSSPEN, 2006.

———. *Skol'ko stoit chelovek.* Moscow: Kolibri, 2018.

Khaustov, V. N., V. P. Naumov, and N. S. Plotnikova, eds. *Lubianka: Stalin i glavnoe upravlenie gosbezopasnosti NKVD, 1937–1938.* Rossiia XX vek dokumenty. Moscow: Mezhdunarodnyi fond 'Demokratiia' (Fond A. N. Iakovleva), 2004.

Khlevniuk, Oleg, V. A. Kozlov, and S. V. Mironenko, eds. *Zakliuchennye na stroikakh kommunizma. Gulag i ob"ekty energetiki v SSSR. Sobranie dokumentov i fotografii.* Moscow: ROSSPEN, 2008.

Kokurin, A. I. and N. V. Petrov, eds. *GULAG: Glavnoe upravlenie lagerei, 1918–1960.* Moscow: Mezhdunarodnyi fond Demokratiia, 2000.

Kosinskii, M. F. *Pervaia polovina veka: Vospominaniia.* Paris: YMCA-press, 1995.

Kul'turno-vospitatel'nyi otdel. *Kanaloarmeitsy plakat.* Dmitlag: Izdanie Dmitlaga NKVD SSSR, 1936.

Kuznetsova, Ina. *Zona miloserdiia.* Moscow: Iz-vo im. Sabashnikovykh, 2005.

Lesniak, Boris. 'Voitsek Dazhitskii (otets Martyn'ian)'. In *Dodnes' tiagoteet. Tom 2. Kolyma,* ed. Semen Vilenskii. Moscow: Vozvrashchenie, 2004.

Lesniak, Boris N. *Ia k vam prishel!* Magadan: MAOBTI, 1998.

Mamuchashvili, Elena. 'V bol'nitse dlia zakliuchennykh'. *Shalamovskii sbornik 2* (1997): 78–88.

Mitskevich, Sergei I. *Zapiski vracha-obshchestvennika.* Moscow: Meditsina, 1969.

Mochulsky, Fyodor Vasilevich and Deborah A. Kaple. *Gulag Boss: A Soviet Memoir.* Oxford & New York: Oxford University Press, 2011.

Modestov, V. K. *Primenenie v bal'neoterapii estestvennykh i iskusstvennykh radioak-tivnykh vod.* Trudy Molot. Med. Inst. Vyp. 20, Molotov, 1941.

Modestov, V. K., P. A. Iasnitskii, and M. A. Rozentul, eds. *Sbornik rabot permskogo otdeleniia Ural'skogo filiala Tsentral'nogo instituta kurortologii.* Perm': Permskoe otdelenie Ural'skogo filiala Tsentral'nogo instituta kurortologii, 1934.

Petkevich, Tamara. *Memoir of a Gulag Actress.* DeKalb: Northern Illinois University Press, 2011.

Pullerits, M. Ia. 'Nemnogo o svoem detstve'. *Kraevedcheskie zapiski [Magadanskii oblastnoi kraevedcheskii muzei. Magadanskoe knizhnoe izdatel'stvo]* 16 (1989): 88–94.

Razgon, Lev. *True Stories.* London: Souvenir Press, 1998.

Rossi, Zhak. *Spravochnik po GULagu.* 2 vols. Moscow: Prosvet, 1991.

Samsonov, Viktor A. *K tebe, Onego, vse puti. Zapiski lagernogo lekpoma, studenta, vracha, prepodavatelia.* Petrozavodsk: Iz-vo Petrozavodskogo univer-siteta, 2000.

————. 'Opyt osvoeniia nachal'nykh osnov meditsiny i prozektorskoi praktiki v usloviiakh Ukhtizhemlaga (vospominaniia)'. *Arkhiv patologii,* no. 1 (1999): 59–63.

————. *Preodoleniia: V nelegkom puti v nauku ot medbrata-zakliuchennogo do profes-sora universiteta.* Petrozavodsk: Petrozavodskii gosudarstvennyi universitet, 2004.

————. *V perezhitom nenast'e: O lagernykh vrachakh i drugikh znakomykh medikakh, a takzhe o zemliakakh-kondopozhanakh, postradavshikh ot repressii 30–40-kh godov (dokumenty i pis'ma iz arkhiva avtora).* Petrozavodsk: Petrozavodskii gosudarst-vennyi universitet, 2001.

————. *Zhizn' prodolzhitsia: Zapiski lagernogo lekpoma.* Petrozavodsk: Kareliia, 1990.

Savoeva, N. V. *Ia vybrala Kolymu.* Arkhivy Pamiati. Vyp. 1. Magadan: AO 'MAOBTI', Obshchestvo 'Poisk nezakonno repressirovannykh', 1996.

Scholmer, Joseph. *Vorkuta.* London: Weidenfeld & Nicolson, 1954.

Shalamov, Varlam. *Neskol'ko moikh zhiznei. Vospominaniia, zapisnye knizhki, perepiska, sledstvennye dela.* Moscow: Eksmo, 2009.

————. *Preodolenie zla.* Moscow: Eksmo, 2011.

————. *Sobranie sochinenii v chetyrekh tomakh.* 4 vols. Moscow: Khudozhestvennaia literatura; Vagrius, 1998.

Shmidt, A. A., ed. *Tsynga i bor'ba s neiu na severe: Sbornik statei.* Moscow & Leningrad: Sanitarnoe upravlenie Gostresta Dal'stroi, Moskva; Biomedgiz, Leningrad, 1935.

Stanislavskii, Konstantin. *Rabota aktera nad soboi v tvorcheskom protsesse perezhiva-niia: Dnevnik uchenika.* 2-e izd. Moscow: Khudozhestvennaia literatura, 1938.

Terent'ev, A. 'Vetlosianskaia slabkomanda'. In *V nedrakh Ukhtpechlaga. Vypusk vtoroi. Malaia seriia,* ed. V. Bulychev, 30. Ukhta: Ukhto-Pechorskoe istoriko-prosvetitel'skoe obshchestvo 'Memorial', 1994.

Triakhov, V. N. *Gulag i voina: Zhestokaia pravda dokumentov.* Perm': Pushka, 2004.

Veresaev, Vikentii. *Zapiski vracha.* Moscow: AST Zebra E, 2010.

Vilenskii, Semen, ed. *Dodnes' tiagoteet: v 2-kh tomakh.* Moscow: Vozvrashchenie, 2004.

Vilenskii, Semen and K. B. Nikolaev, eds. *Souchastniki: Arkhiv Kozlova. Tom pervyi.* Moscow: Vozvrashchenie, 2012.

Vishnia, Ostap. 'Dnevnik Pavla Mikhailovicha Gubenko (Ostap Vishnia)'. In *Pokaianie: Martirolog. T. 8, Ch. 1,* ed. E. A. Zelenskaia and M. B. Rogachev, 419–38. Syktyvkar: Komi respublikanskii blagotvoritel'nyi obshchestvennyi fond zhertv politicheskikh repressii 'Pokaianie', 2005.

————. 'Doktor Ia. P. Sokolov'. In *Pokaianie: Martirolog. T. 8, Ch. 1,* ed. E. A. Zelenskaia and M. B. Rogachev, 357–60. Syktyvkar: Komi respublikanskii blagotvoritel'nyi obshchestvennyi fond zhertv politicheskikh repressii 'Pokaianie', 2005.

————. 'Mens Sana in Corpore Sano'. In *Pokaianie: Martirolog. T. 8, Ch. 1,* ed. E. A. Zelenskaia and M. B. Rogachev, 337–39. Syktyvkar: Komi respublikanskii blagotvoritel'nyi obshchestvennyi fond zhertv politicheskikh repressii 'Pokaianie', 2005.

———. 'Ukhtinskaia tselebnaia voda. Promysel No. II imeni OGPU'. In *Pokaianie: Martirolog. T. 8, Ch. 1*, ed. E. A. Zelenskaia and M. B. Rogachev, 265–71. Syktyvkar: Komi respublikanskii blagotvoritel'nyi obshchestvennyi fond zhertv politicheskikh repressii 'Pokaianie', 2005.

Vnukov, V. A. and Ts. M. Feinberg. *Sudebnaia psikhiatriia. Uchebnik dlia iuridicheskikh vuzov*. Moscow: OGIZ, 1936.

Vogelfanger, Isaac J. *Red Tempest: The Life of a Surgeon in the Gulag*. Montreal & Kingston, London, Buffalo: McGill-Queen's University Press, 1996.

Zhukov, A. Iu. and V. G. Makurov, eds. *Gulag v Karelii. Sbornik dokumentov i materialov 1930–1941*. Petrozavodsk: Karel'skii nauchnyi tsentr RAN, 1992.

Secondary Sources

Adler, Nanci. *Victims of Soviet Terror: The Story of the Memorial Movement*. Westport & London: Praeger, 1993.

Afanas'eva, Tatiana. 'Pisateli Ukrainy na Pechore'. In *Vygliadyvaias' v proshloe*, ed. T. Afanas'eva, 170–6. Pechora: Pechorskoe vremia, 2010.

———, ed. *Vgliadyvaias' v proshloe*. Pechora: Pechorskoe vremia, 2010.

———. 'Vrachi v Pechorzheldorlage'. In *Vgliadyvaias' v proshloe*, ed. T. Afanas'eva, 99–145. Pechora: Pechorskoe vremia, 2010.

Alexopoulos, Golfo. 'Amnesty 1945: The Revolving Door of Stalin's Gulag'. *Slavic Review* 64, no. 2 (2005): 274–306.

———. 'Destructive-Labor Camps: Rethinking Solzhenitsyn's Play on Words'. *Kritika: Explorations in Russian and Eurasian History* 16, no. 3 (2015): 499–526.

———. 'Exiting the Gulag after War: Women, Invalids, and the Family'. *Jahrbücher für Geschichte Osteuropas* 57, no. 4 (2009): 563–79.

———. *Illness and Inhumanity in Stalin's Gulag*. New Haven & London: Yale University Press, 2017.

———. 'Medical Research in Stalin's Gulag'. *Bulletin of the History of Medicine* 90, no. 3 (2016): 363–93.

Applebaum, Anne. *Gulag: A History of the Soviet Camps*. London: Allen Lane, 2003.

———. *Red Famine: Stalin's War on Ukraine*. London: Penguin, 2017.

Asher, Harvey. 'The Soviet Union, the Holocaust, and Auschwitz'. *Kritika: Explorations in Russian and Eurasian History* 4, no. 4 (2003): 886–912.

Badcock, Sarah. *A Prison without Walls? Eastern Siberian Exile in the Last Years of Tsarism*. Oxford: Oxford University Press, 2016.

Barenberg, Alan. *Gulag Town, Company Town: Forced Labor and its Legacy in Vorkuta*. New Haven & London: Yale University Press, 2014.

———. '"I Would Very Much Like to Read your Story about Kolyma": Georgii Demidov, Varlam Shalamov, and the Development of Gulag Prose, 1965–67'. In *Rethinking the Gulag: Identities, Sources, Legacies*, ed. Alan Barenberg and Emily D. Johnson, 220–42. Bloomington: Indiana University Press, 2022.

Barnes, Steven Anthony. *Death and Redemption: The Gulag and the Shaping of Soviet Society*. Princeton: Princeton University Press, 2011.

Baron, Nick. 'Conflict and Complicity: The Expansion of the Karelian Gulag, 1923–1933'. *Cahiers du monde russe* 22 (2001/02): 615–48.

————. *Soviet Karelia: Politics, Planning and Terror in Stalin's Russia, 1920–1939*. London: Routledge, 2007.

Batsaev, I. D. 'Kolymskaia griada arkhipelaga Gulag (zakliuchennye)'. In *Istoricheskie aspekty severo-vostoka Rossii: Ekonomika, obrazovanie, kolymskii Gulag*, ed. V. F. Lesniakov and V. S. Pan'shin, 46–72. Magadan: SVKNII DVO RAN, 1996.

Beer, Daniel. *The House of the Dead: Siberian Exile under the Tsars*. London: Allen Lane, 2016.

Bell, Wilson. 'Sex, Pregnancy, and Power in the Late Stalinist Gulag'. *Journal of the History of Sexuality* 24, no. 2 (2015): 198–224.

————. *Stalin's Gulag at War: Forced Labour, Mass Death, and Soviet Victory in the Second World War*. Toronto: University of Toronto Press, 2019.

————. 'Was the Gulag an Archipelago? De-Convoyed Prisoners and Porous Borders in the Camps of Western Siberia'. *Russian Review* 72, no. 1 (2013): 116–41.

Berdinskikh, Viktor. *Istoriia odnogo lageria (Viatlag)*. Moscow: Agraf, 2001.

Bernstein, Frances Lee. 'Behind the Closed Door – VD and Medical Secrecy in Early Soviet Medicine'. In *Soviet Medicine: Culture, Practice, and Science*, ed. Frances L. Bernstein, Christopher Burton, and Dan Healey, 92–110. DeKalb: Northern Illinois University Press, 2010.

————. *The Dictatorship of Sex: Lifestyle Advice for the Soviet Masses*. DeKalb: Northern Illinois University Press, 2007.

Bernstein, Frances L., Christopher Burton, and Dan Healey, eds. *Soviet Medicine: Culture, Practice, Science*. DeKalb: Northern Illinois University Press, 2010.

Bogumił, Zuzanna. *Gulag Memories: The Rediscovery and Commemoration of Russia's Repressive Past*, trans. Philip Palmer. New York: Berghahn Books, 2018.

Bone, Jonathan A. 'À la recherche d'un Komsomol perdu: Who Really Built Komsomol'sk-Na-Amure, and Why'. *Revue des études slaves* 71, no. 1 (1999): 59–92.

Borodkin, Leonid and Simon Ertz. 'Coercion Versus Motivation: Forced Labor in Norilsk'. In *The Economics of Forced Labor: The Soviet Gulag*, ed. Paul Gregory and Valery Lazarev, 75–104. Stanford: Hoover Institution Press, 2003.

Brandenberger, David. 'Stalin, the Leningrad Affair, and the Limits of Postwar Russocentrism'. *Russian Review* 63, no. 2 (2004): 241–55.

————. 'Stalin's Last Crime? Recent Scholarship on Postwar Soviet Antisemitism and the Doctor's Plot'. *Kritika: Explorations in Russian and Eurasian History* 6, no. 1 (2005): 187–204.

Brovman, G. *V. V. Veresaev: zhizn' i tvorchestvo*. Moscow: Sovetskii pisatel', 1959.

Brown, Adam. '"No One Will Ever Know": The Holocaust, "Privileged" Jews and the "Grey Zone"'. *History Australia* 8, no. 3 (2011): 95–116.

Brown, Kate. *Plutopia: Nuclear Families, Atomic Cities, and the Great Soviet and American Plutonium Disasters*. Oxford & New York: Oxford University Press, 2013.

Bud, Robert. *Penicillin: Triumph and Tragedy*. Oxford: Oxford University Press, 2007.

Budnikova, S. V. 'Nekotorye dannye o repressirovannykh medikakh na Kolyme (po materialam Magadanskogo oblastnogo kraevedcheskogo muzeia)'. In *Kolyma. Dal'stroi. Gulag. Skorb' i sud'by. Materialy nauchno-prakticheskoi konferentsii 13–14 iiunia 1996 goda*, ed. A. M. Biriukov, 46–50. Magadan: Severnyi mezhdunarodnyi universitet, 1998.

Burton, Christopher. 'Soviet Medical Attestation and the Problem of Professionalisation under Late Stalinism, 1945–1953'. *Europe-Asia Studies* 57, no. 8 (2005): 1211–30.

———. 'Vseokhvatnaia pomoshch' pri stalinizme? Sovetskoe zdravookhranenie i dukh gosudarstva blagodenstviia, 1945–1953'. In *Sovetskaia sotsial'naia politika: Tseny i deistvuiushchie litsa, 1940–1985*, ed. Elena Iarskaia-Smirnova and P. V. Romanov, 174–93. Moscow: Variant, TsSPGI, 2008.

Bynum, Helen. *Spitting Blood: The History of Tuberculosis*. 1st edn. Oxford: Oxford University Press, 2012.

Bynum, W. F., Anne Hardy, Stephen Jacyna, Christopher Lawrence, and E. M. (Tilli) Tansey. *The Western Medical Tradition 1800 to 2000*. Cambridge: Cambridge University Press, 2006.

Cameron, Sarah I. *The Hungry Steppe: Famine, Violence, and the Making of Soviet Kazakhstan*. Ithaca: Cornell University Press, 2018.

Canguilhem, Georges. *The Normal and the Pathological*. New York: Zone Books, 1991.

Carnicke, Sharon Marie. 'Stanislavsky: Uncensored and Unabridged'. *TDR (1988–)* 37, no. 1 (1993): 22–37.

Cohen, Stephen F. 'The Stalin Question since Stalin'. In *An End to Silence: Uncensored Opinion in the Soviet Union from Roy Medvedev's Underground Magazine*, Political Diary, ed. Stephen F. Cohen, 22–50. New York & London: W. W. Norton, 1982.

———. *The Victims Return: Survivors of the Gulag after Stalin*. Exeter, NH: Publishing Works, 2010.

Conquest, Robert. *Kolyma: The Arctic Death Camps*. London: Macmillan, 1978.

Conroy, Mary Schaeffer. *Medicines for the Soviet Masses during World War II*. Lanham & Plymouth: University Press of America, 2008.

Davis, Christopher M. 'Economic Problems of the Soviet Health Service: 1917–1930'. *Soviet Studies* 35, no. 3 (1983): 343–61.

———. 'Economics of Soviet Public Health, 1928–1932: Development Strategy, Resource Constraints, and Health Plans'. In *Health and Society in Revolutionary Russia*, ed. Susan Gross Solomon and John F. Hutchinson, 146–72. Bloomington & Indianapolis: Indiana University Press, 1990.

Draskoczy, Julie. *Belomor: Criminality and Creativity in Stalin's Gulag*. Boston: Academic Studies Press, 2014.

Durzan, Don J. 'Arginine, Scurvy and Cartier's "Tree of Life"'. *Journal of Ethnobiology and Ethnomedicine* 5, no. 1 (2009): 1–16.

Engel, Barbara A. *Between the Fields and the City: Women, Work and Family in Russia, 1861–1914*. Cambridge: Cambridge University Press, 1994.

Ertz, Simon. 'Building Norilsk'. In *The Economics of Forced Labor: The Soviet Gulag*, ed. Paul Gregory and Valery Lazarev, 127–50. Stanford: Hoover Institution Press, 2003.

Etkind, Alexander. 'Internalising Colonialism: Intellectual Endeavours and Internal Affairs in Mid-Nineteenth Century Russia'. In *Convergence and Divergence: Russia and Eastern Europe into the Twenty-First Century*, ed. Peter J. S. Duncan, 103–20. London: School of Slavonic and East European Studies, UCL, 2007.

———. *Warped Mourning: Stories of the Undead in the Land of the Unburied*. Stanford: Stanford University Press, 2013.

Ewing, Sally. 'The Science and Politics of Soviet Insurance Medicine'. In *Health and Society in Revolutionary Russia*, ed. Susan Gross Solomon and John F. Hutchinson, 69–96. Bloomington & Indianapolis: Indiana University Press, 1990.

Fedor, Julie. 'Memory, Kinship, and the Mobilization of the Dead: The Russian State and the "Immortal Regiment" Movement'. In *War and Memory in Russia, Ukraine and Belarus*, ed. J. Fedor, M. Kangaspuro, J. Lassila, T. Zhurzhenko, and A. Etkind, 307–45. Cham: Springer, 2017.

Field, Mark G. *Doctor and Patient in Soviet Russia*. Cambridge, MA: Harvard University Press, 1957.

Filtzer, Donald. *The Hazards of Urban Life in Late Stalinist Russia: Health, Hygiene, and Living Standards, 1943–1953*. Cambridge: Cambridge University Press, 2010.

Finnin, Rory. *Blood of Others: Stalin's Crimean Atrocity and the Poetics of Solidarity*. Toronto: University of Toronto Press, 2022.

Fisher, Carl. 'Doctor-Writers: Anton Chekhov's Medical Stories'. In *New Directions in Literature and Medicine Studies*, ed. Stephanie M. Hilger, 377–96. Basingstoke: Palgrave Macmillan, 2017.

Fissell, Mary. 'Making Meaning from the Margins: The New Cultural History of Medicine'. In *Locating Medical History: The Stories and their Meanings*, ed. Frank Huisman and John Harley Warner, 364–89. Baltimore: Johns Hopkins University Press, 2004.

Fitzpatrick, Sheila. *Education and Social Mobility in the Soviet Union 1921–1934*. Cambridge: Cambridge University Press, 1979.

——. *Everyday Stalinism: Ordinary Life in Extraordinary Times: Soviet Russia in the 1930s*. Oxford: Oxford University Press, 1999.

Flige, Irina. 'The Necropolis of the Gulag as a Historical-Cultural Object: An Overview and Explication of the Problem'. In *Rethinking the Gulag: Identities, Sources, Legacies*, ed. Alan Barenberg and Emily D. Johnson, 243–72. Bloomington: Indiana University Press, 2022.

Forsyth, James. *A History of the Peoples of Siberia: Russia's North Asian Colony, 1581–1990*. Cambridge: Cambridge University Press, 1992.

Foucault, Michel. *The Birth of the Clinic: An Archaeology of Medical Perception*. London: Routledge Classics, 2003.

——. *Society Must Be Defended: Lectures at the Collège de France, 1975–76*. London: Penguin, 2004.

Fowler, Mayhill Courtney. *Beau Monde on Empire's Edge: State and Stage in Soviet Ukraine*. Toronto, Buffalo & London: University of Toronto Press, 2017.

Fratto, Elena. *Medical Storyworlds: Health, Illness, and Bodies in Russian and European Literature at the Turn of the Twentieth Century*. New York: Columbia University Press, 2021.

Frieden, Nancy Mandelker. *Russian Physicians in an Era of Reform and Revolution, 1856–1905*. Princeton: Princeton University Press, 1981.

Gavrilova, Sofia. 'Regional Memories of the Great Terror: Representation of the Gulag in Russian Kraevedcheskii Museums'. *Problems of Post-Communism* (2021): 1–15. https://doi.org/10.1080/10758216.2021.1885981.

——. *Russia's Regional Museums: Representing and Misrepresenting Knowledge about Nature, History and Society*. London: Routledge, 2022.

Geizer, I. M. *V. V. Veresaev: Pisatel'-vrach*. Moscow: Medgiz, 1957.

Gentes, Andrew A. *Exile, Murder and Madness in Siberia, 1823–61*. Basingstoke: Palgrave Macmillan, 2010.

———. *Exile to Siberia, 1590–1822*. Basingstoke & New York: Palgrave Macmillan, 2008.

Getty, J. Arch and Oleg V. Naumov. *The Road to Terror: Stalin and the Self-Destruction of the Bolsheviks, 1932–1939*. New Haven & London: Yale University Press, 1999.

Gilley, Christopher. 'Pogroms and Imposture: The Violent Self-Formation of Ukrainian Warlords'. In *In the Shadow of the Great War: Physical Violence in East-Central Europe, 1917–1923*, ed. Jochen Böhler, Ota Konrád, and Rudolf Kučera, 28–44. New York: Berghahn Books, 2021.

Goldman, Wendy Z. and Donald A. Filtzer. *Fortress Dark and Stern: The Soviet Home Front during World War II*. New York: Oxford University Press, 2021.

Goldman, Wendy Z. and Donald A. Filtzer, eds. *Hunger and War: Food Provisioning in the Soviet Union during World War II*. Bloomington: Indiana University Press, 2015.

Grant, Susan. 'Creating Cadres of Soviet Nurses, 1936–1941'. In *Russian and Soviet Health Care from an International Perspective: Comparing Professions, Practice and Gender, 1880–1960*, ed. Susan Grant, 57–76. Basingstoke: Palgrave Macmillan, 2017.

———. 'From War to Peace: The Fate of Nurses and Nursing under the Bolsheviks'. In *Russia's Home Front, 1917–1922: The Experience of War and Revolution*, ed. A. Lindenmeyr, C. J. Read, and P. Waldron, 251–70. Bloomington: Slavica, 2016.

———. 'Nurses in the Soviet Union: Explorations of Gender in State and Society'. In *Palgrave Handbook of Women and Gender in Twentieth-Century Russia and the Soviet Union*, ed. Melanie Ilic, 249–66. London: Palgrave, 2018.

———. *Soviet Nightingales: Care under Communism*. Ithaca & London: Cornell University Press, 2022.

Grebeniuk, Pavel. *Kolymskii led: Sistema upravleniia na severo-vostoke Rossii 1953–1964*. Moscow: ROSSPEN, 2007.

Gregory, Paul. 'An Introduction to the Economics of the Gulag'. In *The Economics of Forced Labor: The Soviet Gulag*, ed. Paul R. Gregory and Valery Lazarev, 1–21. Stanford: Hoover Institution Press, 2003.

Gregory, Paul R. and Valery Lazarev, eds. *The Economics of Forced Labor: The Soviet Gulag*. Stanford: Hoover Institution Press, 2003.

Halfin, Igal. *Red Autobiographies: Initiating the Bolshevik Self*. Seattle: Herbert J. Ellison Center for Russian, East European, and Central Asian Studies, 2011.

———. *Terror in my Soul: Communist Autobiographies on Trial*. Cambridge, MA, & London: Harvard University Press, 2003.

Hardy, Jeffrey S. *The Gulag after Stalin: Redefining Punishment in Khrushchev's Soviet Union, 1953–1964*. Ithaca & London: Cornell University Press, 2016.

Healey, Dan. *Bolshevik Sexual Forensics: Diagnosing Disorder in the Clinic and Courtroom, 1917–1939*. DeKalb: Northern Illinois University Press, 2009.

———. '"Dramatological" Trauma in the Gulag: Malingering and Self-Inflicted Injuries and the Prisoner-Patient'. In *Geschichte(n) des Gulag – Realität und Fiktion*, ed. Felicitas Fischer von Weikersthal and Karoline Thaidigsmann. Heidelberg: Winter-Verlag, 2013.

———. 'Lives in the Balance: Weak and Disabled Prisoners and the Biopolitics of the Gulag'. *Kritika: Explorations in Russian and Eurasian History* 16, no. 3 (2015): 527–56.

———. [Khili, Den.] 'Nasledie Gulaga: Prinuditel'nyi trud sovetskoi epokhi kak vnutrenniaia kolonizatsiia'. In *Tam, vnutri. Praktiki vnutrennei kolonizatsii v kul'turnoi istorii Rossii*, ed. Aleksandr Etkind, Dirk Uffelmann, and Il'ia Kukulin, 684–728. Moscow: Novoe literaturnoe obozrenie, 2012.

———. 'Russian and Soviet Forensic Psychiatry: Troubled and Troubling'. *International Journal of Law and Psychiatry* 37, no. 1 (2014): 71–81.

———. *Russian Homophobia from Stalin to Sochi*. London: Bloomsbury Academic, 2017.

Hechter, Michael. *Internal Colonialism: The Celtic Fringe in British National Development*. London: Routledge, 1975.

Hellbeck, Jochen. *Revolution on my Mind: Writing a Diary under Stalin*. Cambridge, MA, & London: Harvard University Press, 2006.

Holloway, David. *Stalin and the Bomb: The Soviet Union and Atomic Energy, 1939–1956*. New Haven & London: Yale University Press, 1994.

Hooper, Cynthia V. 'Bosses in Captivity? On the Limitations of Gulag Memoir'. *Kritika: Explorations in Russian and Eurasian History* 14, no. 1 (2013): 117–42.

Humphreys, David. 'Challenges of Transformation: The Case of Norilsk Nickel'. *Resources Policy* 36, no. 2 (2011): 142–8.

Hutchinson, John F. *Politics and Public Health in Revolutionary Russia, 1890–1918*. Baltimore & London: Johns Hopkins University Press, 1990.

Iurchenko, V. V. 'K istorii promyshlennogo razvitiia evropeiskogo severa: Proekt ispol'zovaniia ukhtinskoi radioaktivnoi vody v lechebnykh tseliakh (1932–1938)'. In *Liudi v belykh khalatakh*, ed. S. Sapolnova, T. A. Vekshina, and F. G. Kanev, 151–6. Ukhta & Syktyvkar: Komi respublikanskaia tipografiia, 2009.

Jakobson, Michael. *Origins of the Gulag: The Soviet Prison-Camp System, 1917–1934*. Lexington: University Press of Kentucky, 1993.

Johnson, Robert. *Peasant and Proletarian: The Working Class of Moscow in the Late Nineteenth Century*. New Brunswick, NJ: Rutgers University Press, 1979.

Jones, Polly. *Myth, Memory, Trauma: Rethinking the Stalinist Past in the Soviet Union, 1953–70*. New Haven & London: Yale University Press, 2013.

Jones, Stephen F. *Socialism in Georgian Colors: The European Road to Social Democracy 1883–1917*. Cambridge, MA, & London: Harvard University Press, 2005.

Joyce, Christopher. 'The Gulag in Karelia: 1929 to 1941'. In *The Economics of Forced Labor: The Soviet Gulag*, ed. Paul Gregory and Valery Lazarev, 163–87. Stanford: Hoover Institution Press, 2003.

Kaneva, A. N. 'Doktor Viktorov'. In *Problemy istorii repressivnoi politiki na evropeiskom severe Rossii (1917–1956): Tezisy dokladov vserossiiskoi nauchnoi konferentsii*, ed. N. A. Morozov, 35–7. Syktyvkar: Syktyvkar gosudarstvennyi universitet, 1993.

———. 'Doktor Viktorov'. *Ukhta* [newspaper] (23 October 1992): 3.

———. *Gulagovskii teatr Ukhty*. Syktyvkar: Komi knizhnoe izdatel'stvo, 2001.

———. 'Ukhtpechlag: Stranitsy istorii'. In *Pokaianie: Martirolog. T. 8, Ch. 1*, ed. E. A. Zelenskaia and M. B. Rogachev, 77–146. Syktyvkar: Komi respublikanskii blagotvoritel'nyi obshchestvennyi fond zhertv politicheskikh repressii 'Pokaianie', 2005.

Khlevniuk, Oleg. *The History of the Gulag: From Collectivization to the Great Terror*. New Haven & London: Yale University Press, 2004.

Khlevniuk, Oleg and Simon Belokowsky. 'The Gulag and the Non-Gulag as One Interrelated Whole'. *Kritika: Explorations in Russian and Eurasian History* 16, no. 3 (2015): 479–98.

Khlevnyuk, Oleg. 'The Economy of the OGPU, NKVD, and MVD of the USSR, 1930–1953: The Scale, Structure, and Trends of Development'. In *The Economics of Forced Labor: The Soviet Gulag*, ed. Paul Gregory and Valery Lazarev, 43–66. Stanford: Hoover Institution Press, 2003.

Khoroshev, A. F. *Ocherki istorii zdravookhraneniia Magadanskoi Oblasti*. Magadan: Magadanskoe knizhnoe izdatel'stvo, 1959.

Kichigin, A. I. and A. I. Taskaev. ' "Vodnyi Promysel": Proizvodstvo radiia v Respublike Komi (1931–1956 gg.)'. *Voprosy istorii estestvoznaniia i tekhniki*, no. 4 (2004): 3–30.

Kirk, Tyler C. 'From Enemy to Hero: Andrei Krems and the Legacy of Stalinist Repression in Russia's Far North, 1964–82'. *Russian Review* 82, no. 2 (2023): 292–306.

Kolchevska, Natasha. 'The Art of Memory: Cultural Reverence as Political Critique in Evgeniia Ginzburg's Writing of the Gulag'. In *The Russian Memoir: History and Literature*, ed. Beth Holmgren, 145–66. Evanston: Northwestern University Press, 2003.

Kozlov, A. G. 'Dal'stroi kak "kombinat osobogo tipa" i ego rol' v osvoenii severo-vostoka Rossii'. In *II Dikovskie chteniia. Materialy nauchno-prakticheskoi konferentsii, posviashchennoi 70-letiiu Dal'stroia*, 5–29. Magadan: Rossiiskaia akademiia nauk – dal'nevostochnoe otdelenie, 2002.

———. 'Iz istorii kolymskikh lagerei (1932–1937 gg.)'. *Kraevedcheskie zapiski [Magadanskii oblastnoi kraevedcheskii muzei. Magadanskoe knizhnoe izdatel'stvo]*, Vypusk XVII (1991): 61–91.

———. 'Iz istorii kolymskikh lagerei (konets 1937–1938 gg.)'. *Kraevedcheskie zapiski [Magadanskii oblastnoi kraevedcheskii muzei. Magadanskoe knizhnoe izdatel'stvo]*, Vypusk XIX (1993): 17–143.

———. *Iz istorii zdravookhraneniia Kolymy i Chukotki (1864–1941 gg.)*. Magadan: Magadanskoe knizhnoe iz-vo, 1989.

———. *Iz istorii zdravookhraneniia Kolymy i Chukotki (1941–1954 gg.)*. Magadan: Magadanskii oblastnoi dom sanitarnogo prosveshcheniia, Magadanskii oblastnoi kraevedcheskii muzei, 1991.

———. *Magadan: Istoriia vozniknoveniia i razvitiia. Chast' 1 (1929–1939)*. Magadan: SVKNII DVO RAN, 2002.

———. *Magadan: Predvoennoe i voennoe vremia. Chast' 2 (1939–1945)*. Magadan: SVKNII DVO RAN, 2002.

———. *Magadan: Vozniknovenie, stanovlenie i razvitie administrativnogo tsentra Dal'stroia (1929–1945)*. Magadan: SVKNII DVO RAN, 2007.

———. *Ogni lagernoi rampy. Iz istorii magadanskogo teatra 30–50-kh godov*. Moscow: Raritet, 1992.

———. *Teatr na severnoi zemle: Ocherki po istorii Magadanskogo muz.-dram. teatra im. M. Gor'kogo (1933–1953 gg.)*. Magadan: Magadanskaia oblastnaia universal'naia nauchnaia biblioteka im. A. S. Pushkina, 1992.

Kravtsova, Alena and Elena Omelchenko. 'Public Perceptions of Russia's Gulag Memory Museums'. *Problems of Post-Communism* (2022): 1–11. https://doi.org/10.1080/10758216.2022.2152052.

Krementsov, N. L. *A Martian Stranded on Earth: Alexander Bogdanov, Blood Transfusions, and Proletarian Science*. Chicago & London: University of Chicago Press, 2011.

Krylova, Anna. 'The Tenacious Liberal Subject in Soviet Studies'. *Kritika: Explorations in Russian and Eurasian History* 1, no. 1 (2000): 119–46.

Kuziakina, Natalia. *Teatr na Solovkakh, 1923–1937*. St Petersburg: DB, 2009.

———. *Theatre in the Solovki Prison Camp*. Luxembourg & Newark: Harwood Academic, 1995.

Laruelle, Marlene and Sophie Hohmann. 'Biography of a Polar City: Population Flows and Urban Identity in Norilsk'. *Polar Geography* 40, no. 4 (2017): 306–23.

Lifton, Robert Jay. *The Nazi Doctors: Medical Killing and the Psychology of Genocide*. New York: Basic Books, 1986.

Liu, John. 'Towards an Understanding of the Internal Colonial Model'. In *Postcolonialism: Critical Concepts in Literary and Cultural Studies*, ed. Diana Brydon, 1347–64. London & New York: Routledge, 2000.

MacKinnon, Elaine. 'Motherhood and Survival in the Stalinist Gulag'. *Aspasia* 13, no. 1 (2019): 65–94.

Maddox, Steven. 'Gulag Football: Competitive and Recreational Sport in Stalin's System of Forced Labor'. *Kritika: Explorations in Russian and Eurasian History* 19, no. 3 (2018): 509–36.

Mäkinen, Ilkka. 'Libraries in Hell: Cultural Activities in Soviet Prisons and Labor Camps from the 1930s to the 1950s'. *Libraries and Culture* 28, no. 2 (1993): 117–42.

Manley, Rebecca. 'Nutritional Dystrophy: The Science and Semantics of Starvation in World War II'. In *Hunger and War: Food Provisioning in the Soviet Union during World War II*, ed. Wendy Z. Goldman and Donald Filtzer, 206–64. Bloomington: Indiana University Press, 2015.

Markova, E. V. *Gulagovskie tainy osvoeniia severa*. Moscow: Stroiizdat, 2001.

Mason, Emma. 'Women in the Gulag of the 1930s'. In *Women in the Stalin Era*, ed. Melanie Ilic, 131–50. Basingstoke: Palgrave Macmillan, 2001.

McCannon, John. 'Tabula Rasa in the North: The Soviet Arctic and Mythic Landscapes in Stalinist Popular Culture'. In *The Landscape of Stalinism: The Art and Ideology of Soviet Space*, ed. Evgeny Dobrenko and Eric Naiman, 241–60. Seattle: University of Washington Press, 2003.

Mironov, S. P., Iu. L. Perov, V. M. Tsvetkov, and V. M. Iastrebov. *Kremlevskaia meditsina (ot istokov do nashikh dnei)*. Moscow: Izvestiia; Meditsinskii tsentr Upravleniia delami Prezidenta Rossiiskoi Federatsii, 2000.

Morozov, N. A. *Gulag v Komi krae 1929–1956*. Syktyvkar: Syktyvkarskii universitet, 1997.

———. 'Istrebitel'no-trudovye gody'. In *Pokaianie: Martirolog, T. 1*, ed. G. V. Nevskii, 15–237. Syktyvkar: Komi knizhnoe izdatel'stvo, 1998.

Nakhapetov, B. A. *Ocherki istorii sanitarnoi sluzhby Gulaga*. Moscow: ROSSPEN, 2009.

Nakonechnyi, Mikhail. 'The Gulag's "Dead Souls": Mortality of Individuals Released from the Camps, 1930–55'. *Kritika: Explorations in Russian and Eurasian History* 23, no. 4 (2022): 803–50.

———. '"They Won't Survive for Long": Soviet Officials on Medical Release Procedure'. In *Rethinking the Gulag: Identities, Sources, Legacies*, ed. Alan Barenberg and Emily D. Johnson, 103–28. Bloomington: Indiana University Press, 2022.

Obukhov, L. A., K. A. Ostal'tsev, and O. N. Safroshenko. *Khrupkaia letopis': Fotoal'bom. Iz fondov arkhivnogo otdela administratsii Krasnovisherskogo munitsipal'nogo raiona*. Perm': Liter-A, 2012.

Okhotin, N. G. and A. B. Roginskii, eds. *Sistema ispravitel'no-trudovykh lagerei v SSSR, 1923–1960: Spravochnik*. Moscow: Zven'ia, 1998.

Osokina, E. A. *Our Daily Bread: Socialist Distribution and the Art of Survival in Stalin's Russia, 1927–1941*. Armonk & London: M. E. Sharpe, 2001.

Pallot, Judith. 'Forced Labour for Forestry: The Twentieth Century History of Colonisation and Settlement in the North of Perm' Oblast'. *Europe-Asia Studies* 54, no. 7 (2002): 1055–83.

Pereyaslavska, Katya. 'Gulag Art: Elusive Evidence from the Forbidden Territories'. *Art Documentation: Journal of the Art Libraries Society of North America* 30, no. 1 (2011): 33–42.

Pinnow, Kenneth M. *Lost to the Collective: Suicide and the Promise of Soviet Socialism, 1921–1929*. Ithaca & London: Cornell University Press, 2010.

Plokhy, Serhii. *Lost Kingdom: The Quest for Empire and the Making of the Russian Nation, from 1470 to the Present*. London: Penguin, 2017.

Pohl, Otto J. *The Stalinist Penal System: A Statistical History of Soviet Repression and Terror, 1930–1953*. Jefferson, NC: McFarland, 1997.

Poirier, Suzanne. 'Medical Education and the Embodied Physician'. *Literature & Medicine* 25, no. 2 (2006): 522–52.

Pollock, Ethan. *Without the Banya We Would Perish: A History of the Russian Bathhouse*. New York: Oxford University Press, 2019.

Ramer, Samuel C. 'Feldshers and Rural Health Care in the Early Soviet Period'. In *Health and Society in Revolutionary Russia*, ed. Susan Gross Solomon and John F. Hutchinson, 121–45. Bloomington & Indianapolis: Indiana University Press, 1990.

———. 'The Russian Feldsher: A Pa Prototype in Transition'. *Journal of the American Academy of PAs* 31, no. 11 (2018): 1–6.

Rappoport, Iakov L. *The Doctors' Plot*. London: Fourth Estate, 1991.

Rayfield, Donald. *Edge of Empires: A History of Georgia*. London: Reaktion, 2012.

Rogachev, M. B. '"My vynuzhdeny pribegnut' k bor'be": Golodovka politza-kliuchennykh v Vorkute v 1936 godu'. In *Pokaianie: Komi respublikanskii martirolog zhertv massovykh politicheskikh repressii*, ed. G. V. Nevskii and V. G. Nevskii, 95–106. Syktyvkar: Fond 'Pokaianie', 2004.

Ruder, Cynthia A. *Building Stalinism: The Moscow Canal and the Creation of Soviet Space*. London: I. B. Tauris, 2018.

———. *Making History for Stalin: The Story of the Belomor Canal*. Gainesville: University Press of Florida, 1998.

Sapolnova, S. F., T. A. Vekshina, and F. G. Kanev, eds. *Liudi v belykh khalatakh*. Ukhta & Syktyvkar: Komi respublikanskaia tipografiia, 2009.

Shaw, Charles. 'Friendship under Lock and Key: The Soviet Central Asian Border, 1918–34'. *Central Asian Survey* 30, no. 3–4 (2011): 331–48.

Shulman, Elena. *Stalinism on the Frontier of Empire: Women and State Formation in the Soviet Far East*. Cambridge: Cambridge University Press, 2008.

Siegelbaum, Lewis H. 'Okhrana Truda: Industrial Hygiene, Psychotechnics, and Industrialization in the USSR'. In *Health and Society in Revolutionary Russia*, ed. Susan Gross Solomon and John F. Hutchinson. Bloomington & Indianapolis: Indiana University Press, 1990.

———. *Stakhanovism and the Politics of Productivity in the USSR, 1935–1941*. Cambridge: Cambridge University Press, 1988.

Sirotkina, Irina. *Diagnosing Literary Genius: A Cultural History of Psychiatry in Russia, 1880–1930*. Baltimore: Johns Hopkins University Press, 2002.

Slezkine, Yuri. *Arctic Mirrors: Russia and the Small Peoples of the North*. Ithaca & London: Cornell University Press, 1994.

Smele, Jon. *The 'Russian' Civil Wars, 1916–1926: Ten Years that Shook the World*. London: Hurst & Company, 2016.

Solomon, Susan Gross. 'The Expert and the State in Russian Public Health: Continuities and Changes across the Revolutionary Divide'. In *The History of Public Health and the Modern State*, ed. Dorothy Porter, 183–223. Amsterdam: Editions Rodopi B. V., 1994.

———. 'Social Hygiene and Soviet Public Health, 1921–1930'. In *Health and Society in Revolutionary Russia*, ed. Susan Gross Solomon and John F. Hutchinson, 175–99. Bloomington & Indianapolis: Indiana University Press, 1990.

Solzhenitsyn, Aleksandr. *Arkhipelag Gulag 1918–1956: Opyt khudozhestvennogo issledovaniia*. 3 vols. Ekaterinburg: U-Faktoriia, 2006.

Solzhenitsyn, Alexander. *The Gulag Archipelago 1918–1956: An Experiment in Literary Investigation*, trans. Thomas P. Whitney (vols 1 & 2) and H. T. Willetts (vol. 3). 3 vols. London: Collins & Harvill Press, 1974, 1975, 1978.

Staf, Vladislav. 'Local Initiatives: A Historical Analysis of the Creation of Memorial Museums of the Gulag in (Post-)Soviet Russia'. *Problems of Post-Communism* (2023): 1–8. https://doi.org/10.1080/10758216.2023.2166846.

Starks, Tricia. *The Body Soviet: Propaganda, Hygiene, and the Revolutionary State*. Madison: University of Wisconsin Press, 2008.

Stoff, Laurie. *Russia's Sisters of Mercy and the Great War: More Than Binding Men's Wounds*. Lawrence: University Press of Kansas, 2015.

Suny, Ronald Grigor. *The Making of the Georgian Nation*. 2nd edn. Bloomington: Indiana University Press, 1994.

Tarnawsky, Maxim. 'Introduction'. In *Hard Times* by Ostap Vyshnia. London: Glagoslav Publications, 2018.

Taskaev, A. I. and A. I. Kichigin. *Istoriia radiatsionnoi gigieny i radiatsionnoi bezopasnosti v SSSR na primere ukhtinskogo radievogo promysla*. Syktyvkar: Komi nauchnyi tsentr Uralskogo otdeleniia RAN, 2006.

Tepliakov, A. G. *Mashina terrora: OGPU-NKVD Sibiri v 1929–1941 gg*. Seriia 'Airo-Monografiia'. Moscow: Novyi khronograf: AIRO-XXI, 2008.

Thomas, Adrian and Arpan K. Banerjee. *The History of Radiology*. Oxford: Oxford University Press, 2013.

Todes, Daniel Philip. *Pavlov's Physiology Factory: Experiment, Interpretation, Laboratory Enterprise*. Baltimore & London: Johns Hopkins University Press, 2002.

Toker, Leona. *Return from the Archipelago: Narratives of Gulag Survivors*. Bloomington & Indianapolis: Indiana University Press, 2000.

Tolczyk, Dariusz. 'Politics of Resurrection: Evgeniia Ginzburg, the Romantic Prison, and the Soviet Rhetoric of the Gulag'. *Canadian-American Slavic Studies* 39, no. 1 (2005): 53–70.

Trofimenko, I. N. 'Noril'skii ispravitel'no-trudovoi lager': Otbor kontingenta i uroven' smertnosti zakliuchennykh (1935–1950 gg.)'. In *Noril'skaia Golgofa*, ed. O. L. Podborskaia, 30–9. Krasnoiarsk: Obshchestvo 'Memorial'; Regional'noe ob"edinenie 'Sibir'', 2002.

Troubetzkoy, Laure. 'Récits de deux médecins: Veresaev et Bulgakov'. *Revue des études slaves* 65, no. 2 (1993): 253–62.

Tumarkin, Nina. *The Living and the Dead: The Rise and Fall of the Cult of World War II in Russia*. New York: Basic Books, 1994.

Upadyshev, N. V. *Gulag na evropeiskom severe Rossii: Genezis, evoliutsiia, raspad*. Arkhangel'sk: Pomorskii universitet, 2007.

Viola, Lynne. 'The Aesthetic of Stalinist Planning and the World of the Special Villages'. *Kritika: Explorations in Russian and Eurasian History* 4, no. 1 (2003): 101–28.

———. 'The Gulag and Police Colonization in the Soviet Union'. In *Stalin and Europe: Imitation and Domination, 1928–1953*, ed. Timothy Snyder and Ray Brandon, 18–43. New York & Oxford: Oxford University Press, 2014.

Viollet, Catherine. 'L'œuvre autobiographique de Evfrosinija Kersnovskaja: Chronique illustrée du Gulag'. *Avtobiografiя: Journal on Life Writing and the Representation of the Self in Russian Culture*, no. 1 (2012): 223–36.

von Zitzewitz, Josephine. *The Culture of Samizdat: Literature and Underground Networks in the Late Soviet Union*. London: Bloomsbury Academic, 2021.

Vorontsova, I. D. and M. B. Rogachev. 'Neizdannaia kniga ob Ukhtpechlage: iz materialov knigi "5 let bor'by za nedra taigi i tundry"'. In *Pokaianie: Martirolog. T. 8, Ch. 1*, ed. E. A. Zelenskaia and M. B. Rogachev, 163–70. Syktyvkar: Komi respublikanskii blagotvoritel'nyi obshchestvennyi fond zhertv politicheskikh repressii 'Pokaianie', 2005.

Weissman, Neil B. 'Origins of Soviet Health Administration'. In *Health and Society in Revolutionary Russia*, ed. Susan Gross Solomon and John F. Hutchinson, 97–120. Bloomington & Indianapolis: Indiana University Press, 1990.

White, Anne. 'The Memorial Society in the Russian Provinces'. *Europe-Asia Studies* 47, no. 8 (1995): 1343–66.

White, Frederick. *Degeneration, Decadence and Disease in the Russian Fin de Siècle: Neurasthenia in the Life and Work of Leonid Andreev*. Manchester: Manchester University Press, 2014.

———. 'Leonid Andreev's Release from Prison and the Codification of Mental Illness'. *New Zealand Slavonic Journal* 41 (2007): 18–41.

Yeykelis, Igor. 'Odessa Maccabi 1917–20: The Development of Sport and Physical Culture in Odessa's Jewish Community'. *East European Jewish Affairs* 28, no. 2 (1998): 83–101.

Zajicek, Benjamin. 'Soviet Madness: Nervousness, Mild Schizophrenia, and the Professional Jurisdiction of Psychiatry in the USSR, 1918–1936'. *Ab Imperio* 2014, no. 4 (2014): 167–94.

———. 'A Soviet System of Professions: Psychiatry, Professional Jurisdiction, and the Soviet Academy of Medical Sciences, 1932–1951'. In *Russian and Soviet Health Care from an International Perspective: Comparing Professions, Practice and Gender, 1880–1960*, ed. Susan Grant, 97–117. Cham: Springer International Publishing, 2017.

Zavadski, Andrei and Vera Dubina. 'Eclipsing Stalin: The Gulag History Museum in Moscow as a Manifestation of Russia's Official Memory of Soviet Repression'. *Problems of Post-Communism* (2021): 1–13. https://doi.org/10.1080/10758216.2021.1983444.

Zelenskaia, E. A. *Lagernoe proshloe Komi Kraia (1929–55 gg.) v sud'bakh i vospominaniiakh sovremennikov*. Ukhta & Kirov: Blagotvoritel'nyi fond 'Tochka opora'; KOGUP Kirovskaia oblastnaia tipografiia 2004.

Zelenskaia, E. A. and M. B. Rogachev. 'Ukhtinskaia ekspeditsiia OGPU v dokumentakh'. In *Pokaianie: Martirolog. T. 8, Ch. 1*, ed. E. A. Zelenskaia and
M. B. Rogachev, 39–73. Syktyvkar: Komi respublikanskii blagotvoritel'nyi obshchestvennyi fond zhertv politicheskikh repressii 'Pokaianie', 2005.

Zemskov, Viktor N. 'Gulag (Istoriko-sotsiologicheskii aspekt)'. *Sotsiologicheskie
issledovaniia*, nos 6, 7 (1991): 6: 10–27; 7: 3–16.

Zima, Veniamin F. *Golod v SSSR 1946–1947 godov: Proiskhozhdenie i posledstviia*.
Moscow: Institut rossiiskoi istorii RAN, 1996.

INDEX